IMAGES OF BLISS

Images of Bliss

EJACULATION

MASCULINITY

MEANING

Murat Aydemir

University of Minnesota Press
Minneapolis • London

Produced by Wilsted & Taylor Publishing Services
Copy editing by Nancy Evans
Design and composition by Yvonne Tsang

Published by the University of Minnesota Press
111 Third Avenue South, Suite 290
Minneapolis, MN 55401-2520
http://www.upress.umn.edu

LIBRARY OF CONGRESS CATALOGING-IN-PUBLICATION DATA

Aydemir, Murat.
Images of bliss : ejaculation, masculinity, meaning / Murat Aydemir.
p. cm.
Includes bibliographical references and index.
ISBN-13: 978-0-8166-4866-5 (hc : alk. paper)
ISBN-13: 978-0-8166-4867-2 (pbk. : alk. paper)
1. Generative organs, Male—Philosophy. 2. Human reproduction—Philosophy. 3. Ejaculation—Philosophy. 4. Penis—Philosophy. 5. Masculinity—Philosophy. I. Title.

QP255.A93 2007
612.6′1—dc22 2006017450

Printed in the United States of America on acid-free paper

15 14 13 12 11 10 09 08 07 10 9 8 7 6 5 4 3 2 1

"THE HUMAN STAIN,"

she said, and without revulsion or contempt
or condemnation. Not even with sadness.
That's how it is—in her own dry way, that is all
Faunia was telling the girl feeding the snake:
we leave a stain, we leave a trail, we leave
our imprint. Impurity, cruelty, abuse, error,
excrement, semen—there's no other way
to be here. Nothing to do with disobedience.
Nothing to do with grace or salvation or
redemption. It's in everyone. Indwelling.
Inherent. Defining. The stain that is there
before its mark. Without the sign it is there.
The stain so intrinsic it doesn't require a mark.
That stain that precedes disobedience, that
encompasses disobedience and perplexes all
explanation and understanding. It's why all the
cleansing is a joke. A barbaric joke at that.
The fantasy of purity is appalling. It's insane.
What is the quest to purify, if not more impurity?

Philip Roth, *The Human Stain*, 2001

CONTENTS

PART FIVE

LITERATURE

I EXPRESS MY GRATITUDE TO

THE AMSTERDAM SCHOOL

FOR CULTURAL ANALYSIS (ASCA),

which supplied the academic and social context in which this book could be written. Specifically, I consider the school's annual theory seminar, directed by Mieke Bal, as the book's formative background. Mieke Bal and Ernst van Alphen have served as the advisors of the dissertation from which this study grew. They have challenged, pushed, and supported me throughout. I hope the result shows some measure of the formidable academic intelligence they have generously shared with me and reflects some measure of the intellectual enjoyment I experienced in working with them.

M. A.

INTRODUCTION

We all know what male orgasm looks like.

Susan Winnett, "Coming Unstrung: Women, Men, Narrative, and Principles of Pleasure," 1990

Against the general rule: *never allow oneself to be deluded by the* image *of bliss:* agree to recognize bliss wherever a disturbance occurs . . .

Roland Barthes, *The Pleasure of the Text*, 1983

IF RESEARCH RESULTS ARE TO BE BELIEVED, sperm counts in the Western and environmentally polluted world have been on the decrease for some time now. Approximately from 1996 onward, the media have been reporting on the threatening lack of semen with some urgency. In "The Estrogen Effect: Assault on the Male," an episode of the BBC's science series *Horizon* that aired on February 26, 1996, it was reported that sperm counts among young men have been dramatically decreasing over the last decades, while instances of testicular cancer, testicular nondescent, and intersex conditions have been rising simultaneously. The scientists gathered in the program attribute such disturbances to the presence of chemicals in the environment that, because of their molecular shape, act like estrogens on and in the male body.

The chemicals assumed to be responsible, including bisphenol A and various phthalates, are currently widely used in the plastic lining of tin cans and food wrappings. The virtual omnipresence of estrogen-like substances in the environment prompts one of the scientists to proclaim that "we live, in effect, in a sea of estrogens." The statement became the catchphrase for the publicity material advertising and marketing the documentary.

As it happens, living "in a sea of estrogens" also describes the precarious and precious existence of the male fetus while in formation in the uterus. In "How to Build a Man," Anne Fausto-Sterling observes that biologists oftentimes express concern "about how male fetuses protect themselves from being feminized by the sea of maternal (female) hormones in which they grow."[1] Hence, the scientist's statement extends and projects the trope from womb to world. And, whereas the recent environmental history that the documentary traces nostalgically presupposes a clean past when masculinity was still safe from peril, this second allusion to the sea in and from which the masculine subject develops suggests a past that seems always already contaminated.

Though pseudo-estrogens are also associated with rising numbers of breast cancer, the subtitle of the documentary, "Assault on the Male," specifies the "we" in the scientist's statement as "we, men." Additionally, the title personifies the many and diverse molecules doing the damage into a composite character, the agent of the "assault," thus granting it apparent and evil intent.[2] In that way, the program cannot but invoke a story line from an age-old and generic stock: a narrative in which man is faced by a fiend who issues a threat. Finally, the hazard imposed on the male subject is not so much circumstantial, but rather targets the discrete body-shape in which masculinity materializes or incarnates. The documentary makes this disturbing potential concrete by showing pictures of the morphological ravages the molecules have inflicted on male bodies.

Hence, the encircling and formless sea of pseudo-estrogens disrupts masculine morphology itself, rendering it contaminated, undifferentiated, formless. In turn, that threat to the future maintenance of masculine shape is already partially countered by the mythical story form that frames the biological and environmental problem. Consequently, the narrative of man and fiend that the documentary mobilizes both expresses gender anxiety and renders it recognizable and palatable; it suspends and recuperates masculinity in one gesture.

A month earlier, the American men's magazine *Esquire* also reported on the sperm shortage crisis and helpfully spelled out its larger concerns. In the table of contents of the magazine, Daniel Pinchbeck's "Downward Motility" is pitched in no uncertain terms: "Although you may not know it, you're only half the man your grandfather was."[3] Pinchbeck interviews self-described "conservative environmentalist" Gordon Dunhill, who believes that toxic chemicals are also responsible for the decline of the family as well as for causing homosexuality. "Homosexuality is one of the reproductive problems associated with these exposures," Dunhill states (82). Animals, too, are affected. An image of an eagle was accompanied by a text that reads, "Like the countrymen he represents, the national bird is not standing quite so proud these days" (79).

Only when the author receives the results of his own test, taken in the spirit of participating journalism, does the article's sustained ironic and jocular tone subside. For, disappointingly, his sperm count turns out to be only "borderline normal." For *Esquire*, the panic over the decrease in sperm counts fits in with perceived crises of masculinity, heterosexuality, family, and nation, thus associating the issue with the "culture wars" and the "crisis of masculinity," to which many of the publication's pages have phrased ever-ambivalent responses. Hence, the sea of pollutants in which masculinity finds itself at risk of dissolving is not only environmental (the world) and physical (the womb), but also cultural.

From another angle, sociobiologist Robin Baker argues that the issue may not so much be too little sperm, but too much of it. In *Sperm Wars: The Science of Sex*, Baker puts forth the hypothesis that spermatozoa wage a protracted war for the ovum inside the female body. This battle does not play out between cells from the same individual, as in many accounts of reproduction, but between those of competing lovers, who have consecutively ejaculated in the same woman over a period of up to five days. Baker argues that the reproductive organs and chemistry of the sexes have closely adapted to the demands of sperm warfare, and that actual sexual behavior is suited to the practice.

Specifically, the large number of spermatozoa, seemingly excessive in relation to the single egg, are meant to block the advent of the semen of the competing lover. Hence, Baker recycles the common idea of the "war" between the sperm cells and intensifies it by resituating the battle between different men. This rhetoric effectively naturalizes war, a thing of culture, through recourse to evolutionary necessity. Indeed, Baker's coinage of the phrase "sperm war" led the satirical e-zine *FutureFeedForward* to forecast a future news item, dated February 14, 2012, that reports that the RAND Corporation has just released a study identifying "Sperm Warfare tactics as the most 'realistic' threat to the morale of American Troops deployed in forward and danger areas."[4]

Thus, the assault on masculinity issues not only from the sea, the environment, the uterus, and culture, but also from other sperm, other men. Apparently, then, there is not enough masculinity in the world to be shared equally by all men; masculinity is a scarce commodity that must be fought over. The assault or war against sperm and the male body now appear as externalized and projected instances of the violence and rivalry that inhere in the idea of masculinity itself. At the same time, the renewed relevance of war for conception also encloses the too-numerous sperm in a productive economy. For the cells that do not manage to fertilize the egg are made useful after all by their contribution to the battle with the sperm cells from another male individual. This logic of economy and excess cannot but betray a marked anxiety over the elusive numerousness of sperm, which are simultaneously superfluous and scarce.

Ranging from the scientific to the popular, from the serious to the satirical, these examples pertaining to sperm suggest the outline of the cultural background against which semen features, the nebula of anxieties and concerns that it engenders in the world. These concerns coalesce around three densely related issues, which will come up time and again in this study.

The first issue entails the burden of morphology, the necessity to form, maintain, and protect a specifically masculine shape from the dangers that surround it and encroach upon it. It situates sperm in an ambivalent dynamic of solidification and liquefaction, of formation, deformation, and malformation. The second issue centers on economy and quantity, a field of meanings that assigns to the sperm a paradoxical numerousness that oscillates between excessiveness and scarcity. Placing semen on a semantic axis consisting of the oppositions between past and future, retrospection and anticipation, belatedness and precipitousness, the third and final dimension concerns temporality and historicity.

Paradoxes such as these may stand as the enduring symptoms for the long overdue "reckoning with *sperm-fluid*" that Belgian philosopher Luce Irigaray called for. In *This Sex Which Is Not One*, Irigaray questioned

> why sperm is never treated as an object *a*. Isn't the subjection of sperm to the imperatives of reproduction alone symptomatic of a preeminence historically allocated to the solid (product)? And if, in the dynamics of desire, the problem of castration intervenes—fantasy/reality of an amputation, of a "crumbling" of the solid that the penis represents—a reckoning with sperm-fluid as an obstacle to the generalization of an economy restricted to solids remains in suspension.[5]

Irigaray suggests that the consideration of semen *qua* liquid, its treatment as material object, can promisingly intervene in the economy of meaning and gender historically set in place. That economy largely turns on a stark alternation, the one between phallus and castration, between subjectivity and annihilation, in which the former terms can only ever visually appear in the shape of the latter. The phallus can only show itself, become unveiled, as castration and lack; the subject can only recognize itself as annihilated. What cannot maintain solidity might as well not exist.

However, the terms of that predicament, Irigaray proposes, continue to impede the import of the fluid that can only be equivocally generalized in the economy of the phallus. Thus, the alternative between phallus and lack, as well as the critical perspective that that opposition can sustain, cannot accommodate the sperm to which they nevertheless contiguously refer. Together, the mirage of the phallus and the spectacle of castration protect against an even greater apparential specter: the visibility of the quintessentially male substance of sperm in its fluidity.

Because semen cannot be reduced to either the presence or the absence of a solid, it does not fit in the economy that Irigaray identifies. When concretely visible as a fluid object, semen cannot be idealized in a phallic, yet absent, shape. At the same time, the liquid remains too present in its material characteristics to be rendered as castration. Hence, the substance that issues from the solid penis to generate the equally solid product, the child, and that is thus central for the maintenance and reproduction of the economy that, according to Irigaray, gives preeminence to solids, itself does not fit in that economy. Indeed, as a liquid, sperm shares that crucial characteristic with the uterine, environmental, and cultural "sea" that envelops and threatens masculine form. Semen, then, is somehow both central and excessive to the phallic economy, potentially as deforming as it is formative.

Though Irigaray argues that the consideration of liquid semen she deems necessary so far remains in suspension, that suspension has not precluded several other theorists from intimately engaging with the question of sperm, if in a discursive mode more implicit and surreptitious than her forceful "reckoning" demands. Perhaps the impossible place, central and marginal, that semen occupies in the phallic economy of signification and gender also decrees that coming to terms with it is simultaneously long overdue and already happening. Put in suspension, sperm is both studiously ignored and relentlessly questioned.

Even Jacques Lacan, the psychoanalyst who has monumentalized the phallus/lack distinction, offers an account of the phallus that does not remain untouched by the fluid contamination of the sperm. Though Lacan elevates the penis to the status of a master concept for social and psychic life in the phallus, that transformation passes through, and is partially derailed by, the semen he relegates to the margins of his account. From there, it nevertheless infects the effect of meaning that the phallus brings forth as its "bastard offspring." The phallic "image of the vital flow" that Lacan briefly imagines ultimately loops back to "that mark," merely indexed without being named or elaborated upon, that precedes the phallus, thus robbing the concept of its supposedly primary or primordial status. In that way, "phallus" becomes the belatedly privileged name for the seminal mark or trace that precedes and exceeds it (see chapter 2).

Jacques Derrida analyzes the rigidification and solidification of form that the phallus promises not so much as a defense against a castration that is always looming, but rather as a belated protection against the "dissemination" that has already happened. When read as a text on male orgasm, ejaculation, and semen, Derrida's *Dissemination* (1981) emerges as a series of expositions that seizes on many spermatic paradoxes. Derrida dissimulates the "supreme spasm" of orgasm, rendering it as a miming performative rather than an instance of authenticity; designates the impossible number of semen as a "singular plural"; replaces the generative force supposed to inhere in the head of the sperm cell with the unpredictable and disruptive motions of its supplemental tail; and inquires into the "pharmakological" propensity of the fluid that must serve as the conduit for self-same identity (see chapter 9).

If Lacan puts the penis in a vertical hierarchy in which the organ rises to the phallus that simultaneously makes the organ invisible and immaterial, Georges Bataille, through engaging ejaculation and semen, revels in the countermovements that that upward move makes possible. For not only does Bataille reverse the hierarchy, making semen out to be "low" as he mixes it up indiscriminately with urine, saliva, and (menstrual) blood, he also "flattens" the hierarchy on which the genders and these substances are placed. Thus both come to matter, to relate to each other, horizontally and indifferently rather than vertically and hierarchically (see chapter 10).

And, for Roland Barthes, the temporality of ejaculation, when reified as narrative climax, may well procure a pleasure that lends the subject its place. Yet, that pleasure can also be interrupted by a bliss that always arrives either too soon or too late, thus suspending the subject and its place in narrative. Moreover, the switch from pleasure to bliss also enables the semiotic fracturing of the *semina aeternatis*, the common assumptions of thought, into motile *semences* that flick through the text (chapter 8).

In all of these cases, ejaculation and sperm do not feature as the signs for the calibration of meaning and gender, but as the dense and convoluted instances that prevent and preempt both. Indeed, Derrida, Bataille, and Barthes have coined "seminally" overdetermined concepts—dissemination, expenditure, and bliss respectively—that already partially perform the intervention that Irigaray's reckoning with the sperm fluid urges. To further bring out their potential to contribute to that intervention, this study will propose rereadings of the texts introducing and considering those concepts, in which the question of ejaculation, semen, and masculinity is strategically put at center stage.

The paradoxical place of sperm triggers temporalities and visualities, in a word, narratives, other than the ones that the phallus generates. Temporarily, phallic narratives usually recount the immediate switches at which the various meanings that the idol promises tip over to their extreme opposites. Visually, the phallus can only maintain its hold when veiled, to then materialize as castration and annihilation as soon as it is unveiled. Thus, the generic story of the phallus hinges on an immediate and uncompromising either/or alternation between opposites. If not the one, then necessarily and inevitably the other, its logic decrees.

Thus, it is perhaps more correct to say that stories about the phallus only frantically gesture at it, circumscribe it, while the phallus itself remains largely outside the narrative. The phallus resists narrativization. It looms *over* the narrative rather than materializing *in* it. If the phallus is to retain its power, it must stay outside the exchanges of agency, experience, and desire that narrative performs, while yet continuing to serve as their imagined telos, calibration stone, or origin.

But ejaculation forges narrative. As an irreducible happening, bringing about change and consequence, it forces narrators, focalizers, and characters to come up with accounts of what is about to happen, what is happening, and what has happened.[6] Additionally, the sperm, when discharged, presents subjects with a visible and material effect or remainder of the event, which cannot be easily absorbed in the formation or maintenance of identity. In diverse and contradictory ways, the decisive but elusive happening of orgasm and the troubling presence of the viscous trace provoke a flurry of accounts, perceptions, and reactions, attempting to make sense of the event and its effect. As persistent irritants, ejaculation and sperm trigger all kinds of plotting: remedial, recuperative, digressive, questioning, subversive.

Often, narratives that pertain to sperm arrest, flatten out, or quicken the instance of transformation that the phallic stories skip or elide. In temporal terms, sperm stories can thus bring in a host of other relevant differences: between endurance and entropy, motion and stasis, fleetingness and coagulation, instantaneity, iterability, and eternity. Visually, semen similarly invokes dynamic pairs of notions like plasticity and monumentality, solidification and liquefaction, transparency and mottledness, viscosity and elevation, livingness and mortality, becoming wet and going dry, motions upward and downward. Hence, sperm narratives replace the immediacy of oppositions with the temporality of difference. Semen changes the story. By tracing such alternative narratives in various contexts, ranging from Aristotle to the contemporary artist Andres Serrano, from pornography to Proust, and from Lacan to Bataille, the present study attempts to contribute to the reckoning with semen that Irigaray called for.

The narratives that sperm and ejaculation forge are at least double. On the one hand, their narrativization can lead to their reification under the heading of climax, the discrete resolution and culmination of the story at which meaning, identity, and pleasure all come together. That aspect of the narration of orgasm comes to the fore in Peter Brooks's narratology, which privileges what he terms the "significant discharge," as well as in contemporary hard-core pornography, where most sexual encounters close on the so-called cum, money, or pop shot, the image of ejaculation (chapter 5). This mode of telling and showing male orgasm renders it as the pinnacle of narrative and realism, installing specific and predictable meanings at its place.

On the other hand, however, stories of ejaculation often also foreground their own discontents, bringing up doubts and anxieties that qualify the climactic power that is supposed to inhere in, or that is ascribed to, ejaculation. In these narratives, ejaculation is elided, reiterated, or suspended. Rather than serving as the juncture at which the narrative culminates, ejaculation becomes the instance where the story halts, freezes, coagulates, fans out, digresses, or drearily repeats itself. In accordance with the incongruent place Irigaray gives to semen in the phallic economy, ejaculation thus both forces, reifies, and qualifies narrative. In one go, ejaculation demands a story and renders it moot or impossible (see chapters 6 and 7).

The endeavor to think through ejaculation and semen may be overdetermined from the start. In "Conceptions and Contraceptions of the Future," A. Samuel Kimball identifies the "root metaphor" sustaining the approximation of thought and reproduction in the notion of *conception*.[7] Hence, conceiving of sperm, conceptualizing it, cannot but lock the substance in a "conceptive" logic, in which the substance inevitably becomes generative and inseminating, and, hence, masculine, heterosexual, and procreative. "Once the name *concept* arises," Kimball argues, "it is as if thought reaches back behind itself to produce its very advent and subsequent history" (77). Rendering literally what is already metaphorically present in the terms of conceptuality, conceiving (of) semen can only redundantly perpetuate the terms of that history. Can sperm be considered "contraceptively," and if so, how?

In *Male Matters: Masculinity, Anxiety, and the Male Body on the Line*, a book to which I will return shortly, Calvin Thomas brings up Freud's hypothesis that abstract thinking primarily arose "from the patriarchal attempt to establish by conjecture the paternal identification of produced male offspring (for the purposes of bequeathing property) over and against the merely visible or empirical proof of maternity provided by the mother's productive body."[8] Hence, the conceptual thinking that metaphorically privileges semen serves as the speculative means through which the father can claim his son; conceptual, abstract thought ensures that the product mirrors its producer.

At the same time, however, the assumption of conceptuality remains wedded to the concrete, material, visual, and bodily productivity that it rivals and attempts to overrule. And, if the tenor of conceptuality can never entirely substitute the vehicle that forms its ground, then the sperm on which conceptual thinking tropes is ever at risk of becoming contaminated by the metaphor. In its oscillation between metaphoricity and literalness, conceptuality and concreteness, idealization and materialization, semen emerges as the instance where these aspects become entangled with, rather than sharply differentiated from, each other. In its elevating and sublating propensity, sperm reaches above and beyond the bodily productivity from which it originates; yet its viscosity returns a bodily and material *gravitas* to the subject.

Thus, entertaining semen runs the productive risk of bringing to bear on masculine subjectivity the material temporality and visuality that its conceptualization seeks to replace. Moreover, through taking semen as its object, conceptual thinking, in turn, must take into account the considerations of matter, temporality, and visuality that the substance provokes. If semen historically forms the ever-present burden of thinking, then thinking otherwise should precisely take the contradictory position of sperm, both always already a concept, and never entirely divorced from its materiality, as its starting point. Merely the apprehension of sperm in its visibility *qua* liquid suffices to disturb and re-render the conceptual edifice imposed on it.

A spectacular case in point is Aristotle's treatment of semen in *Generation of Animals*. On the one hand, the philosopher argues that semen is the purest of all bodily secretions, so that it can serve as the vehicle for the spirit or *psyche* that gives form to substance. This conceptualization of sperm's generative import requires that the substance cannot be perceived in its concrete materiality, invisibly setting matter into formation within the female body.

Yet, on the other hand, the empirical scientist Aristotle cannot but describe semen in its concrete qualities: it is white, hot, shiny, and foamy. Though delivered as the experiential aspects that indicate its purity, the detailed descriptions of semen that Aristotle offers require its divorce from the reproductive context that lends it its meaning. Hence, they trigger a temporality of entropy in which the seed, cooling down, losing its shine and foam, ultimately reverts to mere matter, adequately compared to a dried-up wad of saliva in the streets. This duplicitous potential of semen comes to the fore when Aristotle compares the fluid with, and distinguishes it from, blood, the stars, and ice, three materializations that the contemporary artist Andres Serrano also imagines in a series of photographs of bodily substances (see chapter 1).

If Aristotle inaugurates the history that conceptual thinking, according to Kimball, cannot but perpetuate, then that history itself now appears as ambivalent, turning on the conceptualization of sperm that cannot leave behind the awareness of its irreducible materiality. Following the reverse materialization of semen in Aristotle's discourse, two concepts from current critical vocabulary enable alternative "conceptions" of sperm. The first is the *abject*. Julia Kristeva uses the term to designate the troubled relationship of the subject to its oozing and secreting body. The abject, Kristeva writes in *Powers of Horror: An Essay on Abjection*, is something that is "[n]ot me. Not that. But not nothing either. A 'something' that I do not recognize as a thing."[9]

In this context, the something of semen is thoroughly ambivalent. Kristeva lists it as one possibly abject substance among others (2, 53). But she also observes that sperm, notably unlike menstrual blood, is not considered to be "unclean" within most religious hygiene rules (71). Thus, sperm may become both dirty, prompting abjection, as well as pure, liable to idealization. Furthermore, Kristeva writes, only through and in orgasmic *jouissance* can the abject "as such" be experienced: "One does not know it, one does not desire it, one joys in it [*on en jouit*]" (9). Hence, sperm can apparently be both clean and dirty, and, moreover, can take part in an immanent rapture that can be "in-joyed," yet not known.

The second (anti)concept is the *formless*. In *Formless: A User's Guide*, Yve-Alain Bois and Rosalind E. Krauss define the term, originally coined by Bataille, as a desublimating gesture or operation of "de-class(ify)ing," a simultaneous "lowering and liberating from all ontological prisons."[10] As the book's introduction clarifies, "It is not so much a stable motif to which we can refer, a symbolizable theme, a given quality, as it is a term allowing one to operate a declassification [*déclasser*], in the double sense of lowering and of taxonomic disorder" (18).

Bois and Krauss also consider one specific substance liable to the operation of formlessness: saliva. The authors quote Michel Leiris, who observes that spittle "lowers the mouth—the visible sign of intelligence—to the level of the most shameful organs" (18). The material qualities of saliva that Leiris summarizes, its inconsistency, humidity, indefinite contours, and imprecision of color, all challenge the mouth as the locus of sublimated speech. Here, Leiris's specific terms, it would seem, are all as appropriate to semen as they are to spittle. Hence, sperm may be the male substance that brings about the threat of formlessness to masculinity's determined maintenance of form. Can sperm lower the penis, and with it, masculinity, in the same way that saliva lowers the mouth? Indeed, semen may form the formless substance that both lowers and de-hierarchizes the phallus/penis. Thus both the abject and the formless suggest ways in which the conception of sperm can be understood "contraceptively": granting a solid, secure shape neither to its material effect, nor to the male body that produces it.

The abject and the formless are both related to the strategic concept of "production anxiety" that Calvin Thomas proposes in *Male Matters*, which I have taken as the recurring thread or line for this study. Broadly, Thomas approaches masculinity as a cultural norm imposed on, or assigned to, the male body. This norm privileges, idealizes, and reifies some aspects of the various heterogeneous processes and energies that that body can, in principle, make available, while repressing others. Masculinity ascribes an intelligible and culturally sanctioned *form* to the male body, which that same body can only partially support. If masculinity must claim the male body as its material and embodied vehicle, then that body can also experience itself at odds with the claim it should ideally and stably substantiate. Therefore, the male body is masculinity's most intimate and threatening "other."

The expression "on the line" in Thomas's subtitle condenses three aspects of his discussion. First, the phrase refers to the discrete boundary lines that masculinity maps onto the male body, the bodily differentiation, hierarchization, or discipline that it mandates. However, the maintenance of the boundary lines drawn up between adjacent and contiguous organs, limbs, and orifices, as well as between their processes and pleasures, also brings about the fear of their overflowing, soiling, or contamination (32). Thus masculinity may find itself "on the line" in a second way: at stake, in peril. Third, the line connotes the traces of writing in, on, and through which the tension between masculinity and the male body, according to Thomas, plays itself out.

As a quasi-bodily or embodied function, writing is both act and appearance, both process and material result, Thomas argues (3). The written line triggers the anxious tension between gender identity and its material self-representation: "[M]asculinity cannot represent its supposedly immaculate self-construction," Thomas writes, "without giving itself over to discursive productions in which the always potentially messy question of the body cannot fail to emerge" (13). Writing condenses the two other meanings of the line: the differentiation that masculinity decrees *and* the contamination through which it puts itself at risk. In writing, then, masculinity becomes graphic in its double sense: both inscribed and bodily explicit, messy. In this specific sense, all writing is "pornographic"; "any *graphos* turns its subject to *pornè* [prostitute]," Thomas quips (26).

To make the tension between body and gender analytically productive, Thomas coins the notion "production anxiety." "I use the word *production*," he explains, "in the sense that Baudrillard develops in *Forget Foucault*: 'to render visible, to cause to appear and be made to appear: *producere*.' The term will designate any process of externalization by which something is made or allowed to appear" (34). Returning to the etymological context of theatrical practice (in its meaning of "leading before an audience," "bringing onto the stage"), *producere* forges the "becoming visible" of (aspects of) the male body in the ways that masculine subjectivity seeks to represent itself. Hence, Thomas argues, the semiotic self-containment that masculinity seeks in representation is ever haunted (or enchanted) by its own "dark incontinence" (16).

The anxiety brought about by the dynamic between necessary self-exposure and its discontents Thomas identifies as specifically modern and modernist, in their broadest senses. His cases ranging from Hegel to Joyce, Thomas cites the masculine paranoia and aggression of many literary modernists as one of his examples (43). "[T]here is a stain on the tain of the mirror stage of modernity," he writes, "a mark or trace that hopelessly fouls the modern metanarrative of man's rational and representational self-possession" (46). That stain, mark, or trace Thomas continuously designates as fecal; shit features as "a sort of crumbling space of morphic indeterminacy" (19). The immaculate self-possession or sublimated form that masculinity seeks out is ever in danger of becoming indiscrete, morphologically indeterminate, by the "excrement" it anxiously produces into visibility. Shit stains the subject.

I want to single out the seminal to continue and supplement Thomas's understanding of masculine production anxiety for two reasons. First, ejaculation and semen seem to me at once more central and more marginal, at once more intimate and more alienated, to the construction of masculinity than defecation and excrement. The former cannot as easily be jettisoned from its self-representation as the latter can. Consequently, the anxieties and ambivalences sperm triggers are that much more acute, and hence, that much more productive. Second, the dread-filled "dumping on the line" that Thomas reads in modernist texts runs the risk of marking and demarcating that line with a vengeance. Yet, to some extent, semen forms the stuff that that line is made of, the *fine*, elemental line that separates masculinity from itself. That seminal trace or line, moreover, still needs to be followed through to its ultimate consequences.

One modernist writer who does so is Proust. In *In Search of Lost Time*, a wet dream featuring a misplaced but generative thigh, a masturbation scene that produces a snail's trail, and an involuntary climax expressing itself like drops of sweat during a wrestling game together form a rich, gossamer textuality. Through it, a formative and transformative subjectivity scrutinizes and tries out various forms of writerly creativity, of being in space, and of relating to other men (see chapters 11, 12, and 13).

Susan Winnett has polemically asserted the familiarity and recognizability of the image of male pleasure: "We all know what male orgasm looks like."[11]

Apparently, we all have an equal share in the generous epistemological availability of male orgasm. However, in *The Pleasure of the Text*, Roland Barthes sheds doubt on the representability and representativeness of what he calls "the image of bliss," singular. That image conforms to the general rule that male pleasure should look masculine: strong, muscled, violent, phallic. However, Barthes cautions, pleasure may also be visible and legible in the disturbances of the rule that links up the body, its pleasurable processes, and the gender assigned to both.[12] Hence, Barthes explicitly leaves open the possibility that male bliss can materialize, become visible and readable, in ways that belie the dominant "image of bliss" under general rule.

Hence my title for this study: *Images of Bliss*, plural. Though the ejaculation of semen is biologically male, that neither automatically means that it is also self-evidently and comprehensively masculine, nor that representations of and reflections on it should always tell the same story, partake of the same imagination, or conform to the same ideology. What happens to the supposedly shared and instantaneous recognizability of male orgasm when, heeding Barthes's warning, we "agree to recognize bliss wherever a disturbance occurs"? Indeed, as Irigaray suggests, the "seminal" may exactly form the necessary but impossible juncture where masculinity differs from itself, where it seeks and fails to claim the material body as its secure vehicle. It is to that differentiality of pleasure that this study attends.

PART ONE

HISTORY, ART

ONE

SEMEN, BLOOD, STARS, AND ICE

Serrano and Aristotle

INFAMOUSLY AND INFLUENTIALLY, Aristotle's *Generation of Animals* of circa 350 B.C. defines the male role in reproduction as active, spirit-bestowing, and formative; the female one, in contradistinction, as passive, material, and formless. Since the female ova are still unknown to him, Aristotle acknowledges and distinguishes between two generative substances, semen and menstrual blood. These two respective fluids largely act and react in accordance with the philosophical and ideological binarism that determines their value—except for the simple fact that the sperm, for all its active, spiritual, and formative propensities, cannot but be *also* a substance. This awkward predicament constantly threatens the gendered and binary opposition that Aristotle's treatise on human and animal reproduction sets up.

Pondering the nature of semen at some length, Aristotle considers semen in close relation to three other entities. The first is blood; its relationship to sperm is threefold. Blood is the raw material for semen. Sperm is distilled or "concocted," Aristotle claims, from blood. Because menstrual blood and semen serve as reproductive substances to a similar extent, they also function as each other's counterparts. In a final twist, they form each other's polar opposites. For, in sharp contrast to blood, only semen transports the spirit or psyche that brings matter to life. Additionally, the spiritual or psychic aspect of semen at one point prompts the philosopher to compare it to the stars, and, at another, to question whether sperm will freeze when exposed to frost in the open air. Hence, Aristotle considers the matter of semen in relation to blood, stars, and ice.

Intriguingly, these three considerations are of great importance in relation to a series of works by the contemporary Cuban American artist Andres Serrano. Serrano's works show semen in a viscous proximity to blood (*Semen and Blood* I and II, 1990), as a quasi-celestial phenomenon comparable to the Milky Way (*Untitled XIV [ejaculation in trajectory]*, 1989), and as a frozen, glacial mass (*Frozen Sperm I*, 1990). Hence, these specific instances of reflection on the relative materiality and immateriality of semen in analogy with blood, stars, and ice provide a point of contact between the ancient philosopher and the contemporary artist. Both are investigating, imagining, and questioning sperm in contrasting yet related ways. This intimate contact urges a close reading of the two in dialogue with each other: Aristotle as illustrated or enacted by Serrano; Serrano as reacting to and against Aristotle; Serrano as provoking a rereading of Aristotle.

Now that the ova have been discovered, thanks to the scientific and empirical attitude he himself originated, Aristotle's treatise and the views it promulgates may well be considered, redundantly, past history. Yet that phrase has a double entendre. Aristotle's work may be condemned to history and seen as obsolete and quaint, but this attitude also puts Aristotle past or beyond historicity, where his thinking can then remain dormant and unchallenged. However, feminist analyses of the ideology and imagination animating contemporary accounts of conception, popular and scientific, have precisely pointed out the tenacity of the Aristotelian view. For example, Emily Martin's "The Egg and the Sperm: How Science Has Constructed a Romance Based on Stereotypical Male-Female Roles" convincingly shows that the distribution of roles assigned to the genders in current textbooks, popular representations, and medical articles remains thoroughly Aristotelian in outlook. They stubbornly characterize *male* as active and formative in generation, and *female* as passive and material, even when new research manifestly counters this view's appropriateness.[1] Apparently, our age is still struggling to come to terms with Aristotle's account of conception, gender, and reproductive substances.[2]

This manifest endurance makes *Generation of Animals*, oxymoronically, present history. Our cultural and ideological history forms exactly the joint that connects Aristotle and Serrano, ancient philosophy and modern art. Despite their separation by time, spatially, horizontally, densely, and tangibly, the two react to each other, stick together, perhaps as intimately and intensely as do the two liquid substances in Serrano's *Semen and Blood I* and *II*.

BLOOD

Two works by Serrano from 1990, titled *Semen and Blood I* and *Semen and Blood II* (Figures 1 and 2) show the two titular bodily fluids in close contact with each other on a dark, transparent surface pane. The encounter is charged with an unbearable tension. The two liquids do not mix, yet they are shown in their closest proximity, their boundaries touching each other, clinging to each other, creating congealing edges and whirls where they

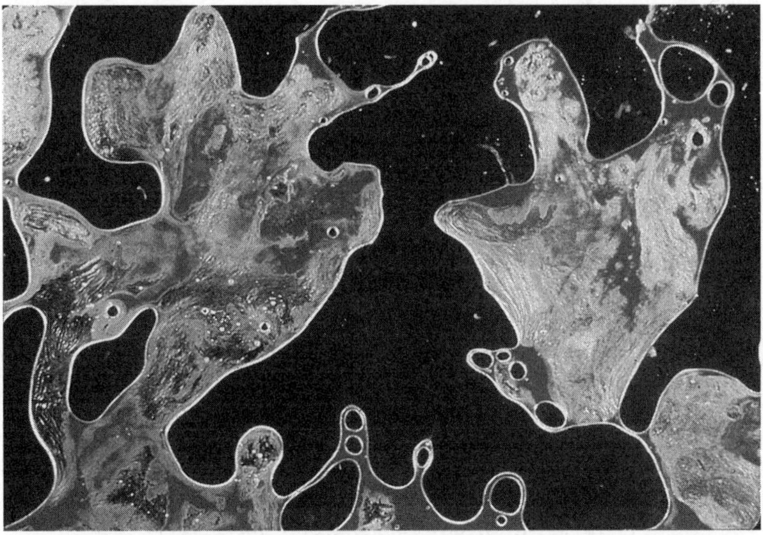

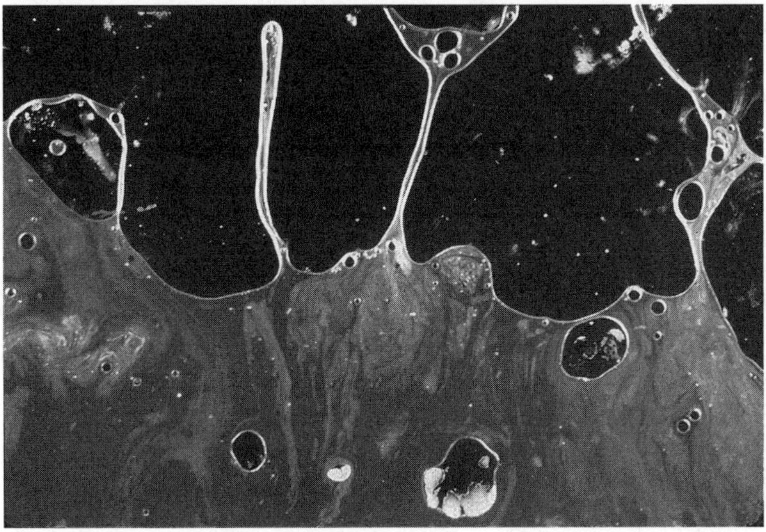

FIGURE 1 (*top*). Andres Serrano, *Semen and Blood I*, 1990. Cibachrome, silicone, plexiglas, and wood frame. 40 × 60 inches. Courtesy of the Paula Cooper Gallery, New York.
FIGURE 2 (*bottom*). Andres Serrano, *Semen and Blood II*, 1990. Cibachrome, silicone, plexiglas, and wood frame. 40 × 60 inches. Courtesy of the Paula Cooper Gallery, New York.

interface. If the two substances fail to amalgamate or mingle, neither can they be said to be separate from each other, as a tangible viscosity keeps them both firmly together, yet apart.

Moreover, both images suggest the temporality of a slow but inexorable process. Something is happening at the cellular level where the two substances meet, cautiously but insistently. The scale of the pictures, then, seems very small. As if looking through an enlarging microscope, the viewer witnesses something that normally remains unseen to the naked eye.

The perceptual plane of the images is horizontal. The viewer is looking at them as if from above, poised *over* the images rather than standing *in front* of them. A strong impression is given that the two substances are not merely perched on the surface and kept in place by gravity; rather, they actively, determinedly, cling to the surface pane. Keeping one's distance from the images becomes difficult: they pull the viewer both over and closer down toward them. As a result, the dynamic of an imperative viscosity at play also bears heavily on the position of the viewing subject.

The contact between these two bodily liquids could take place outside of the body, if one assumes that they are taken out of the body and put under a microscope. Perhaps the images represent cut slices of tissue, positioned on a glass pane or, alternately, flattened between two glass panes. However, the fluids are shown as still alive and active. If not, the blood should have a darker tone and less fluidity; it should be oxidized and dried up. The same goes for the sperm. The question, then, is: for how long can the two fluids remain alive? It is also possible that a photographic microscope has invaded a living body to capture the mysterious process *in situ*. This may indicate that this body is ill, for why else would it submit to such an invasive procedure? Hauntingly, Serrano's blood and semen pictures condense health and sickness, livingness and mortification, thus tuning into the AIDS scare of the time and the social panic that accompanied it.[3]

Finally, the pictures are abstract, or rather, nonfigurative, in the sense that nothing in particular seems to be represented. Their titles, as well as what is generally known from Serrano's manner of working (and from the scandals that accompany it), pledge the representation of actual blood and actual semen. Hence, one sees something that is both matter and form, yet not—as would be the case in an abstract expressionist painting, the art historical genre to which the two photographs clearly allude—matter as sublated or subsumed into form. That move is prevented by the simple knowledge that the matter at stake is not paint, dribbly or not, but body matter. Thus, the works propose a vision of matter that is both nonfigurative and concrete at the same time.[4]

SQUIGGLIES AND CLARET

What Serrano's pictures put before the eye is the viscous proximity of opposites: contagious images of liquids that neither mix nor separate, that may be situated inside or outside of the body, that imply life and death, health and illness, and that compel both abstract and concrete ways of looking. Several clues to a further understanding are found in a recent, commercial, and "low"-culture appropriation of another one of the photographs from the series: the heavy-metal rock group Metallica's use of *Semen and Blood III* for the cover of their CD album *Load* (Figure 3).

In an interview with the band for the Web site Addict.com, reporter Michael Goldberg tries to clarify the signification of the album's cover image. Thematic headings discussed include "sex and violence," presumably to underscore the group's image, as well as "life and death." But then band foreman Kirk Hammett attempts to settle the debate with a statement replete with the tropes of popular art-speak, opening up a new can of worms in the process:

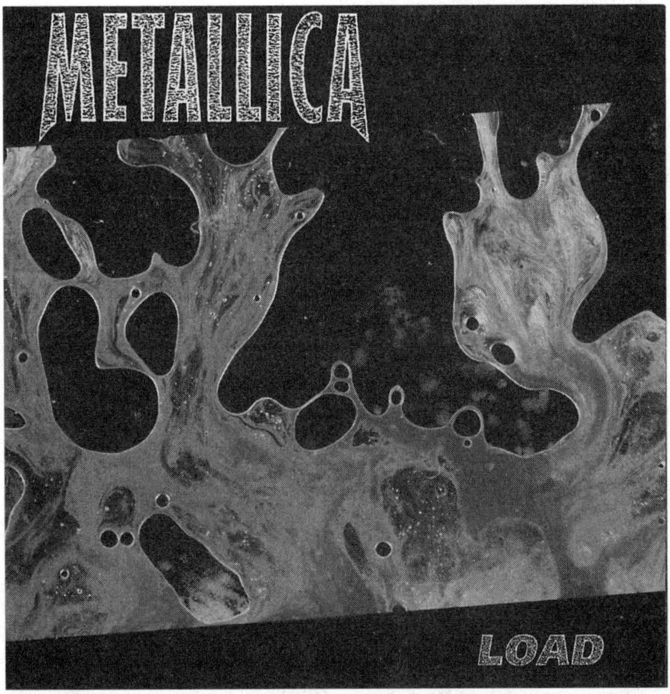

FIGURE 3. Metallica, *Load*, 1996. Album cover. Elektra/WEA.

> I don't really want to get into exploring the deeper meaning of the image only because I don't want people to hear it and get a mindset on it and always see what I get out of that image. I'd rather just explain that it's semen and blood and it's by this guy named Andres Serrano [the 1990 photo of Serrano's semen mixed with bovine blood is titled *Semen and Blood III*] and I think it's a really beautiful abstract image that is open to a lot of interpretation and metaphor.[5]

Hammett's words articulate a familiar series of oppositions that govern the discourse of popular art-reception: preconceived ideas versus spontaneous reaction, depth versus superficiality, literalness versus metaphor, concreteness versus abstraction, and beauty versus ugliness.

The most interesting of these, the seamless juxtaposition of "it's semen and blood" and "it's a really beautiful abstract image," only becomes fully intelligible when the beginning of the interview is taken into account. Hammett's first response was wholly to the point: "squigglies and claret," that is, squirming shapes and the color of burgundy wine. Aptly, these words convey the impression that the ultimate tension and intimacy in the *Semen and Blood* pictures take place between color, as a quality of matter, and shape or form, as a design imposed on matter.

Furthermore, the word used to characterize the shapes, "squigglies," suggests shapes or forms that are not fully formed.[6] Thus, it implies that these forms either are still in the process of becoming, moving to a future state of formation, or are decomposing, breaking down from a previous state of finished formation. Evidently, the intimate tension or conflict that takes place in the two photographs is yet undecided. One may see in them forms slowly emerging out of color, color overruling and reclaiming form, or a temporary stage in an interminable process, moving back and forth. What becomes clear from the operative terms here, form and matter, sperm and blood, is that the discursive background for these images should indeed be the Aristotelian tradition, which associates sperm with form and (menstrual) blood with matter.

What is not discussed in the interview is the title of the album, *Load*. It effectively renames Serrano's *Semen and Blood III*. The new title may suggest a heavy burden or responsibility, a measured task (as in "workload"), or a single charge of ammunition, perhaps continuing the "sex and violence" theme. But "load" is also slang for the ejaculate (as in "dropping or shooting one's load"). Hence, the title suggests an even greater proximity between the two substances: an ejaculation consisting of both semen and blood.[7] This feature, I presume, should indicate an extraordinary intensity rather than illness, or perhaps once more the intimate entanglement of sex and violence, life and death, in the heavy-metal lifestyle. Connotations such as these, because they imagine a coming together of opposites, only work to dispel the tension within the image, which is based on a dynamic of *neither* mingling *nor* separation. The new title *Load* precisely works to "unload" this ambivalence. Then again, the connotation of "viral load," suggestive of HIV infection, immediately makes the Metallica cover uncanny.

Finally, the interviewer's bracketed insertion in the statement suggests that the semen in the image may be Serrano's, but that the blood is bovine. This reference brings up another opposition and another thin boundary: the one between the human and the animal. As Aristotle's title indicates, he treats human and animal reproduction under the same heading, while at the same time distinguishing them. Possibly, the two fluids reacting to each other so intimately and intensely in Serrano's pictures do not belong to the same species.

This poses an anthropic dilemma: if the two fluids are locked in a process of begetting a creature, then what would that be? And, how can the artist's, the exemplary individual's, semen, allegorically possessing his (pro)creative powers, his indexical and material signature, be indiscriminately mixed up with a cow's blood? This questioning of humanity, of humanness, makes something clear about the images that is relevant even without the realization that the blood may not be human: the images are nonhuman in the specific sense that their depiction offers no clue, detail, or perspective that acknowledges or invites human interest—which is different than saying that they are inhumane. Remarkably, there is nothing human in these images of two utterly human fluids.[8]

"AS IT WERE A DEFORMED MALE"

The most pressing and disturbing opposition-put-into-contact in the images is the one between sperm and menstrual blood. Yet there is no explicit indication in the images or their titles of whether the blood is in fact menstrual or bovine blood; or whether, if in fact bovine, the blood comes from a cow or a bull; and, if indeed from a cow, whether it is specifically menstrual blood. Nevertheless, Western culture has a long-standing history of turning the difference between sperm and menstrual blood into an opposition, and of deriving a hierarchy between the sexes from it. That background cannot but impinge on these pictures.[9] It is a history impossible to ignore. The images can be taken up to intervene most relevantly and poignantly in the terms of that history, drawing from it and giving it a new twist.

Aristotle's *Generation of Animals* is one of the earliest and most authoritative instances of that history, coining a phraseology that has endured up to modern psychoanalysis. Because women discharge blood rather than semen, Aristotle characterizes woman as "an infertile male" according to the following rationale: "the female, in fact, is female on account of an inability of a sort, *viz.*, it lacks the power to concoct semen out of the final state of the nourishment . . . because of the coldness of its nature" (1.20). And, in a similar vein: "The reason is that the female is as it were a deformed male; and the menstrual discharge is semen, though in an impure condition; *i.e.*, it lacks one constituent, and one only, the principle of Soul" (2.3).[10]

The burden of binary thinking weighs heavily here. These brief formulations indicate that Aristotle views the two fluids as both analogous and opposed to each other. Since both are equally reproductive substances, they are fundamentally similar. Yet they are also significantly different, while this difference boils down to "one only" thing that is also the all-deciding thing: the respective presence or absence of soul in the matter. In addition, the difference is not so much static but dynamic: the end result of the process of "concocting," the distillation or reduction, in the culinary sense, of nutriment to its final and purest stage.[11] Man and woman, semen and menstrual blood, are the same but different, and this essential difference is, paradoxically, merely a difference of degree.[12] This is why Aristotle is able to place a host of intermediate characters, such as children, old men, fat people, the ill, and eunuchs, on a sliding scale between the two.[13]

The terms of this uneasy constellation are set up in the beginning of the text. There, Aristotle defines male and female as the "principles of generation" (1.2). The male is initially characterized as the "movement" or "efficient cause" of reproduction, the female as its matter. But subsequently Aristotle adds two more definitions that pose an implicit challenge to the first set: male is what generates in another body, female is what generates in its own body (1.2).

This opens up a problem. For, how is the male cause or principle of movement to transport or communicate itself to the materiality of another body, if not by way of a conduit or medium that must also be in some respect material? Hence, the burden of Aristotle's view of semen is to make semen the material medium of transmission for the cause or movement to the matter, while yet insisting that it is something else, something more, than just matter. Sperm must be material in that it communicates, makes contact, and mingles with the substance that forms its counterpart. Yet it must also be something else or more than matter in order to keep up the original distinction between male cause and female matter.[14]

The dilemma becomes acute when Aristotle concedes that the opposing principles, now explicitly put in a hierarchy, should ideally keep separate:

> And as the proximate motive cause, to which belong the *logos* and the Form, is *better* and more divine in its nature than the Matter, it is *better* also that the superior one should be separate from the inferior

> one. That is why wherever possible and so far as possible the male is separate from the female, since it is something *better* and more divine in that it is the principle of movement for generated things, while the female serves as their matter. The male, however, comes together with the female and mingles with it for the business of generation, because this is something that concerns both of them. (2.1)[15]

The exasperation is palpable: if only the two opposing principles could keep well apart. Philosophically and ideologically, that would be preferable, because clearer. However, the business of generation requires a move beyond the outer boundary of "so far as possible," so that the two come together and intermingle on the basis of a common concern. Apparently, reproduction already entails a condition that is less than ideal. Paradoxically, generation both forms the basis, the ground, of Aristotle's distinction between the sexes, and the instance of a mingling or contact that troubles it.

WHY SEMEN MATTERS MORE

At several junctures in the text, Aristotle makes use of arguments to show that the matter of semen is not altogether material in nature. For reasons that will become clear below, I will present them in an ordering that is not present in Aristotle's own exposition. The ten arguments I will distinguish are all present in the text, and they logically cohere under the heading of the problematic (im)materiality of sperm.

Perhaps the most obvious argument Aristotle employs is quantitative. When compared to the quantity of menstrual blood, the quantity of semen seems relatively small. Since the female, Aristotle argues, "must of necessity produce a residue, greater in amount, and less thoroughly concocted," it follows that it "must of necessity be a volume of bloodlike fluid" (1.19). In contrast, the male discharges a secretion that is smaller in quantity and more concocted, and, hence, not quite a "volume" of seminal liquid. Thus, the fact that there is quantitatively less material in the case of semen is taken to prove that it is qualitatively less material in nature.

A second argument is dynamic and temporal. Sperm and blood are differently placed on an axis of progressive refinement of nutriment. The two fluids are both secretions, not waste products, in that they are "a residue of the nutriment" (1.18). Aristotle imagines the whole organism as dynamically transforming food into body matter. At different stages of its completion, this processing produces different bodily substances: "for . . . some of the residues are produced earlier, some later. Nourishment in its first stage yields as its residue *phlegma* and other such stuff" (1.18).

Hence, phlegm is the first residue of food, hardly processed; semen is the final residue, completely concocted; and blood is situated in between these two poles. This placement allows for an unlikely but logical analogy between menstrual blood and diarrhea: "Thus, just as lack of concoction produces in the bowels diarrhoea, so in the blood-vessels it produces discharges of blood of various sorts, and especially the menstrual discharge . . ." (1.20). This last discharge, Aristotle adds, is nevertheless a "natural" one. Menstrual blood is the product of an incomplete cooking process in the body, whereas semen forms the ultimate and final result of that same process.

Third, semen may be material, but, to the substance of the menstrual blood, it communicates or adds not *more* matter to be mingled with it, but the "active and efficient ingredient" that turns, "sets," the blood into an embryo (1.21). The male being active and motive, the female being passive and moved, the semen transmits a spiritual element that gives both movement and form to matter. Semen is regarded as form-giving, and therefore as acting on something else rather than being acted on by something else (1.18). This is why Aristotle sees the male as the cause of generation.

Fourth, even if the pneuma transporting the principle of form travels *to* matter *through* matter, moreover, that matter does not become part of what is materially formed as a result. Twice in a row, Aristotle uses the following simile to explain this: "Compare the coagulation of milk. Here, the milk is the body, and the fig-juice or rennet contains the principle which causes it to set" (1.20)—provided it be understood that the sperm and the fig-juice or rennet do not substantially partake in what is shaped or set into form by them. No more, in fact, than "we should expect to trace the fig-juice which sets and curdles the milk. The fig-juice undergoes a change; it does not remain as a part of the bulk which is settled and curdled; and the same applies to semen" (1.20, 2.3).

Except for the first observation of the relative quantities of semen and menstrual blood, Aristotle's argumentation so far proceeds on the basis of logical categories, such as causality, opposition, and analogy. However, he offers six more indications as to why semen should possess formative spirit or psyche. All of these imply the experiential and empirical perception of its concrete qualities. Hence, the remaining descriptions of sperm all require that it is seen in its material existence. This cannot but imply that, in these cases, the semen is temporarily divorced or cut off from the context of reproduction that determines its status and its function. For once one sees semen, at least long enough to describe it in detail, chances are that it is no longer generative, or will soon cease to be.

To continue, Aristotle observes that semen is white. This color distinguishes it from other bodily fluids, particularly menstrual blood, because white signifies a more advanced, in fact the ultimate, stage of purification of the nutrient. That semen is white applies to "all cases," and, Aristotle continues, Herodotus "is incorrect when he says that the semen of Ethiopians is black, as though everything about a person with a black skin were bound to be black—and this too in spite of their teeth being white, as he could see for himself" (2.2). With respect to bird's eggs, Aristotle decides that the egg white contains the male principle of generation, while the yellow yolk contains the female nutrient or matter, thus distinguishing the "white and pure" from "the yellow and the earthy" (3.1).

The whiteness of the sperm also signifies that it is hot, white-hot. Hot, because the viscous liquid envelops the pneuma that transports the psyche, also named "vital heat," which forms its immaterial aspect. This harks back to Aristotle's distinction between the sexes. Because men are more vigorous and active, more hot, he argues, only male bodies possess the sufficient heat to cook semen out of blood ("male animals are hotter than female ones" [4.1]). Just before ejaculation, the airy, hot pneuma joins the material liquid, so that they can come out together (1.20). Because semen "contains a good deal of hot *pneuma* owing to the internal heat of the animal," the substance is defined as "a compound of *pneuma* and water, *pneuma* being hot air" (2.2).[16]

Additionally, the presence of the hot air inside the sperm not only makes it white, but also causes that white to become shiny. For hot air mixed in with fluids, such as oil, Aristotle writes, lets "the whiteness show through . . . for of course shininess is a quality of *pneuma*, not of earth or water" (2.2).

Another material quality Aristotle observes is sperm's foamy or froth-like appearance. If a liquid is mixed with air by beating or pounding them together, he explains, the liquid thickens, increases in mass, and becomes "foamy." Air is entangled in the liquid, "forced together and compressed" (2.2). This foam increases in fineness in direct proportion to the size of the pockets of air: "the smaller and more microscopic the bubbles are, the whiter and more compact is the appearance of the bulk" (2.2). Again:

> The cause of the whiteness of semen is that it is foam, and foam is white, the whitest being that which consists of the tiniest particles, so small that each individual bubble cannot be detected by the eye. . . . That the natural substance of semen is foam-like was, so it seems, not unknown even in early days; at any rate the goddess who is supreme in matters of sexual intercourse was called after foam. (2.2)[17]

We have arrived at the furthest reach of perceptual scrutiny: Aristotle performing a perception so close up to his object that he is able to make out minute, barely visible bubbles captured in the semen. He must be nearly rubbing his nose in it.

White, hot, shiny, and frothy—the qualities that Aristotle observes in semen all serve to foreground the spiritual or the immaterial quality it contains. At the same time, however, merely noticing these qualities necessitates the careful scrutiny of semen as something that is concrete, material, and visible. This acknowledged visibility takes the substance away from the context of generation in which semen should play the part of a form-bestowing, immaterial, and spiritual principle. A further consequence must be that the sperm goes flat, dries up, in the time it takes to investigate and describe it. Both literally and conceptually, then, semen loses its spiritual status, its life, its livingness, under the philosopher's gaze; Aristotle the ideologue and Aristotle the empirical scientist find themselves at odds. The gap between the two attitudes opens up a narrative of entropy, of living and hot sperm reverting to mere matter, that reaches its ultimate logic in the last two qualities he perceives.

Penultimately, Aristotle notices that sperm changes in appearance once it has left the body. This must imply that the four characteristics observed above, whiteness, hotness, shine, and frothiness, can in fact only be observed momentarily. Outside the body, he notes, semen goes transparent and watery, shedding both its thickness and its whiteness (2.2). Consequently, it reverts to everything that it is not: impure matter. Indeed: "Later, when it has lost its heat by evaporation and the air has cooled, it becomes fluid and dark, because the water and whatever tiny quantity of earthy matter it may contain stay behind in the semen as it solidifies, just as happens with phlegma" (2.2). The same phlegm that served as semen's polar opposite as the first and incomplete stage of concoction now forms a fitting comparison.

However, the ultimate propensity of semen that Aristotle notices appears to serve as the way to counter this vision of the precious liquid dried up like phlegm. Sperm may dry up, but will it freeze? It will not: "watery substances freeze, but semen does not freeze when exposed to frost in the open air" (2.2). The idea that Aristotle may have done the experiment himself adds a note of desperation. The point is that the air, the pneuma captured within the substance, can well evaporate, but cannot turn solid: "this also shows . . . why semen does not freeze: it is because air is impervious to frost" (2.2). Leave it to Serrano to come up with an image to prove otherwise.

THE ILLUSTRATED ARISTOTLE, PART I

Let us imagine a future edition of *Generation of Animals* with "illustrations" supplied by Serrano. What can the *Semen and Blood* images do against, for, and with Aristotle's arguments? What might the philosopher see in Serrano's works? For one, the visual scrutiny that Aristotle carries out on the matter of sperm, yet cannot follow through to the conclusion that *that* is what it is, now materializes in two undeniably concrete images.

Serrano's images put before the eyes what Aristotle seems to deplore: the viscous proximity or spatial intimacy of the two opposed gender principles as embodied in the two liquids that he, at least partially, wishes to imagine and place on opposite ends of a binary scale of values: male and female, sperm and blood, form and matter, spirit and substance, the pure and the impure, human and animal. These opposites touch each other, neither separating nor mixing, yet inexorably interacting. They do not dissolve into each other to form something else; they do not keep apart, either.

Perhaps Aristotle would see the photographs as apt illustrations for either the process of concoction, the separation of semen from the blood that forms its raw matter, or of generation, semen in the process of curdling the menstrual blood that forms its working matter. Whatever process is occurring, however, it is temporarily suspended *in* as well as *by* the images. For what one sees is the processing itself, not its origin, nor its presumed end state. Additionally, the microscopic snapshots give no direction as to which way the process is progressing. Indeed, both substances may be in the process of drying up, dying.

The pictures show the exact edge where the distinction between the two liquids, blood and semen, is losing its shape, its firmness; where the one becomes the other, and vice versa. Hence, the binary boundary between the two itself is shown to be transformative, plastic, morphogenetic. This also means that the opposition between form and matter loses its ground. These "squigglies and claret" show form, color, and matter reacting to and with each other, mutating: badly shaped forms, white-ish and red, composing and decomposing. The white of the semen is going off, becoming off-white. Simultaneously, a velvety sheen extends to both liquids.

Remembering his own observations on the changeability of sperm, perhaps Aristotle would presume that part of the semen has already cooled down, and turned transparent and liquid, like water. That means it would be invisible to the eye against the darkened and transparent pane underneath. Yet, there, tiny pockets of something catch the light. This implies that the semen that is still visible is also in the process of disappearing according to an irregular temporality of entropy, if not for the blood with which it is, at some places more than others, reacting and engaging.

For that must be the final insight that Serrano's pictures offer to Aristotle's investigation into generation, as well as into the gender ideology that it authorizes and participates in: that the substance that Aristotle, and many after him, imagine to possess the principle of life has in fact no life of its own, by itself. Without the blood that generates it, and without the blood that it generates in, the precious liquid, ostensibly so lively, white, hot, shiny, and frothy, steadily and irrevocably goes dead, transparent, cold, dull, and flat.

STARS

Serrano's *Untitled XIV (ejaculation in trajectory)* of 1989 (Figure 4) appears to deliver the visual image fittingly illustrating Aristotle's verbal and conceptual analogy between the substance of semen and the stars:

> In all cases the semen contains within itself that which causes it to be fertile—what is known as "hot" substance, which is not fire nor any similar substance, but the *pneuma* which is enclosed within the semen or foam-like stuff, and the natural substance which is in the *pneuma*; and this substance is analogous to the element which belongs to the stars. (2.3)

Untitled XIV shows a white, or white-ish, jet of semen hurtling through space against a black background. In contrast to the *Semen and Blood* pictures discussed above, this work's perceptual plane is vertical. The viewer observes the quasi-celestial appearance as if positioned from the side. Alternatively, the viewer is situated as if looking upward, observing the phenomenon as occurring in the nocturnal sky, her or his neck craning backward. In both cases, it seems, it is now impossible to look down on what is presented in and by this celestial image. Whereas the previous pictures emphasized not only gravity but also a tangible viscosity, matter clinging to a surface or ground, here seminal matter appears to be shooting through the air of its own accord.

Once again, but in a different way, then, the image forges the anthropic or humanistic dilemma: there is no indication in its framing, figuration, or perspective suggesting that this otherworldly occurrence takes into account the human. It merely and simply happens, irrespective of human interest or existence. Looked at from the side, the picture emphasizes extreme distance, marginalizing the viewer. Looked at overhead, the image dwarfs the spectator, as a huge spatial dimension bearing down on him or her.

With respect to scale, *Untitled XIV* invokes the vast expanse of the cosmos; its black background connotes outer space, in which human beings can only be of little consequence. The stream of semen appears as a galaxy, the Milky Way. At the same time, the knowledge that this huge phenomenon consists of spermatozoa, akin to Aristotle's minute pockets of air captured in the liquid, as well as to Serrano's cellular photography of semen and blood, cannot but prompt the awareness of the very small, the microscopic. Thus, the

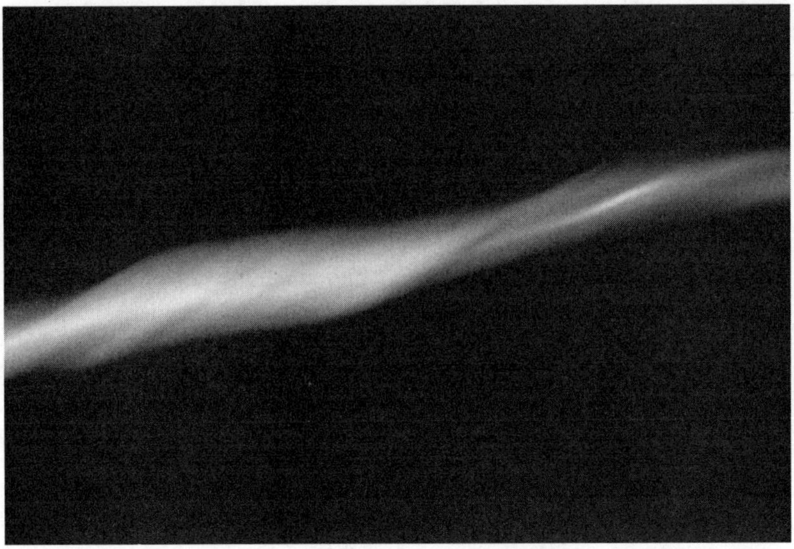

FIGURE 4. Andres Serrano, *Untitled XIV (ejaculation in trajectory)*, 1989. Cibachrome, silicone, plexiglas, and wood frame. 40 × 60 inches. Courtesy of the Paula Cooper Gallery, New York.

viewer's look is effectively sandwiched, bracketed, between two perspectives, both working to qualify the human eye: the infinitely large and the infinitely small.

A similar thing happens for the picture's temporality. On the one hand, it suggests the quasi-eternal temporality of stars, galaxies, and the universe, to which human time is irrelevant. The monumental scale of the work helps to make this eternalizing aspect tangible. On the other hand the image captures a nearly impossible instant: a snapshot, a split-second registration of a moment so fleeting that it cannot endure for another fraction of a second. This makes the work's medium, photography, especially relevant: the infinitesimally short moment of the clicking camera shutter determines the imagery. The image is precariously poised between a before and an after that must be utterly different. Thus, this representation of ejaculation implies the eternal as well as the transitory.[18]

INCONCEIVABLE

The precarious temporality of the ejaculatory moment is comically underscored in an exhibition hosted on the Internet titled *Van Gogh's Ear*.[19] It presents a series of images of objects that refer to well-known art scandals, introduced by supposed curator Jeff Bourgeau. In his introduction, Bourgeau alleges that the exhibition was mounted at the Detroit Institute of Arts in 1999, but was shut down after only four days. Included in the show is a "Masturbation Kit," a plastic bag containing helpful accessories such as a plastic glove, lubricant, and so on. The caption reads:

> Body Fluid #2, 1989. From Ejaculate in Trajectory. Mixed Media. Utilizing this masturbation kit, Serrano was able to over-come [*sic*] inconceivable odds in completing his photo series capturing his own stream of ejaculation in mid-air. Joint gift of the Surgeon General's Committee Against Teenage Pregnancy and the Junior Founders Society.

Indeed, Serrano's *Untitled XIV* and the series of ejaculations-in-trajectory to which it belongs, as well as this exhibit in the show that plays with them, manage to overcome several "inconceivable," nearly impossible, odds. All these take up the various meanings and connotations of the word *conception*.

Van Gogh's Ear displays images of the objects in order to suggest an actual exhibition, supposedly mounted and shut down almost immediately. This brings into play convention, public opinion, and censorship. The masturbation kit cannot be materially perceived where it should have been, that is, in the Detroit Institute of Arts. Hence, *Van Gogh's Ear* points to the "inconceivable" in Serrano's works in its meaning of "unheard of," of a seeming impossibility, something society at large refuses to, or cannot, deal with.[20]

In another meaning of "inconceivable," Serrano's works are hard to conceptualize or understand, since they oscillate between opposing dimensions of time and space, between the eternal and the instantaneous, between the telescopic and the microscopic. Additionally, one may speculate that the images must have been rather difficult to "conceive" in the sense of "to produce" or "to create"—if not, of course, for the prostheses of the camera shutter and the handy masturbation kit supplied by *Van Gogh's Ear.*[21] The kit invokes a particularly awkward and messy production process. Paradoxically, it points out the immaterial, clean, and hygienic appearance of the sticky body fluid in the picture. In that sense, the kit and the image become a wry comment on the necessity and practice of "safe sex."

Finally, the photographs are also "inconceivable" in another sense: the reproductive substance featured in it, captured in mid-air, can no longer generate or impregnate. No doubt this is why the masturbation kit in *Van Gogh's Ear* is sponsored by the Surgeon General's Committee Against Teenage Pregnancy, as the caption quips. But the psychically or spiritually generative, form-bestowing capacity of semen forms exactly the motivation, the ground, for Aristotle's analogy between semen and the stars. The image that so aptly illustrates Aristotle's simile can only dispute the claim that the philosopher wishes to make. If the semen appears star-like, then that is only so because it is divorced from the context of reproduction in which it figures that semen should be star-like. Hence, the visual (Serrano's) and the verbal (Aristotle's) images do not match.

Socially, conceptually, creatively, and reproductively, Serrano's image of ejaculation in trajectory is indeed "inconceivable." That may also be precisely because of the movement, the trajectory, that semen takes part in. The "in trajectory" in the work's subtitle, as well as the appearance of ejaculation as the Milky Way, suggest a road, passage, or journey, motion through space. Yet, because of the image's framing, which cuts off the stream of semen at both ends, the work supplies no clue as to whether this movement travels from left to right or right to left, upward or downward. It merely moves, there is movement, and that is it. Consequently, there is no indication of where this semen will end up once gravity returns. However, the already established separation from the context of generation, so as to enable the sperm to appear in mid-air, hovering and star-like, makes it probable that it will end up in the same way as Aristotle's wad of dried-up phlegm.

Finally, the instantaneous movement of the semen through space causes it to appear in a particular manner. Its hue of white is not pure, smooth, isotopic, or homogeneous. Rather, this specific off-white is opalescent or milky, consisting of internal variations in density, speed, color, and lighting. The seminal jet varies in tone and shine: at some points, it seems more off-white than at others; at some places it reflects the light more prominently than at others. This subtle play with color, light, and shadow suggests an irreducible differentiality within its mass. Twirling around itself, the jet almost looks like a piece of folded cloth being wrung in the air.

If Serrano's *Semen and Blood* pictures put semen in contact with what should serve as its oppositional, binary other in the Aristotelian tradition, this work puts semen in motion so that it becomes other, so that it entangles or folds itself together with its other. Several other interpretations of the textured opalescence of Serrano's "ejaculation in trajectory" are possible. Through Serrano, the "pure" white that Aristotle ascribes to semen will liaise with three other considerations of the significance of white in relation to semen and the stars.

These alternative interpretations come from Georges Bataille's invocation of ejaculation and the Milky Way as mirroring and blurring each other in *Story of the Eye* (1928); from Jacques Derrida's understanding of semen and whiteness in the poetry of Mallarmé as put forth in *Dissemination* (1972); and from Mieke Bal's remarks, following Leibniz and Deleuze, on a "baroque" white in *Quoting Caravaggio: Contemporary Art, Preposterous History* (1999). In each of these three cases, the signification of white, seemingly neutral and bland, will change considerably. Apparently, white is anything but simple.

SOILED WHITE: BATAILLE

As I have indicated, Aristotle views whiteness as the sign of the ultimate stage of purification of matter, which in human generation distinguishes sperm from menstrual blood, and, in birds' reproduction, the masculine "white and the pure" from the feminine "yellow and the earthy" in eggs (3.1). In a different but related tradition, the whiteness of sperm is also taken to prove its provenance from the hard features of the male body, such as marrow and bone, making it, like "liquid bone," impenetrable and unyielding.[22] In both cases, the status of the color white depends on its separation, its discreteness, from what surrounds it and from what it enters into contact with. Bataille argues the opposite: the milky off-white of semen becomes utterly dirty: impure, malleable, commingling, indiscrete.

The following passage, taken from Bataille's *Story of the Eye*, plays out the narrator's own ejaculation and a vision of the Milky Way as reflecting each other. They provoke a mise-en-abyme, "bouncing symmetrical images back to infinity."[23] The fragment is set in a mood of exhaustion and helplessness, shared by the narrator and his two female consorts, Marcelle and Simone. Their state of mind tips over into a suspended animation, an "unreal immobility," a frailty so extreme "that a mere breath might have changed us into light" (41). Then Marcelle falls asleep, Simone pees in her dress, and the narrator comes. "She [Simone] ... made me spurt a wave of semen in my clothes" (42).

This "wave" ushers in a view of the night sky and the Milky Way:

> I stretched out in the grass, my skull on a large, flat rock and my eyes staring straight up at the Milky Way, that strange breach of astral sperm and heavenly urine across the cranial vault formed by the ring of constellations: that open crack at the summit of the sky, apparently made of ammoniacal vapours shining in the immensity (in empty space, where they burst forth absurdly like a rooster's cry in total silence), a broken egg, a broken eye, or my own dazzled skull weighing down the rock, bouncing symmetrical images back to infinity. (42)

The reader will be relieved to learn that the narrator's skull is not about to crack open. However, the effective suspense raised by the possibility that it might attests to the strange approximation and entanglement of perspectives: above and below, usually infinitely distant, are here unbearably close to each other, forcefully bearing down on each other.

From one angle, the low and flattened, and the high are wide apart. The narrator lies on his back, down on the ground, his head resting on a flat rock, staring upward to the sky's "summit." However, from another angle, this distinction is moving and reversing. The rock supporting the head must be "weighed down" by the same head in order to stay put. The temporal contiguity of urine and semen in the preceding text (Simone's urination that instantly prompts the narrator to ejaculate) translates into the spatial commingling of the two in the Milky Way, which consists of "astral sperm and heavenly urine," indiscriminately mixing up the "high" and the "low," generative liquid and waste-product.

On the one hand, the milky and shiny phenomenon flits across a space that is immense and empty, imagined as a "total" absence. On the other hand, this vacuous space is so full that it bursts at the seams, like a broken egg, eye, or skull. From this "breach" or "open crack" in the sky, stuff oozes out like pus to form the Milky Way, which consists of semen, urine, egg white, yolk, vapors, and the inside matter of the brain and the eye.

The passage is followed by a consideration of the favored practice of debauchery by the narrator. It should not, he argues, leave intact "anything sublime and perfectly pure," apparently including the starry heaven (42). For, only people with "gelded eyes," he adds, are able to consider the universe as "decent"; that is why they "are never frightened ... when strolling under a starry heaven" (42). However, the kind of strategic debauchery the narrator wishes to promote soils not only body and thought, "but also anything [he] may conceive in its course, that is to say, the vast starry universe ..." (42). *Conceive*, no doubt, is used here in its double sense of "conceptualize" and "produce." Subsequently, the project of soiling the sublime and the pure is followed through by the connection between the nocturnal sky and menstrual blood: "I associate the moon with the vaginal blood of mothers, sisters, that is, the menstrua with their sickening stench" (42).

Partaking of the ideology that sees menstrual blood as the ultimate abject, this last association is undeniably misogynist. Nevertheless, Bataille's imagination can form a fitting counterpoint to Aristotle's view, for the latter also notes the analogy between the human and the cosmological, not only because he compares the element of semen to that of the stars, *pneuma* to *aither*, but also because he observes and endorses the habit of speaking about the cosmos in gendered terms. People apply gendered terms to the cosmos, Aristotle writes: "in cosmology too they speak of the nature of the Earth as something female and call it 'mother,' while they give to the heaven and the sun and anything else of that kind the title of 'generator' and 'father' " (1.2).

This constellation Bataille works to its limits, soiling and mingling the pure, clean, sublime, paternal, and masculine with its opposites to such an extent that the whiteness of semen is no longer distinct, discrete, or separate from what must be distinguished from it.[24] However, to the extent that this strategy of debauchery depends on that same constellation for its relevant terms, he remains caught up in the ideology that he seeks to dispel. He works it, yet he does not move beyond it. It remains to be seen if the next consideration of semen's whiteness, Derrida's, can do so.

GRAPHIC WHITE: DERRIDA

In "The Double Session," the penultimate essay of *Dissemination*, Derrida offers an extensive analysis of the poetic works of Stéphane Mallarmé. Here, I will only trace it insofar as it addresses the features of whiteness, sperm, and heavenly bodies. "The idea of stars as seeds," Derrida begins, "is a traditional one in poetry."[25] He adds that Mallarmé connects these conventional star-seeds "with male and female milk in association with the milky way" (322). Hence, in Mallarmé, a milky whiteness, semen, and the stars are all closely related to each other.

The milky, starry white and the seminal are directly connected, Derrida argues, sperm simply being described as white, as well as indirectly. Their indirect linkage is established "through the semic constellation of milk, sap, stars . . . or through the milky way that inundates Mallarmé 'corpus' " (267). In the characteristic move of the essay, this seminal "inundation" signifies an excess filling up and drenching of the textual body, as well as its covering, submergence, or blotting out. Hence, seminal white connotes both a hyperbolic presence and an absence. In the course of the essay, these opposites constantly tip over into each other, becoming folded into each other or entangled together.

According to Derrida, Mallarmé's treatment of whiteness has two sides: one thematic and the other typographic. Mallarmé's theme of white, Derrida observes, comprises a series of diverse images and notions, such as virginity, frigidity, snow, sails, swans, foam, curtains, shrouds, milk, stars, sap, and semen. The latter is characterized by Derrida as follows: "SPERM, the burning lava, milk, spume, froth, or dribble of seminal liquor" (266). Yet Mallarmé's poetry also makes specific use of white typographically in the sense that the author's texts frequently leave open intervals and blank spaces, so that the white of the page shines through the words written on it. The point, for Derrida, is that the white (typo)graphic and the white thematic in Mallarmé play on and into each other.

The theme composed of white elements that may add up to an understanding of the work's meaning or content is both enabled and voided by the white graphic. Enabled, because the white of a book's page allows for the white theme to emerge to begin with, granting it its space: "the blankness that allows for the marks in the first place, guaranteeing its space of reception and production" (253). Voided or erased, because a supplementary white, like Tipp-Ex or gum, marks that same page with an active blotting, with "disappearance, erasure, non-sense" (253).

This goes not only for Mallarmé's use of blanks and white spaces as a structuring element in his poetry, but also, even more intimately, for the white that separates the letters of the words on the page, which allows them to appear as discrete, and hence, readable, signs or markers to begin with. Here, white denotes "the carefully spaced-out splitting of the whole," determining the meaning of white "insofar as it refers to the non-sense of spacing, the place where nothing takes place but the place" (252, 257). Without this constituting presence of an absence, the white spacing or spatiality in the text, no text can be readable.

The dependency of the emergence of signification on white spacing also means that meaning can never be sufficiently exhausted or fully accounted for. One may well try to connect the various whites in Mallarmé's text, such as virginity, swans, and shrouds, in a series, and then determine the allegoric significance that governs them, Derrida concedes. However, a single mobile element in the series of whites will invariably "re-mark" on, fold itself into, the whitening textuality that grounds and structures it. Thus, reading cannot progress from one element to another, from one thematic "nucleus" to another, but only trace evasive "theme-effects," unpredictably shifting and moving, multiplying and erasing (250). In one gesture, white enables thematically readable signs to appear, multiplies them, and blots them out.

The thematic whites and the typographic whites fold into each other, erasing markers in some textual folds, and connecting otherwise disparate elements in others. This incessant creasing, folding, and stitching of the fabric determines the text's inexhaustibility with regard to its production of meaning. In Mallarmé, Derrida claims, white always appears in a close contiguity to a series of fabrics, and hence, signifies a "relay through the white canvas or sail, a cloth that is folded and stitched . . ." (260). At these unpredictable relays, folds, and stitches, entirely new meanings may accrue.

In that last sense, white connotes not so much a grounding or blotting absence, but rather a finely textured and multifaceted hyperpresence. Indeed, since white is both no color and all colors put together and mixed up, as well as the color that is best able to reflect light, the reflection of and on white allows these usually opposing perspectives to become entangled. Hence, white, for Derrida, signifies a shimmering multiplicity as well as a potentially endless multiplication of simultaneous possibilities. This is the effect of white that he, at the beginning of the essay and in the "Editor's note" preceding it (173), captures under the heading of "lustre." In Mallarmé's words from "Mimique": ". . . *the perpetual suspense of a tear that can never be entirely formed nor fall (still the lustre) scintillates in a thousand glances . . .*" (quoted in Derrida, 180).

To recapitulate, for Aristotle, the whiteness of semen proves the singular presence of the spirit or soul that inhabits it, which comes from the male, the "superior" and "more divine" gender in reproduction (2.1). Derrida counters this notion of the singular, psychic presence in the milky-white, seminal substance with five alternative readings.[26] First, white may denote the thematic presence of semen in Mallarmé's poetry, but only does so insofar as it is linked up in a series of other whites (milk, fabrics, swans, and so on) that take up, extend, and displace its privilege.

Second, the poetically white appearance of semen is grounded on, inscribed in, a white spatiality, the empty page, which constantly threatens to shine through the—threadbare—markings that make up the text. Third, this white becomes explicitly visible and palpable in the intervals and blank spaces left open in the texts. Fourth, Derrida sees white as an active force of erasure, blotting out or whitening the text. And, fifth, the light-reflecting and -refracting white forms the occasion for an understanding of textuality as intricately textured, folded, faceted, lustrous, and scintillating. Consequently, the distinct white of semen is circumscribed from various sides: it is encompassed by and dissolved into the other whites.

Derrida counters the discrete quality of spermatic white by multiplying it "from within," whereas Bataille counters that same discreteness by mixing it up with the colored fluids, yellowish urine and red blood, usually understood in contradistinction to it. Hence, Derrida can touch the core of the Aristotelian imagination and the tradition it sustains. The "semic," implicating both generation and signification, Derrida argues, is "already swarming"; it is "multiplied from the start" (304). Hence, multiplicity and multiplication do not creep up on an unsuspecting "germ cell previously one with itself"; rather, the ejection "parts the seed as it projects it," inscribing "difference in the heart of life" (304).

For Bataille, space is both totally empty and so full it bursts open at the seams, oozing out matter; for Derrida, space is empty, yet, as such, active, constitutive, and productive. With respect to temporality, Bataille offers two mutually exclusive dimensions, in which the contamination of white semen both has already happened and steadily keeps on happening. Derrida's multiplication from "inside" the opalescent liquid, layering shades of white on white, is originary in the sense of having always already happened, moving incessantly, and also crystallizing in the "perpetual suspense" of the lustre, the liquid tear that neither forms nor falls. Precisely this lustrous and reflective propensity of white is of great importance for the third and last investigation of white that I want to consider.

BAROQUE WHITE: BAL

In *Quoting Caravaggio*, Mieke Bal discusses appropriations and revisions of baroque painting in the contemporary visual arts. To do so, she advances an appropriate mode of analysis that entails the simultaneity, contiguity, or correlation of perspectives usually thought of as distinct or opposed: past and present, fragmentation and totality, color and form, body and soul, interiority and exteriority, surface and depth, large and small. The result is a way of looking at art, contemporary as well as historical, that wavers and vacillates between opposites such as these, which works to transform both the object and the subject of the look.

The chapter called "White Historiography" interprets, among others, several works by Serrano.[27] The "white" of the title refers to the baroque white that Bal, following Gilles Deleuze's reading of Gottfried Leibniz in *The Fold: Leibniz and the Baroque*, understands as both foamy and folded. "Historiography" points to an immanent temporality, in which "forms and things are morphogenetic, producing figures that are found in time," as well as to the interrelated temporality of viewing these timely and changing figurations: the eye bouncing back, flipping between perspectives, being drawn in by the work (Bal, 45, 47).

Baroque white, Bal argues, forms the site where both the stability of the object and that of the subject are challenged. This white is like "foam, like marble chips broken off at rough edges, decomposed into innumerable tiny convex mirrors" (46). It fractures the supposedly smooth materiality of the object, but it also catches the light, mirrors, and reflects back the eye of the beholder (46). Additionally, this eye must negotiate opposing scales by alternating between them: the large and the minute, as in the tiny convex mirrors.

To notice this effect, the viewer must resituate him- or herself closer to the paint, to the matter, and, drawn in, cannot but look again, but now "correlatively" (47). Close-up, the white appears as an intricately textured fabric, a fine and precious skin (52). Finally, the tiny mirrors cannot but distort, enlarge, and deform what they reflect, including the closer look that they compel (50). For Bal, then, white is effectively (inter)active. Owing to its shimmering or scintillating quality, spatially and temporarily, correlatively, white binds together viewer and object, subject and matter.

THE ILLUSTRATED ARISTOTLE, PART II

After these three reconsiderations of white, offered by Bataille, Derrida, and Bal, the specific color of sperm can no longer look particularly smooth, pure, sterile, even-toned, hygienic, immaculate, or neutral. Precisely the opalescence of white, it appears, provokes differentiality, a heterogeneity of perspectives, variations in hues and shades, layers of white on white. When looking again at Serrano's *Untitled XIV* in terms of Bataille, the image now no longer depicts a clean jet of semen shooting through an empty space. Instead, the work represents a space so chock full of matter that it bursts, cracking open and disposing the viscous and thick liquid, oozing out as if from an emerging seam or an infected wound. The shininess of semen that Aristotle notes, linked to the analogously luminescent stars that Bataille rephrases as "vapours shining in the immensity," forms the occasion for the frantic multiplication of reflections between human ejaculation and the Milky Way, "bouncing symmetrical images back to infinity."

Therefore, the simile offers no clear or transparent correspondence between male orgasm and cosmic appearance. Instead, it presents the inexorable blurring and soiling of the two together, the staining or tainting of the reflexive mirror that allowed for the comparison in the first place, through which the two mingle with the menstrual blood and the urine that define them in contradistinction. Hence, Bataille undoes the Aristotelian analogy between the semen and the stars by augmenting it, "bouncing" it, so that it is thrown out of whack.

Look again, together with Derrida. Now, the white of the semen in the image can be seen to "re-mark," to reflect on, the parergonic frame of white that surrounds the image. Only by virtue of that crucial demarcation can the seminal white appear as a relatively discrete appearance—one that nevertheless touches or enters into contact with the grounding white at both ends of the picture, both emerging from it and dissolving into it. Thus, the jet is imbued with the absence it should supposedly fill. Furthermore, the white shape can also be viewed as an uncompleted streak performed by a piece of gum or rubber, blotting away the black of the background that, at some places more than others, nevertheless comes through the white. Once more, this may lead to a consideration of how the Aristotelian imagination has elevated the masculine import in generation, while erasing, blotting away, the feminine input denied a quasi-celestial or semidivine appearance or stature.

Looking closer still, the seminal phenomenon looks like a folded cloth, consisting of layers of fabric, being wrung in the air or hung out to dry. This takes away its movement as well as its momentum. The luminescent piece of cloth, suspended in the air, may indeed provoke a "thousand glances," fracturing the look it compels into many detailed reflections, thus losing sight of the whole, the totality and singularity of spirit that, according to Aristotle, it inhabits and transports.

Look once more, this time with Bal. Featuring the baroque scale-flipping she details, the image can be seen as representing something that is improbably large, like the Milky Way, as well as something small: spermatozoa unseen to the naked eye. This relates back to Aristotle's relative understanding of sperm's whiteness: "the smaller and less visible the bubbles in it, the whiter and firmer does the mass appear" (*Generation of Animals* 2.2). The supposedly pure whiteness of semen is conditional on the scale of the pockets of spirit or air encapsulated in it. The smaller these bubbles, the whiter the semen appears, and the better it reflects the light and the eye, akin to Bal's infinite multitude of tiny convex mirrors captured in the white paint.[28]

Like a fractured distorting mirror, furthermore, the image draws in the male gaze, to then bounce it back, returning it as fragmented, deformed, and enlarged. Hence, it makes both manifest and impossible the masculine imperative that wants to imagine ejaculation on a scale so large, otherworldly, and pure. This out-of-proportion mirroring reflects the disproportionate attention given to semen in patriarchy, its unlikely apotheosis, its elevation to a cosmic scale.

There is one perspective left unconsidered that Aristotle could not but notice: the temporality of entropy that makes semen change appearance over time, the precious substance losing its color and its firmness, going transparent and runny, the heat dying down, the shine turning dull, the froth going flat. In the last work by Serrano that I want to discuss, this material changeability of semen is pushed even beyond the point that Aristotle can consider: semen once more appears as a textured, opalescent white, but now in a frozen state.

ICE

Aristotle asserts, "And this also shows, incidentally, why semen does not freeze: it is because air is impervious to frost" (2.2). In contrast, Serrano's *Frozen Sperm I* (Figure 5) shows a glacial mass of frozen sperm on a dark surface pane. In many ways, it is the "polar" opposite of the previous images. With its horizontal perceptual plane, and its mass of matter frozen in place to the ground, the work leaves behind the alluring and celestial verticality of *Untitled XIV* and returns to the spatial figuration of the *Semen and Blood* pictures. However, whereas the latter depicted the two fluids in an intimate, viscous, and interacting tension, *Frozen Sperm I* offers only the semen that, without the blood that grants it its life, is stuck in a state of immobility and inertia. Instead of the inconceivable instant of the ejaculation-in-trajectory, moreover, this image suggests a materiality without event, all progress or movement being interrupted or suspended. The picture alludes

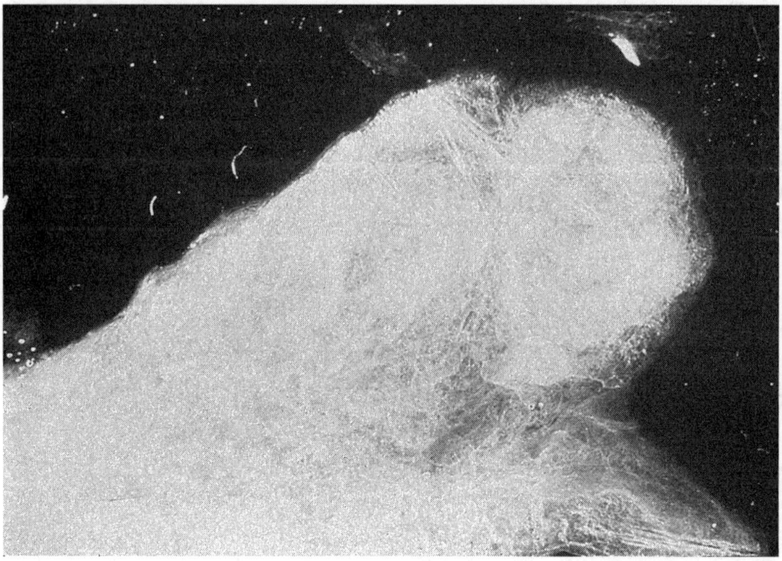

FIGURE 5. Andres Serrano, *Frozen Sperm I*, 1990. Cibachrome, silicone, plexiglas, and wood frame. 40 × 60 inches. Courtesy of the Paula Cooper Gallery, New York.

to an ice age long gone, when slowly moving glaciers covered the earth, an association that relegates the image to a prehistoric past.

Nevertheless, *Frozen Sperm I* partakes of the same kind of scale-flipping that Bal terms "baroque," and that turned out to be relevant for *Untitled XIV* as well as for the two *Semen and Blood* photographs. This image, too, alternates between incongruous perspectives: a satellite view from high up in space, stressing great distance, and a close-up vision of something slight, like a piece of freeze-dried gum. Following up on and extending several of the concerns animating the previous works, it gives them a new twist. Thus a narrative is spinning itself between these three sets of images.

This narrative partakes of the temporality of entropy that I have read in Aristotle's treatise on reproduction. As if depicting the life-cycle of sperm, it moves from the stage of its conception or concoction from the blood that forms its living ground (the *Semen and Blood* pictures) through an intense and fraught moment of trajection or passage (*Untitled XIV*), to end up as rigidly rematerialized, immobile, and inert (*Frozen Sperm I*).

Aristotle, however, refused to acknowledge this last stage, contending that semen, because of the pneuma and the psyche captured inside it, cannot freeze. Instead, he followed his observation of the liquid changing in appearance outside the body—the white turning transparent, its heat going cold, its shine turning dull, its froth going flat—with the vision of sperm as dried-up like a wad of phlegm on the street. Why is that image apparently more attractive to Aristotle than one of frozen sperm? As he argued, the liquid dies down and dries up only *after* the spirit has evaporated, gone elsewhere. Giving up the principle of life, semen reverts to mere matter. Indeed, "Later, when it has lost its heat by evaporation and the air has cooled, it becomes fluid and dark, because the water and whatever tiny quantity of earthy matter it may contain, stay behind in the semen as it solidifies, just as happens with phlegma" (2.2). This explanation saves the spirit from becoming matter.

THE ILLUSTRATED ARISTOTLE, PART III

However, the possibility of semen's freezing, made visibly concrete by Serrano, pledges the enduring imprisonment or entombment of the spirit in glacial matter, hovering inside in a state of suspended animation, not quite alive, nor quite dead.[29] When read in the context of contemporary fears of HIV infection, *Frozen Sperm I* suggests the temporary encapsulation of the fluid's capacity for contamination: solid and immobile, the seed cannot transmit the virus, unless, at some later date, it is thawed again and regains its uncanny force. In an Aristotelian vein, the suspended state of the semen in the image allows for another and final understanding of the white of semen, now considered as icy. If the sperm is indeed frozen, this would mean, in Aristotle's logic, that it has already gone partially transparent and watery. That should be why the ice seems whiter at some places, more transparent and dark at others. Apparently, the sperm is frozen at the exact moment of changing over, of transforming in appearance, of losing its life and becoming dead matter, yet before that process is entirely completed. Hence, the white of the ice is spectral, ghostly.[30]

This puts the semen in a state in between Aristotle's governing oppositions: male and female, spirit and matter, life and death. Also, this threatens the crucial boundaries that Aristotle draws between lifeless objects, plants, animals, and humans. Animals, lacking intellect or reason, nevertheless share with humans the capacity for sense-perception that gives them a qualified access to knowledge, Aristotle claims: "some have more, some less, some very little indeed" (1.23). Though this amounts to little in comparison to humans, to lifeless objects it must seem "a very fine thing indeed." For, "we should much prefer to have even this sort of knowledge to a state of death and non-existence" (1.23). However, this last describes the predicament the precious liquid ultimately falls into in Serrano's photographic series: sperm lying dormant in "a state of death and non-existence."

In the dialogue between Aristotle and Serrano, the principle of life and form that gives sperm its patriarchal accolade, that makes it more than matter, finds its counterpoint in the considerations of semen *qua* substance. The blotchy "squigglies" of semen, the opalescent hue of the trajectory of sperm, the semen entombed in ice, the temporality of entropy, the wad of dried-up sperm—all these visions of semen suggest appearances of the precious liquid as materially formless and changing. The substance that gives both life and form to matter is itself materially shapeless. Hence, it cannot but lack the identity and significance so frantically and determinedly ascribed to it. Indeed, these visions of sperm form the specters that persistently haunt the apotheosis of the semen.

PART TWO

PSYCHOANALYSIS

TWO

IMAGE OF THE VITAL FLOW

Lacan

IF THE PREVIOUS CHAPTER CONCLUDED with semen put into an uncanny, frozen state between life and death, this chapter will cautiously resuscitate the prized liquid back to life. For it is in the shape of "the image of the *vital* flow [*flux vital*] as it is transmitted in generation" that ejaculation momentarily and marginally enters into Jacques Lacan's canonical text on the phallus, signification, and gender.[1] Andres Serrano's *Untitled XIV (ejaculation in trajectory)* (see Figure 4) can as fittingly be taken to "illustrate," to bear on, Lacan's image of ejaculation as it does a specific juncture in Aristotle's treatise on reproduction in the preceding chapter. Indeed, the phrase underscores the same precarious temporality and visibility of male orgasm, which the confrontation between Serrano and Aristotle has sharply brought to the fore.

"[T]he *image* of the vital flow" pledges an uncompromisingly visible appearance of ejaculation. Yet, that promise is instantly revoked by the qualifying "as it is transmitted in generation." Presumably, the flow of sperm must pass imperceptibly within the female body for generation to occur. Doubtlessly, a nongenerative gush of semen that can in fact be fully visible, as in Serrano's "inconceivable" work, cannot but be considerably less vital and lively. Hence, Lacan's image of ejaculation can only be imagined, and not seen in its materiality. As in the case of Aristotle's argument, the perceptibility of sperm would abduct the substance from the context of generation that determines its value, its life.

Moreover, the durative "vital *flow*" conjures up the image of an undeviating and unending source of life and meaning. However, a "punctual" reading of "*as it is transmitted* in generation" ascribes to the flow a precise instant of happening, and hence, an irreducible finality.[2] Thus, a concern for the precise timing of the event of transmission overrules the supposed eternality of the seminal stream. Serrano's subtitle, "in trajectory," highlights the utterly transitory nature of the monumental and quasi-celestial phenomenon that the image depicts. This double tension of visuality and temporality is also readable in the clash of registers in Lacan's phraseology, for the mythopoetic overtones of the "vital flow" and the technical, mechanical resonance of "transmitted" do not quite agree.

Perhaps it is because of those complications that the role of ejaculation in Lacan's essay is so peripheral and tangential. In "The Signification of the Phallus," ejaculation enters the scene only obliquely and is dismissed nearly immediately. The appearance of ejaculation is fleetingly entertained as one of the possible reasons why the phallus must be the chosen signifier of the marriage between *logos* and desire, the connection between language and sexuality. If the ejaculatory image appears to assign a cautious visibility to the phallus, this happens only to be subsequently withdrawn, as Lacan moves on to state as fact "that the phallus can only play its role when veiled" (82).

Put more strongly, exactly the proposition of the visibility of ejaculation works to obscure, to occlude, the function of the phallus-as-veiled, Lacan argues. Hence, the phallus comes to stand at the threshold of visibility and invisibility, as the trope of the veil indicates, and remains untouched by the contradictory image of ejaculation evoked in its proximity. This terse arrangement raises several questions. Why is ejaculation called upon to motivate the selection of the phallus as the "privileged signifier"? What is the precise relation between ejaculation and the phallus? What is the import of ejaculation with respect to the effect of meaning, the signified, which the phallus brands as its "bastard offspring" (82)?

This chapter focuses on Lacan for two reasons. First, Lacan's coinage of the phallus offers a choice opportunity to discuss the congruence of meaning and masculinity. In Lacan's thinking, the phallus rules both the making of gender and the making of meaning in one gesture. What place ejaculation occupies in this alignment of meaning and masculinity, however, is left open for speculation.

Second, the terse and oblique position of ejaculation in Lacan—brought up but not taken up at any length—requires further scrutiny to draw out its possible implications and consequences. Ejaculation can thus be investigated within and from a theoretical framework that only minimally acknowledges it. The noted precariousness of the moment and image of ejaculation forms the guide for my reading. As I will show, a strategic stress on the ejaculatory in Lacan's essay about the phallus can work to displace much of its economy.

NOEUD/NOUS

As I was writing this chapter, I got hopelessly stuck. Of course, the notion that relieved my frustration was that of the "knot." With respect to Lacan, it seems, a twisted sense of irony is never far away, ready to seize one when one is most vulnerable. "We know that the unconscious castration complex," Lacan opens "The Signification of the Phallus," "has the function of a knot [*noeud*]" (75). Castration underlies both the "dynamic structuring of symptoms" and the development of the subject; it also ties the latter together with the former, lending it "its ratio" (75).

Quickly, however, the connecting potential of the knot becomes too tight for comfort, as Lacan reminds us of the fact that Freud suggested "not a contingent, but an essential disturbance of human sexuality" (75). This fundamental disturbance results in "the irreducibility for any finite (*endliche*) analysis" of the effects of the castration complex for both genders. Hence, the knot of castration becomes the primary "point of uncertainty"—the French has *aporie*—that the "Freudian experience" has introduced in our mind (75). The knot of castration, linking up symptomatic and developmental analysis, and granting them a rationale and a structure, is at the same time inexhaustibly irreducible to efforts at its understanding. This knot ties together and twists out of shape in one and the same move.

For an essay entitled "The Signification of the Phallus" that emphatically argues that the phallus is *not* the penis, it is quite surprising, to say the least, that its first sentence should turn on a particular word, *noeud*, which not only means "knot," but also denotes, in French slang, the glans, or head of the penis, and, by synecdoche, "dick" or "knob."[3] This element of the text becomes all the more poignant as soon as one notices another word that echoes it in the essay's last sentence. It is the Greek word for "sense" or "meaning": *nous*. "The function of the signifier here touches upon its most profound relation," Lacan concludes the essay, "by way of which the Ancients embodied in it both the *Nous* and the *Logos*" (85).

The slippage between these two words, "noeud" and "nous," forms an apt example of Lacanian semiosis. It suggests "the effects discovered at the level of the materially unstable elements which constitute the chain of language" (79). The text performs what it preaches; it enacts its own argument. Weighing in as the title's chiasmic counterpoint, the two words come to establish the piece's outer edge or frame. "Nous"/"noeud," "The Signification of the Phallus"/"The Dick of Sense"—the argument begins and ends here, with a pun. Everything else must fall within the scope of this bizarre twist.

In effect, the text speaks in tongues. "Phallus," with its archaic, classical pedigree, is countered by the crude and vulgar "dick" of slang. Vernacular "sense" is upped by the resonant and philosophical "nous." The figure that connects and twists around the title and the frame composed of "noeud"/ "nous" is the chiasmus, a reversal. That rhetorical figure gets its name from the Greek letter chi (X), typographically a cross or knot. Consequently, a reinforced contamination or entanglement of the "phallus" by the "dick" frames a discussion in which it is argued that the phallus is above all not the penis, infecting everything within its scope with the possibility of reversal and traversal.

The entanglement of, or slippage between, different tongues or discourses implies that the essay enacts the mode of semiosis that Mikhail Bakhtin captures under the heading of *heteroglossia*.[4] Meaning "happens" when different registers or languages in a text cross and collide, causing signifiers to bounce off each other. Thus, the phallus only rises to meaning in the close company of redolent signifier strings, like the one that stretches from "noeud" to "nous," and fundamental ambiguities, like the one between "knot" and "dick."

Bakhtin views the genre of the novel as heteroglossia's proper home. Thus, it is not surprising that *noeud*, next to "knot" and "dick," should also denote the "complication," "plot," or "intrigue" of narrative and theater. Therefore, the analysis of the phallic knot must proceed narratively. I begin by attending to the plot's protagonist, which, veiled or not, or rather, precisely *because* it is veiled, nearly obscures all the other characters on Lacan's theoretical stage: the phallus.

THE NAME OF THE PHALLUS

A concept is first and foremost articulated as a word. Since Lacan is often credited with the emancipation of the signifier, let us consider the status of the phallus as a concrete term. What kind of word is "phallus"? It is a translation, and perhaps a bad one. According to David Macey, the French translation of Freud's oeuvre arbitrarily translated German genital vocabulary into *pénis* and *phallus*, leading commentators to imply a meaningful distinction where perhaps none was ever intended.[5] In the authoritative *Language of Psychoanalysis*, J. Laplanche and J.-B. Pontalis cite instances in Freud's oeuvre that cast doubt upon the analytical wisdom of assuming an important distinction between the two.[6]

In addition, the term is a euphemism. Macey also suggests that the French analytical community may have preferred the elegant *phallus* to the more vulgar and medical *pénis* (319). In this sense, the phallus reifies the penis by distancing itself from it. Furthermore, "phallus" is an archaic term, its Greek pedigree granting the concept a classical and conceptual standing. Arguably, any word can turn into a concept when it is translated into Greek. Lacan is much intrigued by the alleged ancientness of the phallus, referring to the "ancients" and to "ancient mysteries" on many occasions ("Signification," 79, 82, 85).[7] Finally, Judith Butler suggests that "phallus" should be understood as a proper name attributed to an organ, thus conferring a linguistic identity and fixity on an otherwise anonymous body part.[8]

As a translation, euphemism, archaism, and a name, the phallus invites many contradictions. For instance, the fixity of the proper name clashes with its translated status. Whereas the archaism promises a mysterious origin preceding proper history, the euphemism points to contemporary social distinction. Apparently, the fact that "phallus" is a single word does not prevent it from featuring in different discourses or uses; this reinforces its heteroglot character. A similar situation holds for the term's various connotations and aspects.

The phallus primarily connotes a nebula of symbolic meanings, like "sovereignty," "power," "wholeness," "authority," and a "transcendental virility." These notions are emphatically not to be imputed to the anatomical penis. "[W]hat is symbolized here," Laplanche and Pontalis explain, "cannot be reduced to the male organ or penis itself, in its anatomical reality" (*Language*, 312–13). According to Lacan, the phallus functions irrespective of anatomy. "[C]linical facts," he claims, "go to show that the relation of the subject to the phallus is set up regardless of the anatomical difference between the sexes" ("Signification," 76).

However, this symbolic view of the phallus does not sit well with Lacan's specific coinage of the concept. Famously, he claims that it is a "signifier" ("Signification," 79–80). The phallus is the signifier of "that mark" [*cette marque*], which itself remains unnamed, unidentified, that initiates the digital or binary chain of meaning, the first blip or one, the first marker of difference, in a potentially endless series of zeroes and ones that will trigger signification (82). In this sense, the phallic signifier is not so much original or primordial, but rather "privileged" in that it forms the dominant way in which the principle of difference is made concrete in a patriarchal culture. Hypothetically, that leaves open the possibility that "that mark" could well be signified differently. In turn, however, the privilege cannot but undermine the phallus's status as a signifier. For the structure of meaning allows for no such exemption, only for relative differences. Dryly, Macey notes that the notion of a "privileged signifier" is a "distinctly unhappy" one within the terms of (post)structuralism ("Phallus," 319).[9]

Next to being privileged, the phallus is something else that a signifier can hardly be. The signifier is defined by a concrete and material perceptibility, whereas the phallus is "veiled." As Lacan claims, "the phallus can only play its role when veiled" ("Signification," 82). This implies that the phallus oversees both meaning and gender, while it recedes from an unqualified visibility, and hence, from its status as a signifier. But even if the observation of anatomy is peremptorily dismissed, a charged visual dynamic of showing and hiding nevertheless returns with a vengeance. Throughout the essay, the phallus appears and disappears, it is veiled and unveiled, it is raised and erased.

As the privileged signifier of differentiation, finally, the phallus also determines gender positions. It does so not in the usual way, in the sense that one gender has the penis and comes to suffer from castration anxiety, while the other lacks the organ and develops penis envy as a result, but rather in the sense that gender relations revolve on the respective positions of "having" and "being" the phallus. Masculinity is reconfigured by Lacan as "having," femininity as "being," the phallus (83). (For more on this dynamic, see chapter 4.)

Its name alluding to different connotations, its meaning implying contradictory aspects—symbol of masculinity and power, signifier of difference, (in)visible, veiled entity, and gender function—the phallus is indeed a *noeud*, a knot. If the concept works, it does so precisely by being less than clear and discrete, by entangling various notions and ideas in a single, tight hold. This also means that it is susceptible to a novelistic, dialogic, or narrative reading, in Bakhtin's vein. For, if the phallus is indeed a discursive *noeud*, it is to be read as such: as a narrative intrigue, plot, or complication.

A narratological perspective on Lacan's essay yields several important opportunities for analysis. First, the lines of thought that are knotted together in an aporetic conundrum or "concatenation" (Lacan's word) under the heading of the phallus may be separated through a narrative analysis, in which the phallus comes to play the role of a complex conceptual character. Second, narratology enables the reappraisal of the essay in terms of the arrangement and movement of different events, characters, and focalizations or perspectives; alternative positions in the struggle for power, for meaning, can become intelligible, as well as the specific and directive slant with which they are presented by the narrator, "Lacan." Finally, the concern for the precarious visibility and temporality suggested by Lacan's figure of ejaculation, "the image of the vital flow as it is transmitted in generation," may move sharply into focus through a narrative analysis. Together, these three possibilities work to give the phallus, supposedly archaic and ancient, and thus before or beyond history, a specific historicity, a "life" story.

True, at first glance Lacan does not seem the storyteller that Freud is. Lacan's penchant is for the abstract, the formulaic, the mathematical. Yet, "The Signification of the Phallus" is thick with narrative promise: an old woman whispering revelations to Daphnis and Chloë (77); the fated discovery of the unconscious and the rediscovery of the "passion of the signifier" in the human condition (76–77); the anticipation that psychoanalysis might "lift the veil from [the function the phallus once] served in the mysteries" (80); the intricate story of the "marriage" of logos and desire (82); tales of appearances and masquerades (84–85).

At many places, the thrust of the essay seems narrative in an age-old fashion: it pledges the unraveling of a mystery, the apprehension of a secret, the answer to a riddle. Man's experience cannot be explained through a recourse to biology, Lacan succinctly argues, "as the mere necessity of the myth underlying the structuring of the Oedipus complex makes sufficiently clear" (75). Less clear, however, are the precise narrative or mythical trajectories that move through the text and, consequently, the question of in what way and to what extent the meaning of the phallus can or should be fathomed narratively.

Ejaculation plays a crucial but unclarified part in the "theoretical fiction" of Lacan's essay.[10] It does not form the climactic outcome of the story; that position is taken up by the emergence and calibration of the phallus as a master concept. For Lacan, ejaculation commands neither a concept, nor an uncompromising image. Nor does it bear a proper name, euphemistic, archaic, or otherwise. Nor is it in any way privileged as a relevant symbol, signifier, or gender pivot, even though the phrase "vital flow" seems thick with mythopoetic imagination. If ejaculation is veiled, as the phallus is, it is veiled with an effectivity that nearly removes it from the theoretical scene altogether.

Nevertheless, ejaculation is part and parcel of the argument in "The Signification of the Phallus." Not only is it briefly considered as one of the propositions grounding the phallus as the signifier that organizes language and sexuality, it also comes back into focus when the effect of meaning, the signified, is described as the "bastard offspring" of the phallus (82). Indeed, Lacan theorizes the occurrence of meaning through a scene of procreation that should put ejaculation, the "flow" or "transmission" of semen, at center stage. Furthermore, the fact that this progeny is characterized as "bastard," in the sense of both "illegitimate" and "hybrid," might well indicate the extent to which both meaning and sperm escape the phallus that spawns, marks, or brands them. To prepare for a narrative reading of "The Signification of the Phallus," the next section will inquire into the framing, the setup, that determines the story of the phallus.

THE STORY'S SETUP

The central events recounted in the essay are the veiling and the subsequent *Aufhebung* or sublation of the phallus. However, these two related events can only be understood if their embedding frames are taken into consideration. As mentioned above, the first relevant frame is made up of the chiasmic link between the title of the essay and the two related words from its first and last lines: "The Signification of the Phallus" and "The Dick [*noeud*] of Sense [*Nous*]." Forming the outer edge of the text, this frame inflects everything within its scope with the possibility of recontamination and reversal. In that way, moreover, Lacan impedes the understanding of the penis in its anatomical "reality." Apparently, signification relates to the alternative of "dick" and "phallus." Both terms are replete with extra or excessive connotations that preclude neutrality or a quasi-medical objectivity.

As a second frame, a chiasmus also characterizes the overall movement of the essay. The text performs a marked move off course, a steady lapse away from its stated aims. "The Signification of the Phallus" starts off with the unambiguous claim that the unconscious castration complex, in and through which the phallus functions, is crucial for the formation of the subject. Without the castration complex, Lacan argues, the subject "would be unable to identify with the ideal type of his sex, or to respond without grave risk to the needs of his partner in the sexual relation, or even to receive adequately the needs of the child thus procreated" (75). Hence, castration and phallus are initially called upon to warrant "ideal" gender positions, heterosexuality, reproduction, and child care. These norms also underlie the dominant stories of our culture.

Although the essay's opening gesture anticipates a happy ending to the development of the subject, if only the consequences of the castration complex are sufficiently taken into account and worked through, this promise manifestly fails to be kept at the end of the essay. By then, Lacan has moved far beyond sexual ideality. Rather than normative gender, heterosexuality, reproduction, and child care, Lacan at the end entertains respective theorizations of male and female homosexuality; quaint notions of why frigidity in women is better tolerated than impotence in men; the claim that "ideal or typical manifestations" of gender behavior are "entirely propelled into comedy"; and the twin observation that women may vanquish their "essential" attribute of masquerade, and that "virile display itself appears as feminine" (84–85). The reversal in perspective that separates the essay's ending from its beginning is quite staggering. The whole argument falls within the reach of this second, uprooted frame of a slippage.

What has happened in between the beginning and ending of the essay to garner such dire consequences? Granted, the middle part of the text sees the emergence of desire as "paradoxical, deviant, erratic, eccentric and even scandalous" (80). Yet, that in itself does not account for the essay's massive move astray. At the heart of the essay, in the core of the twisted "noeud," something of a fundamental nature must have happened to bring about such a stunning lapse.

The third and last frame to consider is less easily recognizable and localizable. It concerns idiom, the rhetorical strands the essay returns to over and again. Even when he addresses diverse matters, the narrator "Lacan" often uses the same words and figures, sometimes accompanied by their German equivalents to signal his indebtedness to Freud. These come together in three distinct but closely related tropes. The first one entails a rhetoric of upward and downward motion (for instance, the lifting and drawing of the veil, the *Aufhebung* of demand and the phallus, the *Erniedrigung* of the satisfactions of needs and of love in men).

The second trope concerns a vocabulary of appearing and disappearing (for example, the "other scene," the phallus veiled and unveiled). The third one is a rhetoric of movement forward and backward, primarily of time (for instance, "deferred action," the "return" to Freud, the "retreat" of the discovery of the unconscious). In these strands of rhetoric, one might well suspect the diagrammatic presence of the penis under and in the text's lines, moving back and forth, up and down, appearing and disappearing. Perhaps, then, the text itself works as a veil to obscure the subrhetorical presence of the penis. Hence, the third frame of the text, suggested by the idiomatic recurrences that imply the plasticity and motionality of the penis, calls for a reevaluation of the moment of veiling and unveiling, the first event of the story. What is going on under the Lacanian veil? The plot thickens.

GRAPHIC CONCATENATION: WHEN PHALLUS MEETS SIGNIFIABLE

The specific passage I want to submit to a narrative close reading narrates the twin events of the veiling and unveiling, and the *Aufhebung*, or sublation, of the phallus, its coming into being as a concept. It also includes Lacan's ejaculatory oxymoron. Because of the fragment's philosophical complexity, in which Freud meets Saussure and Hegel, another aspect of the text's heteroglot discursivity, the precise implications of these events are not easily grasped. That is why I quote the passage in full below, with the addition of paragraph numbers and some of the original text in French between square brackets:

(1) The phallus is the privileged signifier of that mark [*cette marque*] where the share of logos is wedded to [*se conjoint à*] the advent of desire.

(2) One might say [*On peut dire*] that this signifier is chosen as what stands out most easily [*le plus saillant*] seized upon [*attraper*] in the real of sexual copulation, and also as the most symbolic in the literal (typographical) sense of the term, since it is the equivalent of

the (logical) copula [*copule (logique)*]. One might also say that by virtue of its turgidity [*turgidité*], it is the image of the vital flow as it is transmitted in generation [*l'image du flux vital en tant qu'il passe dans la génération*].

(3) All these propositions merely veil [*voiler*] over the fact that the phallus can only play its role as veiled [*voilé*], that is, as in itself the sign of the latency [*latence*] with which everything signifiable [*tout signifiable*] is struck [*frappé*] as soon as it is raised (*aufgehoben*) to the function of signifier.

(4) The phallus is the signifier of this *Aufhebung* itself which it inaugurates (initiates) by its own disappearance. This is why the demon of *Aidoos* [*Scham*, shame] in the ancient mysteries rises up [*surgit*] exactly at the moment when the phallus is unveiled [*dévoilé*] (cf. the famous painting of the Villa of Pompeii).

(5) It then becomes the bar [*la barre*] which, at the hands of this demon, strikes [*frappe*] the signified, branding it [*le marquant*] as the bastard offspring [*la progéniture bâtarde*] of this signifying concatenation [*sa concaténation signifiante*].

Thick with conceptual, philosophical language, this fragment does not seem particularly narrative at first sight. The fifth paragraph performs the circled return of the first. Both the notions of the "mark" [*cette marque*] and the connection or "wedding" [*se conjoint à*] of paragraph one reappear in the last [*le marquant, concaténation*]. However, something must have occurred, since the fifth paragraph witnesses the birth of the "bastard offspring" of meaning.

Moreover, the phallus, described as the "privileged signifier" in the first paragraph, and circumscribed in the second paragraph in tangible, linguistic, typographical, and visual terms, reenters the scene in its capacity of the semiotic bar; that is, *after* having been veiled and *aufgehoben*. Hence, a decisive, transformative, and consequential event has in fact transpired. The phallus has made something happen, the generation of meaning, and something has happened to the phallus. Initially, it is the signifier of "that mark"; later, it is doing the "marking" itself.

The first paragraph links or "marries" *logos* and desire, language and sexuality. This connection is underpinned by the word that states it. "Conjonction" [*se conjoint à*] translates as "meeting," "wedding," "coitus," and linguistic "conjunction." As a reading instruction, the word invites a double reading of the whole passage in both marital or sexual and linguistic terms. The intimate entanglement of the two domains is followed up by terms such as "sexual copulation," the "copula" or copulative verb, "generation," and the final "concatenation." Many of the words used play into this double register. *Copula* refers to the verb function or to the logical joint or hyphen between two terms, as well as back to the "copulation"; *turgidity* to the swelling of the penis and to a writing style that is rigid and "not flowing"; and the *bar* to a "rod," a typographic "line" or "stripe," and to "deletion" or "erasure."

The double entendres on "marriage," "copulation," and "conjunction" prompt two consequences. The opening line ushers in a *graphic* reading of the fragment in the double meaning of that word: *both* as explicitly and visibly sexual *and* as linguistic and typographic. Ironically, the same passage that is so much about veils and shame is also suggestive to the ~~point~~ of being lewd. In addition, the emphasis on conjunction and the dialectic of *Aufhebung* forge the consideration of a second, antithetical agent, besides the phallus, to take part in the event. Glossed over to the point of being nearly invisible, "everything signifiable" is the likely candidate for that position; this signifiable is "struck" [*frappé*], or rather, more graphically, "thrusted into" or "fucked" by the phallus. Hence, the first paragraph proposes the occurrence of meaning as understood in linguistic and sexual dimensions, and as playing out between two characters or agents, between phallus and signifiable.

As Lacan goes on, the second paragraph considers three proposals as to why the phallus must be the selected signifier of the marriage between sexuality and language. They are preceded by a strongly qualifying "one might say" [*on peut dire*], as if to caution that the narrator might not be prepared to espouse or validate them unequivocally.[11] The first proposition is based on tangibility. As a kind of stick figure, the phallus stands out [*le plus saillant*] as what is most easily grabbed [*attraper*] in copulation. Curiously, the phallus must be the privileged signifier because of the supposed tactile preponderance of the penis during coitus—surely a matter of perspective.

The second proposition compares the coital tangibility of the penis to the linguistic copulative verb, which relates subject to predicate, or to the hyphen that connects yet separates two terms in logic (as in "A-B"). That latter possibility is brought up by the addition of the specifying "logical" [*logique*]. Moreover, the hyphen can indeed serve as "the most symbolic [equivalent] in the literal (typographical) sense of the word" of the outstanding and graspable qualities of the phallus. More so than the verb function, the hyphen is a specifically typographical signifier.

After considering the election of the phallus in tangible, linguistic, and typographical terms, the third proposition centers on visibility. Now the phallus is preferred as "the image of the vital flow," motivated by its "turgidity." Ejaculation figures as a rigid jet that passes [*passe*] between two people or entities in reproduction, thus referring back to the copulation and to the connecting potential of the hyphen and/or the copulative verb.

The three propositions that Lacan entertains seem scarcely coherent and relevant. Yet they become instantly comprehensible once they are viewed in relation to the semiotic bar, which makes its appearance in the last paragraph. Transcribed as a thin line that divorces signified from signifier, and that puts the latter *over* the former—"S–s," signifier over signified—the ultimately separative bar is preceded by a triple consideration of the *connecting* potential of graphic markers like the line, stripe, hyphen, or dash. The penis sticking out, the typographical hyphen, the image of the rigid flow—these are all presented as material, tactile, and perceptible lines that join participants, people, or terms.

Therefore, the whole paragraph acquires coherence if one is prepared to see the three quaint propositions as verbal circumscriptions of one visible signifier, simply, a line, the mark of "conjunction" and "concatenation," be it in marriage, copulation, language, or logic. This mark, initially called upon to join different entities, will later "strike" [*frapper*] and separate again. If the passage is indeed burdened with the verbal transcription or circumscription of the visual, typographical signifier of the line or stripe, then the narrator "Lacan" works both angles of its figuration: it joins and disjoins, connects and disconnects, attaches and severs, marries and divorces.

I have dwelled upon this typographical reading of the second paragraph to suspend and delay a more obviously narrative way to read the three propositions. They can also be viewed as the stereotypical narrative of male sexuality: from erection (the penis sticking out [*le plus saillant*]), to copulation, to ejaculation [*flux vital*]. Therefore, the second paragraph graphically moves back and forth between, and thus entangles, the concretely penile and the typographic.

BASTARD OFFSPRING

In the third and fourth paragraphs, the previous three evocations of the line are promptly dismissed. Tangible, typographic, linguistic, and visible, they obscure, with their material and sensory perceptibility, the fact that the phallus can only perform its genuine role when it is surreptitiously withdrawn from all further sight and contact. Once veiled, the phallus becomes the obscure sign of the *Aufhebung* of "everything signifiable" to the position of signifier. It can only become this negative sign, the sign of an absence, by receding from its earlier propositions. To partake in the *Aufhebung*, the signifiable is "struck" with "latency." In the fifth paragraph, a signified is generated from this dormant potential, struck by the phallic bar as the bastard offspring of the encounter between phallus and signifiable. I presume that the narrator implies here that the potential for meaning must be manipulated by the principle of differentiation in order to produce a signifier that, in turn, triggers a signified. In that way, the phallus must vanquish its former capacity to join terms in favor of the function of differentiation.

Yet, in step with the double entendre of the reading instruction, the scene of *Aufhebung* can also be read graphically, a possibility that persistently shimmers through the rhetoric of the passage, ranging from the marriage of the first line to the appearance of progeny in the last. *Aufhebung* entails the simultaneous elevation and disappearance of the phallus. In other words, it becomes erect and penetrates, strikes, or fucks the signifiable.[12] As a result, the signifiable is invested with a "latency," a temporal and visual interval. Since *période de latence* means "incubation period," the connotation of pregnancy seems particularly apt. Reappearing, the phallus finally becomes the *barre*, at once the semiotic function of differentiation and a "rod." Finally, the "bastard offspring" [*progéniture bâtarde*] is born.

It appears that the story line underlying the psycho-semiotic theory is indeed the oldest story of patriarchy: an active, masculine principle forces meaning out of a passive, feminine material, itself predominantly dormant and latent. The narrative forms a sarcastic term-for-term parody of the romantic promise of the wedding and the ostensibly espoused ideals of gender, heterosexuality, reproduction, and child care. In this way, Lacan continues his opposition to the tendency to put one's psychic trust in what he calls genital "tenderness" and "maturation" to harmonize and fulfill the subject. However, in doing so he wittingly or unwittingly reiterates a story line that is thoroughly sexist and heterosexist in its implications.

However, the bastard child of meaning is not the only entity being conceived here. The passage also witnesses the birth, the coinage, of a concept, the phallus, in its final and proper shape. This implies that the concept itself is caught up in the generation of meaning, its product rather than its origin, and can only be conceived as such through its encounter with the signifiable. It is only with child, so to speak, that the phallus achieves its ultimate functionality.

Aufhebung proposes a triple semantic register: elevation, erasure, and reserve. The sublated term lifts up, cancels out, and saves the preceding ones in a new synthesis. The first two implications are clear. Erasing the former penile connotations, the phallus raises an organ to the stature of a semiotic and philosophical master concept. As the new concept, however, the phallus figuratively retains many penile characteristics. *Aufhebung* articulates erection and penetration; the phallus as *barre* is also a "rod"; it maintains its capacity to "strike" [*frapper*]; and the effect of meaning is described as "offspring."

The appropriation of a concept that promises a higher synthesis in order to perform and illustrate the irreducible split between, and simultaneity of, the penis and the phallus is something of a rhetorical masterstroke. For, the veiling and elevation of the phallus ultimately leads right back to the dismissed penis, or rather, to the "dick" [*noeud*] of meaning. As in a magic trick, the drawing of the veil anticipates a surprise. What will appear as it is lifted again may be either a graphic signifier, a concept, or a body part; indeed, a bunch of flowers, a white rabbit, or a decapitated assistant. What seems to have disappeared for good, however, are the feminine signifiable and male ejaculation.

THE MAGICIAN AND THE VEIL

The transformative power of the veil points to the magician, the performing narrator, "Lacan," who wields it. As I have suggested, the story of the birth of meaning and the calibration of the concept that produces it are intertwined or concatenated. So, what good does it do the magician or narrator to draw the veil during his performance?[13] I want to consider several explanations of that move.

First, the whole passage works to obscure an entirely different understanding of privilege, which Lacan delivers scarcely two pages before. The three reasons why the phallus should be the chosen signifier replace an earlier account of the notion of privilege. Here, it is constituted by the subject's "demand" in its address of the Other.[14] Hence, the privilege does not so much follow from the imagined characteristics of an organ, its ancient stature, or its charged veiling, but rather from a plea issued to it. "Demand constitutes this Other," Lacan argues, "as already possessing the '*privilege*' of satisfying needs, that is, the power to deprive them of the one thing by which they are satisfied" (80, emphasis added).

Next to privilege, the notion of *Aufhebung* is already present in this earlier account as well: "Hence it is that demand cancels out (*aufhebt*) the particularity of anything which might be granted by transmuting it into a proof of love, and the very satisfactions of need which it obtains are degraded (*sich erniedrigt*) as being no more than a crushing of the demand for love" (80–81). Additionally, pregnancy is already at the scene. Through demand the mother becomes "pregnant" [*être grosse*] with the Other or "other scene" (80).

The repetition of these three elements—privilege, *Aufhebung*, and pregnancy—in the quoted passage on the generation of meaning and the emergence of the phallus indicates that the earlier account of privilege should bear on the phallus as well. The two accounts mirror each other. Thus, it must be the address of a demand that turns the penis into the phallus, which then returns "crushed" as mere penis. In the later fragment, moreover, it is the narrator himself who issues the demand to the penis with his veil, working to draw in or hook the reader in a joint call for the penis to be the phallus. Indeed, the trick with the veil forces the reader to forget or ignore the earlier account of what constitutes privilege. His or her attention has become focused on the veil, on what has disappeared and what will reappear, and no longer on the hand that performs the veiling; the standard manipulation of attention that enables magic to take effect.

Lacan suggests the earlier account of privilege with regard to the "primordial relation to the mother" (80). Yet the mother has almost completely disappeared in the later passage, another function of the veil. "[E]verything signifiable" is immediately struck and raised to meaning. Throughout the fragment, the narrator's focus is persistently on the phallus, so that its necessary and essential antagonist is obscured. This slanted narration starts with the alleged tactile preponderance of the phallus in copulation, continues with the coining of the turgid *flux vital* as the only element in generation worth mentioning, and concludes as the phallus brands meaning as its offspring, while the maternal signifiable does not stake its claim. However, ejaculation is not presented as the high point or end point to this masculinist perspective, as one would perhaps expect.[15] Notwithstanding that, the signified is affirmed as being conceived out of a "signifying concatenation," and not from some autogenerative effort of the phallus.

The temporal progression of the passage appears swift and immediate. The respective stages follow one another in due course. But the dexterity of the hand that works the veil cannot entirely conceal the fact that a lengthy temporal pause or delay takes place, as suggested by the word *latency*. That word invokes the deferral, return, retreat, or reserve, which Lacan entertains throughout the essay. Even the phallus becomes the sign of this latency when it disappears behind the veil. Therefore, the phallus is visually lost for a considerably longer period of time than its swift unveiling suggests. Narratologically, the period of latency, incubation, or pregnancy is told with a minimal summary that is on the brink of an ellipsis.[16] Yet another function of the narrator's play with the veil, then, is that it allows him to skip over the durative power of the latency nearly completely, but not quite. The smooth veiling and unveiling allows for a timing or pacing of the story of generation that practically jumps over the delay or interval that it cannot but factor in.

Nevertheless, the signifiable apparently exerts a staying power from inside its near elision. For one wonders why meaning should be a "bastard," a child out of wedlock or a hybrid. Perhaps the phallus and the signifiable are in fact unmarried, though the passage begins with a wedding. More probably, the progeny of meaning is able to move astray when, during the interval of latency, the phallus is held in abeyance. That is why the child of meaning can escape the phallus that spawns it. Meaning, according to Lacan, emphatically does not arrive in the shape of the requisite "good son," who will continue "the name of the father." Thus, the phallus strikes the newly born meaning in an attempt to bring it under a control that is in fact already lost. In the interval of the latency, the phallic seed gets lost. That is why meaning cannot but be heteroglot.

The final function of the veil that I want to suggest has to do with the displacement of ejaculation. The second paragraph puts forth the turgid "image of the vital flow" as one of the propositions conducive to the privilege of the phallus. In the fifth and last paragraph, progeny sees the light of day. So, what has happened in the middle part? The passage juxtaposes two incomplete narratives of ejaculation. They fail to fully incorporate ejaculation, while at the same time motioning in relation to it, toward it, or around it.

As I have suggested, the second paragraph narrates the standard procession of masculine sexuality: from erection to copulation to ejaculation. But then the story abruptly arrests, so that the ejaculation can continue happening, and thus maintain its turgidity and vitality. The image of ejaculation that endures is the one of Serrano's ejaculation-in-trajectory. Poised as an unbending and forceful stream, solid, stationary, and eternal, ejaculation continues endlessly. If this first narrative arrests the completion of climax, the second one skips to the ultimate effect without offering a retroversion or flashback of what must have happened before. The fifth paragraph stages the juxtaposition of the phallus and the progeny of meaning, which cannot but imply that the "vital flow" must have achieved generation, and therefore, ended. Hence, Lacan's two story lines break apart at the exact instance of the ejaculatory happening: the one moving forward without ending it, the other moving backward and around it without telling it. Ejaculation "happens" at the precise breach of these two story lines.

Ejaculation must have occurred at the moment when the veil was drawn. This strategic veiling enables ejaculation to live on as turgid, even if the "transmission in generation" would require it to give up that virtue. Also, the veiling glosses over the moment of ejaculation itself. Nearly erased from the narrative, it makes way for the culmination of the birth of meaning and the calibration of the phallus as a semiotic function. In that way, finally, the veil allows for the investiture of the kindled demand in the penis/phallus rather than in ejaculation.

Right within the heart of this intrigue, however, two temporal instances move the whole story off course, and can be called upon for a critique from its inside. These are the ellipsis of the latency and the displacement of ejaculation. Both are utterly crucial for an account of a production of meaning that is couched in terms of conception. Marginalized to make way for the phallus, they nevertheless influence the story's outcome. The alienation of the semen during the period of latency or pregnancy turns the conceived meaning into a bastard, whom the phallus cannot entirely control. Thus they cause the staggering move off course of the essay from sexual ideals, heterosexuality, and child care to the comedy and masquerade of gender and homosexuality. Meaning is a bastard, because the phallus cannot vouch for it.

The bathetic lapse from mythopoetic "vital flow" to "bastard offspring" takes place, then, because of the rerouting of semen through the signifiable's latency. It points to the simple fact that the spurt of semen cannot transmit directly to what it generates, but must go through a temporal and visual delay. Nevertheless, the temporalities of pregnancy and ejaculation remain readable, precisely, in Lacan's oxymoronic image of ejaculation. Indeed, "the image of the vital flow as it is transmitted in generation" is itself arguably a bastardized or hybridized form. For it concatenates the female and durative aspect of pregnancy with the male and punctual aspect of conception, both of which the narrator "Lacan" cannot quite account for, suggesting simultaneously, impossibly, an eternal "flow" and an instantaneous "transmission."

Hence, the veil in the passage occludes the earlier account of privilege as the effect of an addressed demand, the position of the mother or the signifiable in the generation of meaning, the interval of latency or pregnancy in which the phallic semen moves astray, and the precarious instantaneity of ejaculation. But the veil in the hands of the narrator, drawn and withdrawn with deliberate effort, can perhaps also be seen as the sign of an awkward self-consciousness.

SHAME AS AWKWARD SELF-REFLEXIVITY

At two places, Lacan's essay suggests that the subtle and sophisticated trick with the veil may be something of a mixed blessing. The first concerns shame. As Lacan writes, "the demon of *Aidoos* [*Sham*, shame] in the ancient mysteries rises up exactly at the moment when the phallus is unveiled" (82). Hence, he ascribes a feeling of shame to those who witness the anxious unveiling of the phallus, with the reader of the essay presumably among them.

Immediately, however, the demon takes over for the narrator, replacing the veil in the latter's hands by the bar in his own ("at the hands of this demon"), effectively disowning the narrator. The bastard offspring of meaning arises from the administrations of this demon. Initially ascribed to the onlooker, the sense of shame thus applies back to the narrator himself, the magician who manipulated and handled the veil so dexterously, who is now left standing empty-handed. Hence, shame comes to infect both the observer and the performer, the reader and the narrator. The result of this magic trick is not so much the triumph of a stunned surprise, but rather an inchoate sense of shame that starts to circulate between its participants.

This shame can be read as a minimal articulation of an awkward self-awareness as the phallic trick comes to an end. It suggests the effort of the veiling and unveiling, as well as a disillusionment over the double result, the bastard of meaning and the concept of the phallus. Moreover, it again moves the penis to the fore at the precise moment when the phallus is calibrated as a semiotic master concept; the Greek word *aidoion* means "private part." Apparently, phallic meaning and gender revolve on a sense of self-consciousness and shame that can only be obliquely addressed. Now that the *Aufhebung* of the phallus is completed, what ultimately rises is merely a self-reflexive awareness of shame, linked to the penis. This affect challenges the ostentatious success of the conceptual trick.

The second trope casts more doubt on the narrator, "Lacan." The short, penultimate paragraph of the essay reads, "The fact that femininity takes refuge in this mask, because of the *Verdrängung* inherent to the phallic mark of desire, has the strange consequence that, in the human being, virile display itself appears as feminine" (85). How can these words not apply to what the narrator has been doing throughout the essay? For the penis and the male body have in fact "taken refuge" in the masquerade of the veil. And, the "strange consequence" is that the narrator's game of "now you see it, now you don't," of showing and hiding, teasing and withholding, starts to come across as a *feminine* striptease act, especially if one infers a male viewer or reader. Apparently, the exposition and exposure of the phallus and masculinity must take up the veil, conventionally a feminine accessory. The same veil that should have saved masculinity from its visual and temporal, its narrative, trouble, makes it appear as feminine instead.

Ejaculation and semen are at once central and marginal to Lacan's conceptual and copulative account of the production of meaning. The "image of the vital flow" is displaced and discredited, though the central and privileged phallus brands and claims the effect of meaning as its seminal offspring. Simultaneously, the phallus is merely the signifier of something else: "The phallus is the privileged signifier of *that mark* where the share of *logos* is wedded to the advent of desire" (emphasis added). Hence, "that mark," not the phallus, is the instance where *logos* and desire become originally concatenated. Consequently, "phallus" can only be the belated name for a marking that precedes and exceeds it.

That mark, pointed at without being named, identified, given a referent, or ascribed a concept, can, in principle, be anything, an advantage that the phallus does not have. However, the rhetoric of the essay suggests its linkage to sexual substances, and the essay's convoluted treatment of ejaculation warrants the implication that it can be a trace or smear of sperm. It is the formless stain that the veil and the phallus cannot sublate or hide. Indeed, "that mark" is analogous to the wad of entropically material, dried-up phlegm in Aristotle's treatise. In the wake of Lacan's oxymoronic narrative of ejaculation, centering on the incongruous juxtaposition of the vital flow and "that mark," the following two chapters will present case studies of the masculine appearing in and beyond the context of Lacan's understanding of masculinity and visibility.

THREE

ANAMORPHOSIS / METAMORPHOSIS

Ambassadors

THE PREVIOUS CHAPTER HAS SHOWN that the bleak economy of the phallus and castration, subjectivity and annihilation, that Lacan advocates finds its counterpoint in the densely visual and temporal narratives of the veil, pregnancy, and ejaculation. Indeed, Lacan is as famous for his work on visuality, on the look, the gaze, and the screen, in *The Four Fundamental Concepts of Psycho-Analysis* as he is for the essay on signification and the phallus. Taking up the precarious temporality and visuality of the image of the "vital flow" and the haunting presence of the stain of "that mark," this chapter inquires into the dynamic of masculine visibility by putting a male look at the penis and the male body at center stage.

Such a look triggers and articulates anxious concerns about the organ's apparentially unstable stature and its capacity to "morph" temporally into different shapes. Since the full realization of the penis in climax immediately gives way to the organ's reverting to what Lacan terms its "less developed state," that capacity is relevant for ejaculation. Ejaculation brings a temporal finality to bear on the stature of masculinity that Lacan is hard-pressed to acknowledge, linking the instantaneous and the durative in the "image of the vital flow as it is transmitted in generation." Additionally, the possibly seminal "that mark," where language and sexuality become entangled with each other, may haunt the form that masculinity can or should take with the specter of formlessness. Therefore, the penis and ejaculation can bring in morphological possibilities and considerations that the economic alternative between the phallus and castration cannot; the "image of the vital flow" and "that mark" bring to bear a visible, morphological trouble upon masculinity that the smooth and stable phallus attempts to overcome.

I will start with Lacan's apparent delight in the stretched image of erection in *Four Fundamental Concepts*. Subsequently, I will discuss, critique, and extend Lacan's reading of the two powerful men who make their rigid, phallic appearances in Hans Holbein the Younger's *The Ambassadors* (1533). Appearing on the cover of several editions of Lacan's work, this painting to some extent has been rebranded as a Lacanian one, as much as it is Holbein's, serving almost as the logo of the theoretical enterprise.[1] However, this re-authorization or incorporation of the painting may well favor some of its aspects more than others, so that its potential to nuance Lacan's project becomes subdued. Hence, this chapter proposes an analysis of *The Ambassadors* both within and beyond the scope of the Lacanian frame.

DELICIOUS GAME

In the section on visuality in *Four Fundamental Concepts*, Lacan is again fascinated by visual trickery. However, this time the ploy is performed not with the magician's veil, but with the device of anamorphosis. Because of a simple, noncylindrical anamorphosis, Lacan explains, an image on a flat surface projects on another, oblique surface "a figure enlarged and distorted."[2] "I will dwell, as on some delicious game," Lacan continues, "on this method that makes anything appear at will in a particular stretching" (87).

One sees it coming. The willful stretching of any indiscriminate object or image seems insufficient, if not moot, for explaining the delight of the game. Yet Lacan's fascination for the anamorphic device becomes clear when he focuses attention on the plasticity of the penis, the organ's propensity to enlarge and distort. "How is it that nobody has ever thought of connecting this . . . with the effect of an erection?" he asks. "Imagine a tattoo traced on the sexual organ *ad hoc* in the state of repose and assuming its, if I may say so, developed form in another state" (88).

At stake, then, is erection, the extension of the penis between formlessness and its "developed" state, its ambiguous posture within the visual. That this observed plasticity should offer such an unqualified delight, however, seems less obvious. True, enlargement may be the benefit of the game, especially when it can be executed entirely "at will." But anamorphosis also distorts, though that second effect is partially revoked when Lacan substitutes the image of the penis for the one of the tattoo inscribed on it. Only through erection, the tattoo reaches its true form, its visibility and readability. If the implication is that the penis, too, acquires visual identity and intelligibility only in its erect shape, then the delight of the game rests solely on the will that controls it. That is why I suspect an anxiety over the visibility of the penis to motivate the game, one that perhaps makes masculinity particularly vulnerable.

Lacan's initial delight quickly turns out to be little more than a setup to wrong-foot the reader. For he concludes that the viewer encounters not so much a grandiose and controllable erection, but rather his own castration in anamorphic imagery; in Lacan's words, "something symbolic of the function of the lack, of the appearance of the phallic ghost" (88).

The perspectivism that anamorphosis plays with and deforms, Lacan explains, is congruent with the construction of the Cartesian subject as a central "geometral point" (86). As research into the perfection of painterly perspective progressed, he speculates, the sixteenth century became equally enchanted with the distortion of vision, as if an acute awareness triggered doubts about the position of centrality and mastery that the subject came to occupy within the newly invented field of perspectivized vision (87).[3] In contrast to perspective, anamorphic representation does not offer the viewer a central position from which to behold and oversee the visual world. Instead, the viewer's position becomes slanted, oblique, awkward. What is distorted, then, is not only the image, but also the subject's look. Somehow, this distortion is connected to the plastic visibility of the penis, its duplicitous potential to inflate and deflate, its capacity to pose and to be in repose, its vacillation between different states.

That the organ's changeability should be a matter of concern is no surprise, since the development of the subject, its coming into being as such, relates to a crucial penile disappearance act. At moments in the "infantile monologue" during the stage of language acquisition, Lacan notices syntactical games centered on an "unconscious reserve" (67–68). In turn, this reserve is connected to a traumatic "nucleus," which proceeds from what Lacan terms "the encounter with the real" (53, 69). This confrontation with the real Lacan calls *tuchè*, Greek for "fate" or "coincidence" (69). It is variously characterized as an "accident," a "traumatic" event, a "shock," an "obstacle," and a "hitch" (53–60).[4] This accidental but essential encounter is initially unwelcome to the subject, Lacan goes on, because it refers to the so-called primal scene: the picture or scenario the child observes, infers, or fantasizes of the parental coitus (69–70).[5]

Note the backtracking and tiered linearity of Lacan's argument. It traces a diachronic genealogy or psychic history, which, after an extensive series of steps, ultimately arrives at a stage designated as primal or original. Each aspect or term relates back to an earlier and more primordial one: from the child's monologue to reserve, to nucleus, to the encountered real, to the primal scene. This narrative of origin, moreover, explains and substitutes for the temporally nonlinear and dwelt-upon game of anamorphosis, which turns on the steady oscillation of stretching and contraction.

That the primal scene is originally unwelcome and traumatic for the child is for Lacan not merely a fact, but a "factitious fact, like that which appears in the scene so fiercely tracked down in the experience of the Wolf Man—the *strangeness* of the disappearance and reappearance of the penis."[6] Apparently, the child is unable to come to terms with the encounter with this piece of the real, and this inability is what determines its subjectivity, or rather, subjectivity *per se*. For the syntactical games that characterize the period of learning to speak emerge precisely as an enduring attempt to overcome the confrontation with the visual fate of the paternal penis, similar to the way in which the *fort/da* game struggles to overcome the visual absence of the mother. In this sense, the penile disappearance triggers and facilitates the acquisition of language and subjectivity; signification emerges as a defense against the "strangeness" of the disappearance and reappearance of the penis.

Such a "syntactical" or *fort/da* game Lacan plays, too, with anamorphosis, with the image of the penis and the tattoo. Yet, where the child's play is ridden with anxiety and trauma, Lacan's own game is exhilarating and delightful. Lacan can be taken to contrast the phallic stretch or alternative between the anamorphic image of erection and the lack or castration that appears as "the phallic ghost," with the traumatic strangeness of the (dis)appearance of the penis, whether this occurs in copulation or, presumably, through the organ's inflation and deflation. Apparently, beyond the terrible opposition of the phallus and castration resides a dimension stranger still: the visual, *meta*morphic plasticity of the penis itself. Hence, the alternative of the phallus/castration is countered by the alterity of the penis. It is tempting to infer that this alterity propels and motivates the charged dynamics of phallus and lack to begin with. Brought up by the Wolf Man, the metamorphic strangeness of the penis, of the alien and alienable of the male body, contaminates the bleak opposition between phallus and castration, power and annihilation, life and death, with changeability and variability.

In the meantime, something odd has happened with respect to the understanding of castration on the part of psychoanalysis. In the usual account, the development of gendered subjectivity is prompted by a sudden peek at the supposedly glaring difference between the sexes: the "absence" of the penis on the female body. Yet here Lacan suggests a different account of the genesis of the castration complex. It does not so much follow from the (male) look at the anatomy of the other sex, but rather from a look at gender equals, be it from the observed or imagined (dis)appearance of the penis of the father in the primal scene, or from the (dis)appearance of the erection of the subject himself. Consequently, a differentiality immanent in man, or between men, is pushed to the fore.

COOL MEN

Lacan's optical playfulness turns spooky, the atmospheric temperature of the text moving down a peg or two, as he moves on to discuss Hans Holbein's double portrait of Jean de Dinteville (to the left) and Georges de Selve, known as *The Ambassadors* (Figure 6). In the foreground, the oil painting shows an anamorphic skull, only recognizable in its proper proportions from an oblique angle.[7] The two male dignitaries pose, "frozen, stiffened in their showy adornments," Lacan notes, surrounded by objects that symbolize the arts and sciences of the time: compasses, globes, books, a sundial, a lute (88).[8]

Authority and wealth are called into question by death already lurking at the scene. "All this shows that at the very heart of the period in which the subject emerged and geometral optics was an object of research," Lacan

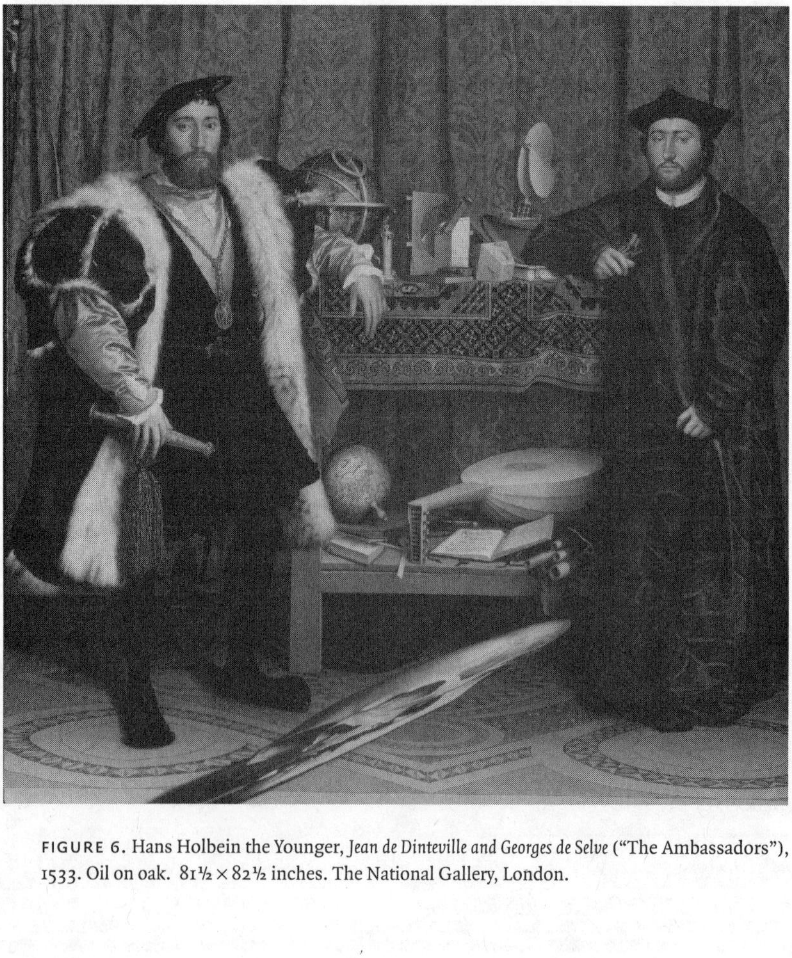

FIGURE 6. Hans Holbein the Younger, *Jean de Dinteville and Georges de Selve* ("The Ambassadors"), 1533. Oil on oak. 81½ × 82½ inches. The National Gallery, London.

claims, "Holbein makes visible for us here something that is simply the subject as annihilated—annihilated in the form, that is, strictly speaking of the minus-phi [–Φ] of castration" (88–89). The embodied form that masculinity can take in Lacan's interpretation of the painting switches from the phallic, the stiffened postures of the two men, to castration, the annihilation of form that the skull suggests. In that way, the anamorphic dimension of the alternative between phallus and lack, power and annihilation, seems accounted for. However, that leaves open the accompanying, metamorphic strangeness or alterity of the male appearance that Lacan also intimates. Can *The Ambassadors* propose a masculine morphology that cannot be reduced to *either* the phallus *or* the minus-phi?

Undercutting Lacan's ghostly reading of the painting, Willibald Sauerländer remarks on the particular "chilliness" that emanates from Holbein's oeuvre in "The Art of the Cool." This mood he perceives in the impersonality of Holbein's art, in its impenetrable or discreet attitude, and in the atmosphere of mortality that surrounds the portraits. Though Holbein dispenses with the conventional *memento mori* iconography of the Middle Ages, Sauerländer argues, death is nevertheless apparent as engraved on the faces of the sitters, suggesting "the coldness of death in Holbein's portraits from life."[9] These two qualities, the cold atmosphere of mortality and the displacement of the usual icons of death, culminate in the face of death in *The Ambassadors*, simultaneously positioned frontally and marginally.

In *The Threshold of the Visible World*, Kaja Silverman clarifies and extends Lacan's interpretation. With its empty sockets, the skull leers at the viewer, turning him or her into "the being looked at." "[R]ather than positing us as viewer," Silverman writes, the painting "puts us in the 'picture.' The presence of the death's head thus marks the alterity of the gaze in relation to our look, and our emplacement within the field of vision."[10] Refusing to be apprehended in a single grasp, *The Ambassadors* splits apart the subject who beholds it.

In contrast to the rest of the image, the skull is rendered anamorphically. It requires the viewer to give up his or her position directly in front of, and at a secure distance from, the work, the usual position for viewing a perspectival image (177). Adopting an oblique angle to the painting, the viewer immediately receives the skull's grin, which repudiates the mastery that the central perspective promises to the viewing subject.[11] Two mutually exclusive systems of intelligibility compete, one perspectival, the other anamorphic, and work to suspend the subject.

These two systems are also thematically at odds. The perspectival look aligns the viewer, Silverman continues, with the knowledge, power, and wealth that the ambassadors embody, underscored by the social distinction of their clothing (176). Yet, the anamorphic look reveals the status of both the ambassadors and the viewer who identifies with them to be idle and transient in the tradition of *vanitas*. This second look debunks the worldview that perspectival representation and viewing imply, which Silverman specifies as "the dominant fiction" still prevalent today:

> The upper portion of *The Ambassadors* shows us more than Holbein's "world." It also shows us our own. In addition to earthly accomplishment, the painting validates "masculinity," "whiteness," "monarchy," and "God," and it places all of these terms in a close metaphoric relation with each other. In so doing, it also effects that equation upon which the dominant fiction still depends, and upon which our sense of "reality" is consequently most dependant: the equation of the penis and phallus. (179)

As long as the viewer remains directly in front of the work, the painting exercises its reality effect and allows the viewer to believe that the phallus and the penis are one, and that the penis wields real power in the world (179). Once the observer moves to the side to meet the skull's eyes, the phallus tips over into its opposites of castration and annihilation.

In his reading of the painting in *Ways of Seeing*, John Berger adds the two historic ideologies sustaining the series of equations that determine the worldview that, according to Silverman, links up monarchy, whiteness, divinity, masculinity, and the penis/phallus, namely, capitalism and colonialism. Generally, Berger claims, the template for the genre of oil painting to which *The Ambassadors* belongs "is not so much a framed window open on to the world as a safe let into the wall, a safe in which the visible has been deposited."[12] Berger argues that a specific way of seeing the world, determined by new attitudes to property and exchange, has found its most insidious and alluring expression in the genre.

Oil painting displays buyable, exchangeable things, or commodities. The viscous materiality of the new painting technique lends the genre the ability to visually render the "tangibility, the texture, the lustre, [and] the solidity" of the exhibited objects; "It defines the real as that which you can put your hands on," Berger writes (88). Additionally, the instruments on the top shelf in the painting are used for navigation, and hence, to Berger, suggest the slave trade, global commerce, and colonization. The hymnbook and the treatise on arithmetic on the table refer to the aggressive conversion of the colonized to Christianity and to the Western practice of accounting (95).

Berger is an astute observer of the stance of the ambassadors, of their "presence as men," as he puts it (94). Confident and formal, rigid in their postures, the men show a "curious lack of expectation of any recognition"

(94). The two ambassadors are not only "cool" in the sense of chilly or mortal, as Sauerländer suggests, but also in the second sense of the word as "composed" or "imperturbable." Their gazes "aloof and weary," Berger continues, the ambassadors "wish the image of their presence to impress others with their vigilance and distance" (97). This need for distanciation, according to Berger, follows from the rise of individualism, which promises equality while simultaneously withdrawing its concretization by making actual equality inconceivable.

The vapid stares and the self-enclosed postures of the ambassadors allow the viewer to slip into their positions as if into an accommodating garment, without any obstacles that could trigger dialogue or critique. "The fact that the scene is substantial, and yet, behind its substantiality, empty," Berger suggests, "facilitates the 'wearing' of it" (102). Only the ephemeral and empty-eyed skull intimates an alternative optic, one not driven by the urge to possess and control all that is made tangible and visible (91).

To Lacan, Silverman, and Berger, geometral perspective offers no natural vision of the world, but a way of seeing that entails a specific ideological understanding of the world and the subject, as phrased in Cartesian, phallic, capitalist, colonialistic, and individualistic terms. To those ideologies, the anamorphic skull serves as a haunting counterpoint. As argued above, however, Lacan brings up a second dimension of alterity, besides castration and annihilation, in the direct vicinity of his reading of *The Ambassadors* in *Four Fundamental Concepts*. He locates that potential in the metamorphic strangeness of the male body and the penis. Consequently, this potential can bring up the temporality and historicity of the body, its variability, *within* the terms of the framing ideologies rather than from a position relatively marginal to them, as the skull does. The appearance of embodied masculine power may be internally, intimately, burdened by that strangeness at precisely the stance where it seems most convincing.

In the perspectival representation the work offers, Silverman views the coherence of what she calls the dominant fiction, which matches whiteness, masculinity, and divinity to the phallus. Such a vision of the world should display integrity and stability. Two details counterbalance that order, however, and suggest a dominance already under strain even before the anamorphic, castrating vision is entertained. One of the books on the table is authored by Luther. Additionally, the lute has one broken string, the iconographical symbol for "discord." In *Holbein's Ambassadors: Making and Meaning*, Susan Foister, Ashok Roy, and Martin Wyld argue that the painting represents a "floating, fallible" world caught up in historical upheaval.[13]

Furthermore, the two systems of intelligibility that Silverman distinguishes, perspectival and anamorphic, seem internally split as well. The painting's perspective, to begin with, is at its most obvious in the floor mosaic, which is rendered by the slanted and receding lines of perspective in the expected manner, as well as in the relative positioning of the left-hand ambassador's feet upon it. Yet this spatial organization is closed off or foreshortened by the heavy curtain drawn just behind the two figures. As a result, there is no horizon, spatial vista, or vanishing point to complete the perspective of the painting. The effect is a claustrophobic flattening or shrinkage of the space where the men stand.

Moreover, the skull, though positioned outside the usual perspective, acquires a hyper-perspectival 3-D motility through anamorphosis, which makes it seem to fly outside the painting's frame and into the space between it and the viewer. Thus, the spatial world in which the ambassadors strike their poses and into which the viewer enters is precarious and reversible rather than stable. As a result, the distinction between perspective and anamorphosis becomes precarious.

This cannot but bear on the stance of the ambassadors, on their "presence as men," as Berger puts it. Indeed, as I have mentioned above, the two men come across as "cool" in both senses of the term. First, in Sauerländer's sense, they emanate a chilly mood of mortality, the same aspect that Lacan observes in the men's "frozen" postures, which to him suggest castration, death, and annihilation, a phallic ghostliness. Moreover, the emphasis on the men's rigid, formal poses brings in Lacan's delicious game, the device of anamorphosis playing with the "state of repose" and the "developed form in another state" of the penis (*Concepts*, 88). The game suggests a temporality and variability as inherent to the postures, however rigid they may seem. Hence, the temporization of vision that Silverman ascribes to the movement back and forth between the painting's perspectivized and anamorphic dimensions must also apply to the motility of the men's postures.

Second, they appear as "cool" in the contemporary sense of seeming unaffected yet utterly confident, of being impressive without apparent effort, as Berger suggests (albeit without using the word). This second meaning of coolness points to a specific modality of the self-display of masculinity, of appearing as recognizably masculine without trying too hard, without the effort tainting the projected image. Condensing the mortal and the apparitional or apparent, Lacan's "phallic ghost" suggests both those meanings of "cool." Sharing a vapid stare, a rigid bearing, and a general attitude of self-possession, the two ambassadors appear as equally cool, equally masculine. If they are understood to serve as the exemplary representatives of an emerging class or gender, or of the nexus between the two, then the men can participate in that project to a similar extent.

However, the similarity of the general attitude of the two cool men immediately becomes uncanny as soon as one notices the extreme similarity of their faces. Indeed, they largely have their facial hair and features in common, strangely so for a double portrait. Are these men not so much colleagues, fellow ambassadors, but rather brothers, twins, or clones? Furthermore, the genre of portraiture makes clear that the ambassadors do court the look of the viewer, demanding his or her acknowledgment, even if the idiosyncrasies of their faces seem to have been erased.

Thus, what the painting offers up for the viewer's recognition is not so much the coolness that the two men have in common, nor the lack of individuality in their faces, but rather the obvious differences in the way the two men are dressed. *The Ambassadors* is fashion portraiture, portraiture through costumes. This aspect of the image corresponds to the notably intricate elaboration of surfaces and fabrics in the painting. As Berger points out,

> Except for the faces and the hands, there is not a surface in this picture which does not make one aware of how it has been elaborately worked over—by weavers, embroiderers, carpet makers, gold smiths, leather workers, mosaic-makers, furriers, tailors, jewellers—and of how this working-over and the resulting richness of each surface has been finally worked-over and reproduced by Holbein the painter. (*Ways of Seeing*, 90)

The Ambassadors plays on, and plays with, a series of relative similarities and differences between the two men, pertaining to their attitude, their poses, and their costumes.

Even without taking the annihilating skull into account, then, the supposedly monolithic and phallic perspective that *The Ambassadors*, in part, represents turns out to be heterogeneous. This world is not so much threatened by death or castration but by life, by living history. While the external world of the painting is in motion and out of joint, its internal space is so claustrophobically foreshortened that the two men nearly lose their footing, their spatial bearings. Crucially, the apparent awareness and weariness that accompany the men's cool deportment revolve on similarities and differences between the two men, and not between the men taken together, and the ultimate other of death. Indeed, the castration and annihilation that Lacan views as the exemplary truth of the painting effectively obliterate the differences between the two men.

Once the pathos of death has been brought up, it is easy to forget that the effect of ghostliness that Lacan describes specifically pertains to masculinity, both in his argument and with respect to his chosen object, *The Ambassadors*. In this sense, the painting may enable a vision that undermines the Lacanian reading in which to-be-seen automatically spells death and annihilation. After all, this equation can follow only from the rigorous maintenance of an ideological gender binary: whereas men practically die when they are looked at, when they emerge in the picture, women are as good as dead unless they are seen.

TWIN AMBASSADORS

Recently, *The Ambassadors* has been restored. The British Broadcasting Corporation (BBC) broadcast a documentary, *Restoring The Ambassadors*, about the process and the controversy that surrounded it.[14] The assembled team of art historians made two remarkable discoveries. The skull's nosebone does not fit the anamorphic projection of the image. It is thought to be the result of a previous effort at restoration. X-rays revealed the lingering presence of several other nosebones under the presently visible one, all wrong in some way or other, but not the original nosebone as presumably painted by Holbein. To meet the challenge, the investigating team brought in a real skull and painted in a correct—correctly distorted, that is—nosebone from its example, facilitated by photography and computer-animation techniques.

However, such a recourse to reality was unavailable in the case of another missing part. The restorers discussed the probability that the ambassador on the left was originally endowed with a codpiece.[15] This ambassador's crotch area appears to have been painted over, though curious folds and creases have stubbornly remained. The team compared the figure with other, similar paintings featuring codpieces, but ultimately declined to put in a restored one.[16]

The latter, aborted attempt at restoration cannot but direct attention to the crucial role fabrics, folds, and upholstery play in the picture, overdetermined by the worked-over quality, the attention to surfaces in the painting, that Berger detects. Rather than entering into the discussion of whether or not a codpiece should be there, I want to stress what occasions the debate in the first place: the posture and dress of the left-hand ambassador. The stubborn folds and creases of his costume, I propose, can be taken to allude to the function of the veil and anamorphosis in Lacan's work. Indeed, those two optical games both suspend and charge, re-emphasize, the contours of male visibility. Such a perspective, at first sight, does not seem to involve the other, right-hand ambassador. His physical form in general and his crotch area in particular do not appear to partake of the game, delicious or anxious, of making appearances, of revelation and distortion. Hence, this contrast constitutes a marked difference between the fellow dignitaries, who seem otherwise so alike.

When I first saw a reproduction of *The Ambassadors*, what struck me was not so much the fleeting skull, which one would expect to command all attention. Rather, my eyes started to switch back and forth between the men's faces, as if to seek out an individuality in them that seems conspicuously lacking. Though the men are endowed with respective names and functions, the similarity of their facial features threatens their individuality, perhaps even the generically individualizing conventions of portraiture. Yet the missing individuality of the ambassadors can be found elsewhere: in their respective outfits, postures, and gestures, which turn out to be not so alike as initially appears. Hence, I propose two supplemental or complementary lines of inquiry to bring out these differences: the first centrifugal, the second comparative.

Two elements in the painting are marked by the decisive attempt to flee its center, to become and remain marginal. The first of these is the skull. Indeed, one can easily imagine a more conventional version of the work in which the skull, as the requisite iconographical sign for the notion of *memento mori*, would inhabit the same space as the men—centrally positioned on the table, for example—to burden the men with the reminder of transience. Instead, the skull nearly seems to flee the entire scene. In that sense, the skull is connected to another element that seems almost ridiculously centrifugal. In the far upper left corner of the painting, the curtain is drawn a little to the side, partially revealing a small crucifix. Again, one would expect this religious symbol to be given considerably more size and prominence. In their shared marginality, the skull and the crucifix establish a new and diagonal frame through which to survey the scene, with the two ambassadors captured within its hold.

At first sight, the crucifix and the skull convey opposing attitudes to mortality: death vindicated versus death victorious. If the skull is there to remind us of the imminent reality of death within life, the crucifix promises the mercy of an afterlife of the soul.[17] However, this initial and obvious opposition is complemented by another one that reverses its values. Whereas the crucifix shows the viscerality of the body in Christ's suffering, the bald skull has lost all flesh. Hence, I take this diagonal frame as signaling the concern for the substantiality, the materiality, the fleshiness of the male body. That this burden of the flesh not only frames the scene but also punctures and weighs down on it is indicated by another detail. The badge on the cap of the left-hand ambassador repeats the symbol of the skull. This internal repetition of one end of the diagonal frame makes the consideration of the metamorphic potential of the flesh integral to the scene.

As I have argued, the juxtaposition of the similarities and differences between the two men triggers a reading that does not so much alternate between power and its demise, between phallus and castration, as Lacan's interpretation does, or between mortal life and eternal afterlife, as brought up by the conventional interpretation of the skull and the crucifix. Rather, it vacillates between the relative and respective presences of the male figures "as men." Such a reading recalls the child's game of "spot the differences."

SPOT THE DIFFERENCES: EMBARRASSING EMBRASSE

The two men stand in front of an intricately pleated and heavy curtain, which alludes to the same dynamic of exposure and hiding that underlies Lacan's delicious games with the veil and with anamorphosis. However, this curtain, figuratively speaking, seems to be down or drawn closer to the figure at the right to a relatively greater degree, and up or withdrawn from the one on the left. The left-hand dignitary spreads his legs apart, and his hands extend away from the body. Consequently, his black doublet protrudes from the space between his opened thighs. His openness is further emphasized by the framing lines of white fur, and by the v-necked doublet that shows his red shirt, which is slashed at his upper chest and the wrists to reveal a white undershirt. Both are mirrored by the position of the necklace with its central medal suspended just above the man's crotch.

In sharp contrast, the right-hand ambassador poses with his legs together; his posture is considerably more rigid. His arms move toward each other and remain close to the body. The adorned but severe, massive purple-brownish coat is kept in place at his lower body by the grip of his left hand. The cramped grip of both his hands, the right one holding a glove, is betrayed by the whiteness of his knuckles, thus contrasting his closed fists to the more relaxed and open gestures of his counterpart's hands. A white collar closes off his upper body.

So, if the two men show off their phallic positions of power and knowledge, they cannot be seen to do so in the same way. The doubling and layering of fabrics—from curtains, to garments, to undergarments, to skin—suggest ways of charging and hiding the visibility of the contours of the male body. Where one ambassador seems responsive to the delight of the game with regard to both his pose and his outfit, teasingly both covering and stressing his genital area where originally there may have been a conspicuous codpiece, the other ambassador only shows a prim resolve in showing off masculinity through hiding the male form with the firm hold of his left hand.

These differences between the two men set the stage for a recognition of the metamorphic alterity to or internal differentiality in masculinity as implicitly suggested by Lacan. The staff that the left-hand ambassador holds in his hand points straight to the wrinkled fabric that both covers and accentuates his genital region. Moreover, noticing the staff, one cannot fail to see the suspended tassel, curtain holder, or *embrasse* that hangs under the staff alongside the figure's leg. In the specific context of Lacan's reading of the painting in *Four Fundamental Concepts*, the staff and the *embrasse* can be taken together to imply the alienating potential for shape-shifting that the penis has, its variability between erection and deflation. A look at Titian's portrait of Charles V supports that connotation (Figure 7). Not only does that painting depict the dagger and the tassel in the same suggestive figuration, but it also adds in the missing codpiece, and even a pointing finger.

If this generic cousin is any indication, not only does the left-hand ambassador play with the possible emergence of the penis in the picture, but the figuration of his accessories also hints at the strangeness of what such a visualization would bring to bear: the unstable posture of the penis in the field of vision between disappearance and appearance, formlessness and

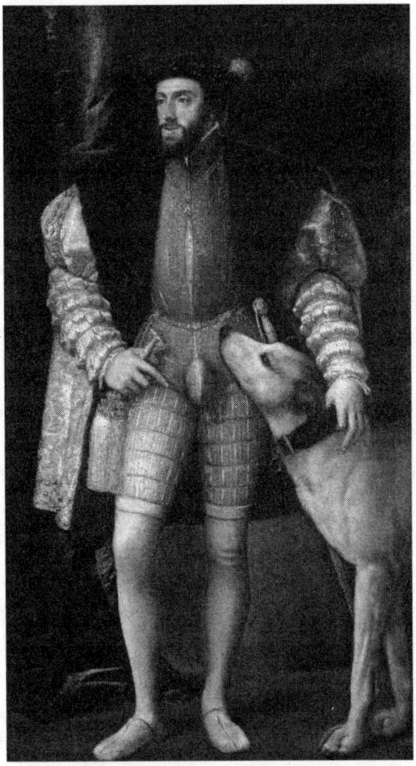

FIGURE 7. Titian, *Charles V with Hound*, 1533. Oil on canvas. 75⅝ × 43¾ inches. Museo Nacional del Prado, Madrid.

"developed" form, between pose and repose. In the final analysis, it is this variability, I contend, that motivates and grounds the centrifugal frame that establishes a concern for the flesh of the body, as well as the bleak alternation of phallus and castration that Lacan entertains. It suggests a *vanitas* that is particularly male. Indeed, the limp *embrasse* promises a certain embarrassment.

MAN IN BLACK: MELANCHOLIA AND EMPIRE

The appearance of the fellow ambassadors as uncannily similar, as virtual twins or clones, suggests they feature in the mode of signification that Lacan terms imaginary. Indeed, Lacan remarks on the function of the "double" or *Döppelgänger* in his essay on the mirror stage.[18] The placement of the image in the imaginary order allows for a perspective in which the two men, in some capacity or other, mirror each other.[19] In the mirror stage, the child "mis-cognizes" its specular equivalent and takes it on as a *Gestalt*. The subject assumes a stable and whole identity, Lacan argues, "in a contrasting size [*un relief de stature*] that fixes it and in a symmetry that inverts it" (2). Rigidified and unified, the mirror image suggests an apparential stature that is wholly at odds with the turbulent drive motility, the insufficiency of motor control, and the fragmentation that the child, according to Lacan, is actually experiencing.

When seen against the background of Lacan's mirror stage, the two portrayed ambassadors come to serve as the juxtaposed and outfolded mirror images of each other. Whereas the left-hand dignitary betrays the motility, lack of motor control, and resulting fragmentability of the body that characterize the child before the mirror in the erectile figuration of his staff and the *embrasse* or tassel, the ambassador to the right offers the fixity, unity, rigidity, and mastery that the mirror image promises—provided the penis remain outside of the picture. Whereas Lacan considers the imaginary as a necessary stage that should largely be left behind and overcome in the development of the subject, Holbein shows the two positions, before and in the mirror, as simultaneously and equally persistent. Hence, the penis cannot take part in the rigidification of form that the mirror pledges.

Additionally, the hyperbolically worked-over or showy accoutrements of power, wealth, function, profession, and rank of the ambassadors can now be understood to function as the symbolic attempt to overcome the imaginary sameness, to the point of collapse, brought about by the mirror. Indeed, the men differ from each other only with respect to their accessories, utterly conventional and arbitrary signifiers. Hence, they establish a secondary differentiation, next to gender, between men, between gentlemen.

The elision of the troublesome and metamorphic penis in the figuration of the right-hand ambassador must come at a price. In *Bodies That Matter*, Butler proposes that any awareness of the body, of its outline as a whole and of its distinction into related parts, is the result of "a theatrical delineation or production of the body, one which gives imaginary contours to the ego itself, projecting a body which becomes the occasion of an identification which in its imaginary or projected status is fully tenuous" (63). This theatrical formation of the body, Butler adds, results from the iterative enactment of cultural prohibitions and ideals.

While the phallus to some extent functions as an "idealization of anatomy," Butler also inquires into what might be lost through such an idealization: "What is excluded from the body for the body's boundary to form? And how does that exclusion haunt that boundary as an internal ghost of sorts, the incorporation of loss as melancholia?" (62, 65). Viewed in this vein, Holbein's skull operates as such an internal ghost, possessing the scene with melancholia over what masculinity must lose, exclude, to acquire an intelligibly visual shape, to strike a pose. Thus, *The Ambassadors* becomes a picture of mourning.[20] This mourning, however, does not so much pertain to castration, to the loss of the phallus, as Lacan would have it, but rather to the loss of the penis *to* the phallus. It is because of the phallus that the penis becomes ghostly. Hence, the real ghost of the phallus is not castration, but the strange and metamorphic variability of the penis.

Furthermore, the distinction between the two men in the painting can also be taken to suggest a historical change. Showy versus diffident, dressed up versus dressed down, the two respective outfits may imply the historic development of masculine power from its feudal and aristocratic mode to the modern one. In the former, power is personal, spectacular, charismatic, and embodied; in the latter, it is institutional, self-effacing, functional, and bureaucratic. According to John Harvey in his book *Men in Black*, the modern sense of masculine dressing for power, with its values of "self-effacement and uniformity, impersonality and authority, discipline and self-discipline, a willingness to be strict and a willingness to die," is indicative of the maintenance of imperial order.[21] Such a reading, moreover, makes Lacan's understanding of masculinity as veiled specifically modern, and hence, historically specific.

Perhaps this historical shift brings with it a change in concomitant modes of perversion as well. The appearance of modesty might well cover up for perversion, whereas showing off, the reveling in display, might as well obscure the fact that there is little to show, that it is all show and nothing more. One can speculate that the "modern" ambassador on the right keeps his heavy coat closed in the front of his body because he is in fact stark naked underneath. Meanwhile, the left side and "aristocratic" dignitary seems protected from such a sudden and complete disclosure because of the layering of the several garments of his outfit. Hence, the left-hand ambassador comes across as a stripper, ready to engage in the game of dispensing with layer after layer of clothing, whereas his colleague on the right appears in the shape of a possible exhibitionist, a flasher, ready to bare all in a single gesture. Yet the *embrasse* that suggests a curtain call, a *démasqué*, if only it were to be pulled, can be found on the left.

The possibility for such a queer curtain call is followed through in John O'Reilly's *A Vanitas* (Figure 8). The artist and model appears to take a break from the making of the *vanitas* painting that is positioned to the side, with the skull used for modeling placed on the table to the right. Coolly yet vulnerably, O'Reilly strikes a pose. His arms extend, the robe is slipping off his body. No ghost appears.

Just as the phallus does, ejaculation indexes the penis. But whereas the phallus inevitably mobilizes the binary opposition between either penis or annihilation, either totality or castration, in which economy the one constantly tips over into the other, ejaculation, brought up by the terse juxtaposition of the phallic vital flow and the formless "that mark," puts the penis in a morphological dynamic that cannot be reduced to such either/or alternatives. What emerges in Lacan's arguments on anamorphosis and *The Ambas-*

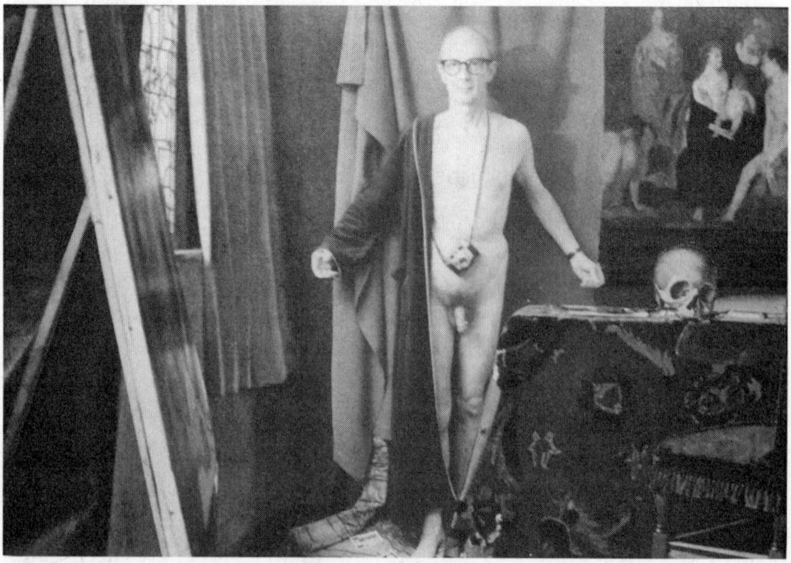

FIGURE 8. John O'Reilly, *A Vanitas*, 1985. Polaroid and half-tone montage. $3\frac{3}{4} \times 5\frac{3}{8}$ inches. Courtesy of the Howard Yezerski Gallery, Boston, Massachusetts.

sadors is a formation of masculinity that factors in its bodily vulnerability, plasticity, and variability. From a phallic perspective, that potential can only be evaluated as haunting, threatening: the strange ghost that the "phallic ghost" removes from view. However, the playfulness of the ambassadors' dress-up games and O'Reilly's compelling self-exposure suggest that the production, in Thomas's sense, of the male body "in the picture" may be as enchanting as it is haunting.

FOUR

THE PARTING VEIL

Angel in the Flesh

CONNOTING PORTENTOUS IDEAS such as progress, reason, genius, modernity, and humanity, Leonardo da Vinci's *Vitruvian Man* is among the most cited images of Western culture (Figure 9). Originally the drawing served to illustrate a passage from Vitruvius' *De architectura*, which rationalizes the ideal geometric proportions of classical architecture through a recourse to the human body.[1] Additionally, *Vitruvian Man* is linked to the mathematical problem of squaring a circle. Since it is specifically, and not coincidentally, a male body that supplies those inquiries with their visual image and vehicle, one might well speculate that the burden of the image is in fact the exact reverse: to calibrate the male body in terms of geometry, architecture, and mathematics; to impress ratio and rationality on the male body, and to render it intelligible in those terms.[2]

Like the ambassadors in the previous chapter, the male figure in *Vitruvian Man* strikes a pose. Yet, unlike Holbein's painting, there seems to be little acknowledgment of the apparitional specter that haunts the posturing of masculinity. The penis may be in the picture, but the figure's face remains impassive, his deportment cool, his stance frontal and solid. Apparently, the production of the penis into visibility does not necessarily bring up anxious intimations of castration and annihilation. Neither, for that matter, does it offer a sense of delight or playfulness.

The male figure appears to be animated in the sense that he jumps from one position to another, but altogether the image is devoid of animation, perhaps in accordance with this man's serious and rational function. Additionally, there is no diagonal line or frame bearing on the figure, as is the case in *The Ambassadors* (see Figure 6), so that the horizontal/vertical organization of the image remains securely in place. Only the rendering of the feet gives this male figure a slight measure of substance and motion, which hesitantly direct him outside the framing circle and square that almost totally imprison him.

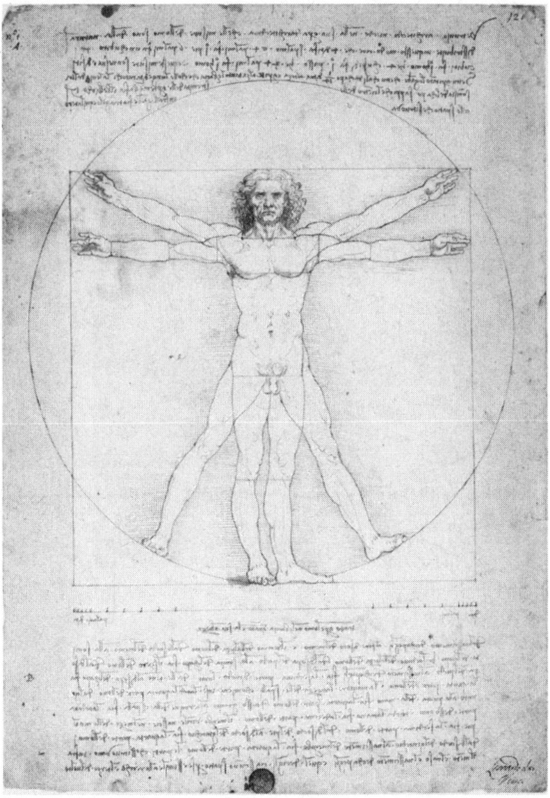

FIGURE 9. Leonardo, *Vitruvian Man*, 1492. Pen, ink, watercolor, and metalpoint on paper. 13½ × 9⅝ inches. Galleria dell'Accademia, Venice.

However, the animation of desire is alluringly present in two other works by Leonardo. In *John the Baptist* (1513–16) (Figure 10) and in the controversially attributed *Angel in the Flesh* (Figure 11), the diagonal lines made up from the positions of the shoulders, faces, smiles, and fabrics prompt the address to and the seduction of the viewer.[3] Furthermore, the *Angel*'s gossamer veil, which reveals a crude caricature of the penis underneath—Lacan's "dick" or *noeud*—and the *Baptist*'s raised finger, which promises a privileged or transcendental meaning, together suggest a reading in terms of Lacan's duplicitous use of the notion of *Aufhebung*, as both elevation and erection. In turn, the analogy between the finger and the penis is, in the *Angel*, countered by the figure's fleshy breast. The many similarities and dissimilarities between the two images once again invite the comparative interpretation of "spotting the differences."[4]

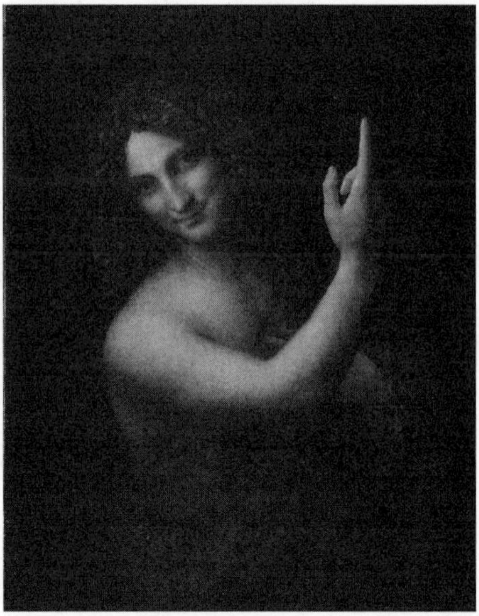

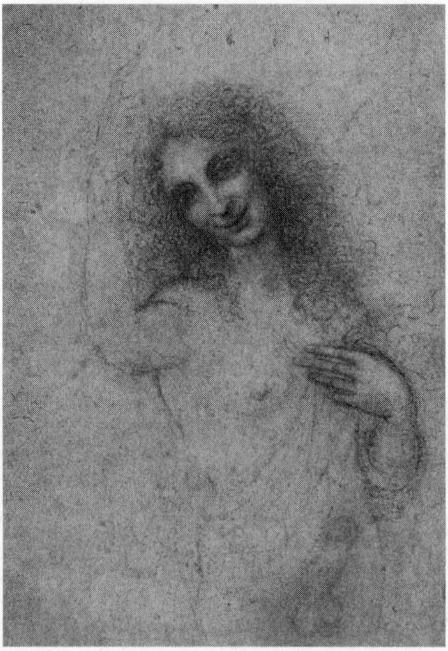

FIGURE 10 (*top*). Leonardo, *John the Baptist*, 1513–16. Oil on wood. 27 3/16 × 22 7/16 inches. Musée du Louvre, Paris.
FIGURE 11 (*bottom*). Leonardo, *The Angel in the Flesh*, 1513–15. Stone chalk or charcoal on rough blue paper. 10½ × 7¾ inches. Private collection, Germany.

Following up on the entropic narrative of semen in Aristotle, the precarious visibility and temporality of Lacan's "vital flow," the persistent presence of "that mark," and the strange and metamorphic plasticity of the penis in *Four Fundamental Concepts* and Holbein's *Ambassadors*, I provide such a reading in this chapter. The specific aspect of the appearance of masculinity under consideration is twofold. First I will inquire into masculinity's dependency on address, the look of the second person that the representation of masculinity must capture and enlist. For the precision-calibrated investiture of demand in the penis, kindled by the veil, makes the phallus, rather than ejaculation, the chosen signifier in Lacanian theory. Hence, this chapter inquires into the workings of addressing and being addressed by the male body, particularly into the dynamic of distinguishing between the body and its parts, and of determining what part or aspect of the body—penis or ejaculation—will garner meaning.

Second, the veil and address also concern the parting and partitioning of the male body, the relationship that holds between its unified form and its privileged or discarded parts or aspects. On the one hand, the phallic form of masculinity can only become imaginarily whole on the condition that the metamorphic penis stays outside the picture. On the other hand, masculinity must invest itself in the same organ for its shape to become intelligible and recognizable. In this vein, the architecturally and geometrically unified bodily form of the *Vitruvian Man* may find its illuminating counterpart in *The Angel in the Flesh*, where the angelic flesh materializes in both the prominent penis and the breast.

THE SPECTER HAUNTING MALE MORPHOLOGY

The second chapter of Judith Butler's *Bodies That Matter*, titled "The Lesbian Phallus and the Morphological Imaginary," starts with a critical return to Freud's essay *On Narcissism: An Introduction* of 1914. According to Freud, Butler explains, the subject's erotogenic awareness of the body and its parts is triggered and facilitated by sensations of pain and illness. Since the subject's ego, however, is first and foremost "the projection of a surface," Butler argues, painful and pleasurable signals can only become epistemologically accessible in relation to the imaginary construction of bodily surfaces and outline.[5]

What kind of incentives and constraints allow the bodily to come to matter, to achieve an imaginary form? Holding Freud true to his claim that to speak of sexuality through and as illness is "symptomatic of the structuring presence of a moralistic framework of guilt," Butler concludes that the body materializes, shapes into being, as the embodiment of cultural prohibitions, as the result of "forcible effects of . . . regulatory power" (63–64). Hence, the body becomes intelligible only as the materialization of power.

In step with the notion of gender performativity she espouses, the metaphor Butler uses to indicate the imaginary delineation or production of the body is a theatrical one (63). However, this sense of the theatrical is not so much expressive, active, or original, but conventional. The "apparent theatricality," she writes, "is produced to the extent that its historicity remains dissimulated (and, conversely, its theatricality gains a certain inevitability given the impossibility of a full disclosure of its historicity)" (12–13). Thus, the body is produced into intelligibility by the iteration of historically established, yet ahistoricized codes, moves, gestures, rituals, steps, rites, turns; that is, by embodied "quotes."

Yet precisely because the morphological establishment of a proper body is entirely dependent on the force of the power that issues its constraints and prohibitions, Butler leaves open the possibility that alternative kinds of bodies, improper bodies that do not "matter" much, can be theatricalized at the edge of possible experience. "[B]ecause prohibitions do not always 'work,' that is, do not always produce the docile body that fully conforms to the social ideal," she argues, "they may delineate body surfaces that do not signify conventional heterosexual polarities" (64).

In the course of Freud's argument on narcissism, Butler detects an odd slide that specifically pertains to the male genitalia. Initially, she suggests, Freud singles out the penis as the prototype for the effect of erotogenic awareness of the body. But subsequently the penis is recategorized as one example among many others. Ultimately, Freud is forced to conclude that erotogenicity is in fact "a general characteristic of all organs" (61). In that way, "the temporal or ontological primacy of any given body part is suspended," Butler claims, for to "be a property of all organs is to be a property necessary to no organ, a property defined by its very *plasticity, transferability,* and *expropriability*" (61).

Making the most of the double meaning of *property* as both "attribute" and "possession," Butler then brings this insight to bear on the Lacanian formula for masculinity of "having the phallus":

> In effect, the "having" is a symbolic position which, for Lacan, institutes the masculine position within a heterosexual matrix, and which presumes an idealized relation of property which is then only partially and vainly approximated by those marked masculine beings who vainly and partially occupy that position within language. But if this attribution of property is itself improperly attributed, if it rests on a denial of that property's transferability . . . ,

> then the repression of that denial will constitute that system internally and, therefore, pose as the promising spectre of its destabilization. (63)

Paradoxically, the formation of a properly masculine body depends on the possession of an attribute that resists it with impropriety and expropriability, and that haunts the vanity of such an attempt like a specter. The organ that must be possessed, owned, in order to be masculine, instead possesses or haunts masculinity like a ghost.

That the figuration of masculinity cannot own (up to) the penis is signaled doubly in *The Ambassadors*, both in the ghostly and anamorphic skull that according to Lacan conveys castration and death, and in the figuration of the dagger and the tassel that invokes the plasticity of the penis. That painting also brings in the constitutive involvement of the audience, of the viewer. Indeed, to coin performativity and theatricality as concepts for the understanding of gender, as Butler does, cannot but raise the question of the audience to the theater performance. Holbein's painting makes clear that it matters a great deal where the viewer stands, literally, in relation to the posturing on display.

For the significance of the scene largely depends on the viewpoint that the observer is led to adopt, be it perspectival, in which the viewer is slotted in the geometric arrangement that lines up the penis with the phallus, with worldly power; anamorphic, in which the viewer recognizes his or her castration in the skull's grin; or comparative, in which the viewer's look moves between the two male figures, and is forced to recognize the potential for metamorphic alienation of the penis in the figure on the left.

Butler's account of the performative formation of the body's imaginary form stands at the crossing of speech act theory and the Lacanian mirror stage. Both those theoretical frames consider the second person, the listener or viewer, as essential rather than accidental to the effect of meaning. In the mirror stage, the "miscognition" of the child is affirmed by the look of the caregiver who supports it in front of the mirror, and who joins its jubilation. In speech act theory, illocution or force and perlocution or effect largely depend on the response of the person who listens. Her or his response decides whether the speech act of the subject is either felicitous or misfiring. Hence, it is imperative to account for the function of the audience in relation to the performance of gender.

As I have argued in chapter 2, Lacan suggests not one, but two different accounts of what constitutes the privilege of the phallus. In the first, the stature of the phallus is made rhetorically probable by considering a series of penile qualities, the alleged ancientness of the phallus, and its charged veiling and subsequent revelation in the narrative. But in the second account, the phallus's privilege follows from the demand that the subject addresses to the penis, thus impregnating it with added meaning, relevance, and value. As it turns out, Lacan suggests several ways in which the meaning of the gendered body depends on the structural polarity of address and response.

OTHERING THE BODY: A COMEDY

In "The Signification of the Phallus," Lacan states his understanding of what he terms "the Other." Situated at the collapse of language and the unconscious, the Other is a dimension alterior to, yet constitutive of, all possible subjectivity and signification. However, throughout the argument, this linguistic and extra-psychic Other is also repeatedly considered as an instance of address. Hence, the Lacanian Other starts to oscillate between the impersonal and the personal, the abstract and the concrete.

The "passion for the signifier" that Freud intuited *avant la lettre,* Lacan begins, does not imply a culturalist or social view of language ("Signification," 78–79). Rather, he claims, "[i]t is a question of rediscovering in the laws governing that other scene [*ein andere Schauplatz*] which Freud designated, in relation to dreams, as that of the unconscious" (79). In that sense, these linguistic and unconscious "laws" precede the social and cultural world that the subject inhabits.

Note the theatrical, spatial, visual, and temporal implications of "that other scene." Yet, Lacan subsequently abridges "that other scene" to "the Other." That notwithstanding, he continues to refer to it as a *place.* Once the subject speaks, she or he calls upon this "very place," the unconscious as ruled by the linguistic laws of substitution and combination, of metaphor and metonymy. "[W]hether or not the subject hears it with his own ears," Lacan writes, he or she finds his or her "signifying place" in this spatial and theatrical dimension of alterity (79). And because of the subject's necessary recourse to this elsewhere, she or he is no longer the grammatical subject of her or his speech: it is not an "I" who utters language, but an "it" [*ça*] that speaks both to and through "me."

Hence, all that can be meaningfully articulated in speech depends on "that other scene" appealed to by the subject, who becomes its object rather than its subject, the addressee of meaning rather than its sender. More precisely, the Lacanian Other both is addressed by the subject and in turn addresses the subject, so that the latter becomes split between the grammatical positions of the first and the second person, between "I" and "you."

Lacan does seem intent upon maintaining a level of topographical abstraction, even though the structure of addressing and being addressed would in fact imply a sociocultural dialogue. However, the shift from "that other scene" to "the Other" can also be understood to signal the extent to which this elsewhere, the linguistic and unconscious dimension of spatial alterity, is always already personified because of the subjective appeals issued to it.

This slippage between, on the one hand, the topographically abstract and the alien, and on the other hand, the intersubjective and personifiable connotations of the Other, cannot be entirely prevented by that term's capitalization and definite article. Hence, Lacan suggests a double move with respect to otherness. On the one hand, Freud's originally indefinite "*ein andere Schauplatz*" becomes an impersonal or third-person place because of Lacan's reworking of it as "*that* other scene." On the other hand, because of the appeals addressed to it, that same scene becomes reworked as a personal other, who is liable to second-person investment.[6]

That second and personal reading of otherness is underlined when Lacan moves on to the polarity of address and response, which is "manifest in the primordial relation to the mother" (80). Here he distinguishes between need, demand, and desire as distinct modes of address. Need deviates into the demand for what he terms the proof of love, because of its introduction in the linguistic structure of appeal and response (81).

As the subject must appeal to the other scene in its speech, owing to "the putting into signifying form as such" of the subject's impetus, and owing to "the fact that it is from the place of the Other that his message is emitted," the uttered need turns into something else and something more than a simple request for its satisfaction. For, even when the request is in fact fully granted by the subject who is addressed—here, the mother—the offered gratification falls in "some way short" of the demand for the collapse of the dialogic structure the subject was forced to enter to begin with (80). Hence, demand, too, oscillates between another subject, the mother, and the Other in the address it enacts.

Demand cannot be met by any kind of gratifying response, since that would call for "a presence or an absence" that the Other cannot deliver. For the Other is itself responsible for the suspension or splitting of the subject between the positions of the first and second person. But, in turn, this Other itself splits apart between the second person, who is the object of the address of demand, and the other scene that forms the detour of speech. The resulting frustration, Lacan claims, translates into desire. The demand that the two others or the double Other cannot meet endures as a residue of affect, which is invested in another person, the object of desire. In that way, impersonal Other and personal other become entirely entangled. Through desire, the stage of "that other scene" becomes inevitably peopled with actors.

That duplicity designates the sexual life of the subject as enigmatic,

Lacan continues, since it signifies otherness to him or her "twice over" [*doublement*]: as "a demand made on the subject of need, and as an ambiguity cast onto the Other who is involved" (81). Hence, desire, according to Lacan, can best be seen as a form of personification. Indeed, it personalizes the Other in the shape of another person, who becomes burdened with the demand for love. This rhetoric of personification is given a surprising slant when Lacan moves on to the relation between the genders.

"Let us say," he proposes, "that these relations will revolve around a being and a having" (83–84). Masculinity is configured as "having the phallus," femininity as "being the phallus." However, another modality immediately intercedes in this crisp distribution of values:

> This follows from the intervention of an "appearing" which gets substituted for the "having" so as to protect it on one side and to mask its lack on the other, with the effect that the ideal or typical manifestations of behaviour in both sexes, up to and including the act of sexual copulation, are entirely propelled into comedy. (84)

With this intrusion of appearances, masks, and comedy Lacan polemicizes against his adversaries. Throughout the essay, he reproaches them for "normalizing the function of the phallus," for worshipping "the virtue of the 'genital,'" and for partaking in a moralizing trend of "genital oblativity . . . to the tune of Salvationist choirs" (78, 81). Interestingly, though, he also distances himself from the opening claim of his own essay, where he ordains that, without the castration complex, the subject would remain "unable to identify with the ideal type of his sex" (75). By now, that opening move starts to come across as comical, as tongue-in-cheek. The performance of ideal or typical gender manifestations, Lacan suggests, should be met with bemusement or outright laughter.

Additionally, the recalibration of the genders in relation to the phallus as a matter of making hilarious appearances brings the constituting involvement of the second person, audience, or viewer to the fore. It does so by signifying otherness twice over. For the respective positions of being and having the phallus can only be accredited in the eyes of the second person. In a synecdochal logic, the relations to be signified are usually phrased as follows. The masculinity of having the phallus is affirmed by someone else's desire for the subject's penis, a part of the body. In contradistinction, the femininity of being the phallus is avowed by someone else's desire for the whole body.

Thus, gender is ultimately conferred on the subject's body by the rhetorical habit of the beholder, decided by his or her predisposition to prefer either a *pars pro toto* or a *totum pro parte*. Moreover, since the phallus is not the penis, and since the modality of appearing overrules the having in the case of masculinity, as Lacan argues, the synecdochal dynamic of part/whole substitution leaves open the possibility that *another* part than the penis can well be invested with a *pars pro toto* desire.

In addition, the first and second person of desire are firmly locked into a dialogue or exchange that forces these positions to switch irrespectively of what gender the subject embodies before he or she enters into desire. If the second person is constituted as *having* the phallus by the first person's *pars pro toto* desire, then it automatically follows that the first person constitutes him- or herself as *being* the phallus in the second person's eyes, as well as vice versa. Desire can only be "suffered," Lacan claims, in relation to a signifier that is alien to the subject (83).

The polarity of first and second person of desire, and the possibility of role switching that this entails, Lacan explains, prevents the subject "from being satisfied with presenting to the Other anything real it might *have* which corresponds to the phallus—what he has being worth no more than what he does not have as far as his demand for love is concerned, which requires that he *be* the phallus" (83). Having only accounts for something in relation to a second person who must be; being only accounts for something in relation to a second person who must have; and the first person will switch values accordingly.

Hence, the phallic making of gendered bodies results from the constitution of the subject in its entry into the polar structure of the address, both issued at and by the other, the resulting alternation between first and second personhood, and the shifting of personifying and synecdochal desires. This comedy of role-playing makes the signification of the phallus theatrical and performative, in Butler's vein. Yet, as I argue in the next section, that theatrical potential may already be betrayed by Lacan's or the narrator's own performance with the veil in "The Signification of the Phallus."

THE DEICTIC VEIL AND THE PHALLUS/PENIS

A dogged discussion bears heavily on the concept of the phallus: does it or does it not ultimately refer to the penis? Kaja Silverman and Daniel Boyarin propose quite different understandings of the crucial role that is played by the Lacanian veil in relation to the phallus/penis, in a disagreement that proves highly instructive.

In *Male Subjectivity at the Margins*, Silverman makes full use of the analytical distance between penis and phallus. The "equation of the male sexual organ with the phallus" is at stake in the ideological belief commanded by what Silverman terms the dominant fiction of patriarchy. Yet the incommensurability of the phallus and the penis is nevertheless readable in the cracks and fissures that appear when the dominant fiction is put under historical strain, thus laying bare the lack that the symbolic order installs in both sexes as the condition of subjectivity.[7]

In "The Lacanian Phallus," however, Silverman strikes a note of caution with regard to maintaining a strict distinction between the two. Conceding that the difference between phallus and penis has been beneficial to contemporary theory, teaching "that the male sexual organ can never be equivalent to the values designated by the phallus, and that consequently all subjects might be said to be castrated," she warns that

> the metaphorics of veiling and unveiling deployed by Lacan ... suggests that it may not always be politically productive to differentiate sharply between penis and phallus. To veil the phallus in this way is to permit it to function as a privileged signifier, as Lacan himself acknowledges.[8]

Silverman implies that the very distinction between penis and phallus works as a veil, which allows for the latter term's privilege.

This is exactly the charge that Daniel Boyarin makes against Silverman. "The dominant fiction of gender (and thence of so much else)," Boyarin argues, "is not of an equation of the penis with the phallus but of a split between them."[9] Precisely the distinction between the two, "the separation of masculinity from the embodied male body," allows for the reification of the phallus as the pinnacle of power, potency, and sovereignty (52). Hence,

> it is precisely the "veiling" of the phallus, this very amnesia, the hiding of the emblem from explicit representation ... that has most enabled it to do its cultural work, while remaining itself immune, as it were, to further "history." (50)

Cut loose from the body and immunized from history, the phallus easily achieves transcendence. The concept may be strategically deployed to debunk the penis, and thence the contingent powers of patriarchy, but it is the split between the two that allows the phallus to come into being in the first place.[10] Hence, Boyarin's veil points to the hiding and forgetting of the real penis, which to him only needs to become visually explicit to bring down the phallus from its quasi-metaphysical pedestal.

As soon as the distinction between phallus and penis rigidifies into a clear opposition, it would seem, it yields two equally unproductive effects. On the one hand, the phallus, when detached from the male body, can reign supreme, uncontaminated by that body's contingency and historicity. On the other hand, the penis, if detached from the phallus, promises to be accessible in its pseudo-objective, anatomical, or historical reality. One may get to know the penis for what that organ really is, and recognize it in its true shape. However, that latter move is effectively prevented by Lacan, as he sets up the alternation between exalted phallus and vulgar dick or *noeud*, and not one between mythical phallus and objective penis. There must be another way out.

After conceding that the sharp distinction between phallus and penis is not always politically productive, Silverman moves on to trace instances in Lacan where both terms slip into each other. Hence, Boyarin's criticism is not entirely warranted. Silverman observes that the phallus is often contaminated by the visual. In a manner akin to the mirror stage, the phallus entertains iconic and indexical relations with an idealized image of the penis. "This double motivation not only links the phallus closely to the penis," Silverman writes, "but it distinguishes the phallus emphatically from the linguistic signifier, which conventionally entertains an arbitrary relation both to the signified and to the referent" ("The Lacanian Phallus," 90).

Furthermore, she remarks that, even in its most abstract appearances, the phallus turns on the "opposition of tumescence and detumescence" insofar as it impossibly promises to fill in and fill up lack (93). This problem prompts Silverman to coin a supplemental distinction between two different kinds of phalluses: "whereas the imaginary phallus is a signifier of wholeness and sufficiency, the symbolic phallus is a signifier of what every fully constituted subject has surrendered" (92). To conclude, she notes that there exists "a good deal of slippage" in Lacan, both between penis and phallus, and between the phallus in its symbolic and in its imaginary capacity. However, this "good deal of slippage" seems precisely the point, so I would hesitate to set up a second distinction to remedy and clean up the initial one between penis and phallus. Do we really need another phallus?[11]

Both Silverman's and Boyarin's readings focus attention on the veil. To Silverman, the veil is responsible for the sharp distinction between penis and phallus, and enables the latter term's privilege over the former. For Boyarin, the veil alludes to the forgetting and obfuscation of the historical penis. However, I would argue to the contrary.

For *veiled* does not mean *invisible*. In one and the same gesture, a veil *both* suspends, defers, *and* charges the difference between visibility and invisibility. The veil cannot draw a clear demarcation line between perceptibility and imperceptibility, or between phallus and penis, because its effects depend on the texture of the fabric, and on the specific moments at which it is drawn and withdrawn. Indeed, the veil makes those differences material rather than conceptual. It makes the distinction between phallus and penis *matter* to the precise extent that that difference is itself *material*, and thus indiscrete. As a taunt or tease of sorts, the veil suggests not so much the occlusion of the penis or the discrete differentiation of the penis/phallus, but rather the heightened and emphasized play with the male body and its visibility.

Moreover, the veil suggests a dynamic that problematizes, but does not abolish, the logic of distinction underlying the discussion, by charging the difference between the two terms with seduction; that is to say, by making that difference indiscrete, qualified, tenuous, and fragile, materially thin or thick, flattening or creasing. Finally, the veil can be taken up to shift the debate from referentiality—does the phallus refer to the penis?—to another modality of signification: deixis. For the veil can only work in an intersubjective relationality between the first person who wields it and the second person who watches and responds, who reacts to its performative effects.

Indeed, the Lacanian veil proposes a semiotic model in which referentiality and deixis become entangled or enfolded. Initially, the veil blocks and prevents referentiality. Meaning cannot be based upon the thing to which the sign refers, since that object is withdrawn behind a shroud. The veil not only makes the referent disappear, but also simultaneously triggers and kindles the desire for reference, for what has just disappeared behind or underneath it. Hence, in one and the same gesture of veiling, referentiality is both preempted and recharged. The debate concerning the phallus/penis distinction plays exactly into that double movement. The veil also reframes this double referentiality in a deictic setup: someone is doing the veiling and someone else is watching. If not, there would be little point in veiling and unveiling anything. In that way, the viewer or the second person comes to partake of the effect of the veiling that is performed. This deictic semiotic of the veil I want to bring to bear on Leonardo's images.

EVERY TEMPTATION

The two works by Leonardo, *John the Baptist* and *The Angel in the Flesh*, are replete with deictic signs: looks, smiles, gestures. This abundance raises the question of whether the two elements most conducive to a Lacanian reading, the fleshy penis and the privileged meaning that the fingers promise, could or should be implicated in the extensive elaboration of deixis in their direct vicinity. Since at least two art historical commentators have felt themselves to be strongly addressed by the images, I begin my interpretation with their reactions.

"*John the Baptist* leads to every temptation," Serge Bramly notes in *Leonardo: Discovering the Life of Leonardo da Vinci*. For Bramly, the painting paradoxically procures an excess of affect over a minimum of signification:

> accessory detail and anecdote are reduced to a minimum: a dark background replaces the landscape, and there is no color apart from the transparent gold of the lighting on the face: one can appreciate the painting without being obliged to decipher it—the

> beauty, the smile, and the gesture immediately appeal to the emotions. There is nothing to *read*. Nothing in it suggests the terrestrial life of the saint who lived like a hermit on the bank of the Jordan and who is usually represented as gaunt and wild in aspect; this work asks simply to be experienced emotionally.[12]

Apparently, the painting cannot be read inter- or pretextually: the male figure only nominally features as John the Baptist ("Nothing in it suggests the terrestrial life of the saint"). Neither can it be easily viewed iconographically, as the requisite details are brought back to a bare minimum (the reed cross and the tunic). Since the figure is not placed in an identifiable setting or landscape, narrative reading will not do either. Finally, the image cannot be read stylistically, because the only color present is a transparent glow. The only thing left is its emotional and seductive appeal, its temptation. Bramly cites Jules Michelet, who writes, "This canvas attracts me, overwhelms me, absorbs me; I go toward it in spite of myself, like the bird toward the snake" (261).

Yet the reading that Bramly does offer is nevertheless narrative in the biographical sense. He views *John the Baptist* as the climax of the artist's accomplishments. Between the lines, the tempting force of the artist's last work now becomes clearer:

> Leonardo set out to disturb and trouble the emotions. He had progressively purified the syntax of his work throughout his career, finally reaching one supreme emotion that contains all others—and since some element of his sexuality crept into it, reason cannot always resist the overwhelming impression it conveys. (264)

The argument is remarkable in its meandering. The progressive purification leads to "one supreme emotion," which, though all-containing, nevertheless excludes "some element of his sexuality." That element then creeps back in to contribute to the "overwhelming impression" of the work.

Bramly's commentary suggests that the alleged foreclosure of readability prepares the ground for the affective exchange that goes on between work and viewer. Ironically, the force of that affect becomes most clear in Bramly's own way of dealing with the suggestive sexuality of the *Baptist*. While Bramly's ambivalence may be taken to emphasize the painting's strong appeal to the viewer, such goodwill is more difficult to maintain in the case of a recent response to *The Angel in the Flesh*.

Writing in *The New York Review of Books*, art historian Henri Zerner objects to the inclusion of the drawing in an exhibition on Leonardo at the Boston Museum of Science. Noting that the "bizarre drawing" is not uncritically established as Leonardo's, Zerner argues that there are plenty of other and authenticated studies for the lost work of *The Angel of the Annunciation;* "a striking conception," Zerner specifies, presumed to represent "Gabriel [as] facing the viewer who is thereby put, so to speak, in the shoes of the Virgin Mary." Our drawing, however, strikes Zerner quite differently:

> In the drawing exhibited ... Gabriel has been turned into some kind of hermaphrodite freak by the addition of an erect penis and a female breast. Is it possible that such a weird image is by Leonardo? Even if we assume that the drawing is authentic, we still want to know whether it has been tampered with by a later hand.[13]

The questions can only be rhetorical. Hence, Zerner resists the supplementarity of the penis, the breast, and the "later hand" to the authenticity of Leonardo. But the supplementarity of these body parts—penis, breast, and hand—may exactly be the point.

Nevertheless, Zerner's article offers ample opportunity for a less dismissive engagement with the work. Attributing to Leonardo a visual epistemology, in which the eyes can grasp and record the world, he also attends to two counterpoints to such an endeavor present in the artist's work. According to Zerner, Leonardo did not see the novelty of linear perspective as a straightforward set of rules and procedures. Instead, the painter attempted to understand the tension between what he called artificial perspective and the "physiology of visual perception," or "natural" perspective. "He investigated, for example, the 'distortions' in an image caused by the artist's working on a flat surface, while the retina, on which the image forms in the eye, is curved," Zerner writes. Hence, Leonardo may have been as intrigued by visual—that is, anamorphic—distortions as Lacan would be in a later age. Zerner remarks on the artist's passion for draperies, for a *chiaroscuro* of textile folds that create the impression of volume, which brings to mind the workings of the Lacanian veil.

In the reticence, ambivalence, and disgust articulated in Bramly's and Zerner's reactions, the works' address of the critical eye becomes that much clearer. Apparently, the painting and the drawing put their viewers in shoes that not everyone likes to wear. Hence, the male figures in the two images point not only to heaven, but also to the viewer.

SMILE AND BREAST: DOUBLE-CROSSING GENDER

In *John the Baptist* and *The Angel in the Flesh*, the vertical lines are supplemented and countered by diagonal bearings or leanings. Whereas the former indicate reference, the latter engage the viewer deictically. In the *Bap-*

tist, the intricately curled hair of the figure and the heavy tunic form a threshold of visibility. Light and vision disappear into their meandering contours. They create an impression of volume and three-dimensionality, which is otherwise lacking because of the darkened and flattened background. Robbing the painting of a deep spatial perspective, the background relegates all attention to the figure who steps into the light at the painting's front.

Together, the hair and the robe frame the diagonal lines that are made up of the figure's smile and the bare shoulder, both offered up to the viewer. In turn, those diagonals set off the vertical lines of the cross and the raised finger. The cross is emphatically thin and elongated. According to tradition, it is made of reed. Largely in the dark and barely perceptible, the cross prepares for the raised and slightly elongated finger. It receives the light from one side, and forces the viewer's attention on the detailed rendering of the Baptist's fingertip and the nail.

The *Angel* retains much of the *Baptist*'s formal arrangement. However, the focal point of the finger is now rivaled by the figure's conspicuous and cartoonishly rendered penis, pushing up against the diaphanous veil that is the obligatory remainder of the Baptist's tunic. In turn, the penis is set off by the androgynous breast of the figure. Akin to the *Baptist*, the verticality of the penis and the finger is complemented by the diagonal lines of the veil's folds and the breast.

Because the vertical fingers in both images point outside the frames without the thing pointed at being present, these gestures come to suggest meaning *per se*: signification happens, occurs, just above the *Baptist*'s slender fingertip. Hence, the *Baptist*'s and the *Angel*'s raised fingers can be read to invoke an ultimate meaning, a transcendental signified as ordained by God, a gesture that the viewer is invited to join. But where the *Baptist*'s lower body is invisible because of the heavy tunic and lack of illumination, the *Angel* produces into visibility the concrete signifier that underpins the elevation of meaning in the shape of the penis.

In the figuration of the fingers and the penis, similarly vertical and turned upward, one may recognize the move of phallic meaning from the tangible, visible, and material signifier, toward its elevation or *Aufhebung* into a near-divine signified. Yet here that move seems to work both ways: from signifier to meaning and back again. This motionality also partakes of the double and ambivalent referentiality that was suggested by the semiotic model of the veil. Although the *Baptist* suspends the penile referent from sight with the heavy and dark tunic, the promise of its eventual reappearance is kept in the *Angel*. The veil both blocks and recharges referentiality; it both hides and reaccentuates the penis. Indeed, the only difference between the phallus and the dick or *noeud* is the gossamer-thin veil.

The model of the veil suggests that the play of reference be situated within a frame of deixis, a performance of addressing and being addressed. The frontal position, the turned head, the ingratiating smile, and the offered bare shoulder in the *Baptist* all engage the viewer. Those signs invite or enlist the second person to join the manual gesture of the figure. Hence, one may read the finger as an appeal to the symbolic Other or other scene. To a decisive extent, the *Baptist* implies that meaning will arrive from somewhere else, from outside the frame.

Addressing that Other together with John forces the viewer to enter into the structure of polarity in language, and in turn to be addressed from that other place. Signification, then, cannot be exhausted or saturated in the personal exchange between the image and the viewer. The Other is indexically "present" as the dimension of constituting alterity. Yet Lacan also intimated that the appeal for meaning issued to the Other quickly entangles itself with the address of needs, demands, and desires toward another person, the second person. So, if the *Baptist* and the *Angel* solicit the viewer in the joint recognition of the Other, he or she may in turn invest the figure with desires of his or her own.

Another form of otherness that Lacan considered is the structural necessity of the look of a second-person viewer to affirm the appearance or comical performance of gender ideals. In this respect, Leonardo's images become troublesome. As Bramly indicates, the figure of the *Baptist* does not comply with the image of John as an old and gaunt hermit. Moreover, one may well suspect *Mona Lisa*–like qualities in the figure's face and his smile. Leonardo's *Baptist* is invested with a poignant beauty and androgyny. Consequently, it is difficult to decide *what* gender should be affirmed. This complication becomes more distressing, and thus more productive, in yet another modality of othering: the synecdochal alienation of gender in the exchange of desire.

According to Lacan, as I have argued, gender is caught up in a reversible polarity of first and second person. Having the phallus must be affirmed by a second person's desire for a body part, usually the penis; being the phallus must be affirmed by a second person's desire for the body's whole. But in order to perform such a validation, that second person must switch values accordingly: "If I am to affirm your having, then I must be," and vice versa. In that sense, the ambivalence or androgyny of the figures comes to apply to *the viewer*. Seductively, they address the viewer, who must return the gesture, but without much clarity as to the positions to be taken up. To push the point, the *Angel* even adds another private part to supplement the penis, the figure's breast, to enable more than one synecdochal move between part and whole to take place.

The *Angel* lacks the requisite reed cross that the *Baptist* carries over his shoulder. However, a cross-like figuration of gender seems to arrive in its place. It entails the crossing of the masculine, vertical lines of the penis and the hand pointing upward, and the feminine, horizontal line consisting of the other hand that points at the fleshy breast. That latter line is hidden, veiled, by the Baptist's gesture, which works to obscure the other hand and the figure's chest. Hence, gender is, as it were, double-crossed in the *Angel*. In one human figure, the genders come to bear on each other in the intersecting shape of a cross, traversing the desire for distinction and demarcation.

Double-crossed, moreover, because the straight lines burdened with gender, horizontal or vertical, feminine or masculine, are bisected by the queer and diagonal lines that shape the figures' address to the viewer: the slanted head, eyes, smile, shoulders, and the folds of the gossamer veil. These diagonal, deictic lines come to inflect straight gender lines.

One of these diagonals consists of the famous Leonardo smile, which Freud connects to the mother.[14] That smile is recognizable in the faces of both the angel and the Baptist. In *Male Subjectivity at the Margins*, Kaja Silverman enlists Freud's biographical essay on Leonardo to account for a specific form of male homosexuality, which she terms the Leonardo model. Silverman reads a first clue in an added note to *Three Essays*. There, Freud considers the possibility of a homosexuality in which the subject identifies with the mother, and loves his object as what he once was in relation to her (367). That form of homosexuality, as Silverman explains, Freud imputes to Leonardo.

But as Silverman then points out, the bird fantasy that forms the kernel of Freud's analysis does not square with its logic. In the fantasy, an infant is visited in his cradle by a bird vigorously tapping the child on its mouth with its tail. Freud's model would require that the subject features as the maternal, actively loving bird, in a scene condensing breast-feeding with fellatio. Nevertheless, Freud concludes that Leonardo plays the part of the child in the cradle, being administered to by the bird.

Seizing on the critical leeway thus offered, Silverman decides on the structural reversibility of Leonardian homosexuality. The subject *either* identifies with the mother and desires what he once was in relation to her, *or* identifies with what he once was in relation to the mother and desires someone else in her place (371). These positions of desire and identification continue to complement each other. To Silverman, the mouth is an "ideal locus" for the Leonardo model of homosexuality, because it is both a "privileged site of maternal care" and suggestive of the oral sexuality that underpins the model in accordance with the tail-flapping bird (372).

The fact that the maternal smile features on a male figure in the *Baptist* and the *Angel*, then, indicates the degree of identification of the subject with the mother, or rather, the mutual absorption of the two positions. That way, the smiling mouths of the Baptist and the angel intimate the jubilant moment of the imaginary sharing of the gift of love. The subject is *both* the subject *and* the object of the smile. Those positions are equally available and reversible. The viewer can either receive the smile, or insinuate himself into the picture to bestow it, or move between the two options. This promise of reciprocal and interchangeable validation, I contend, is responsible for the strong emotional appeal of the *Baptist*.

Besides a maternal and an erotic site, however, the mouth is also the locus of speech. Small wonder, then, that both the Baptist and the angel do not directly point at the viewer, but at the symbolic elsewhere or other scene that intervenes within the exchange of smiles. If the smile pledges a mute and imaginary wholeness or presence to circulate between the first and second person, the raised finger calls upon the Other for semiosis to recommence.

I started this chapter with Butler's claim that our sense of our bodies is the result of a theatrically and performatively produced morphology, the arrangement of an outline, surfaces, and a proportional relation between whole and parts. In a paradoxical contrast to castration logic, Lacan specifies the femininity of being the phallus as the effect of the second person's *totum pro parte* desire. Congruently, the masculinity of having the phallus turns out to be the result of the second person's *pars pro toto* desire.

Hence, masculinity cannot but be at grave risk of overinvesting in the possession of the part, and consequently of losing control over the whole. That is ultimately why the part must not be shown all too prominently, the final reason for the veil. Yet that veil itself is also responsible for the parting of the male body, for the privileging of one specific part over the whole. Between the elevating verticals of the penis and the finger, and the engaging and deictic diagonals of the breast, the hand, the folds, and the shoulder, the veil, thin or thick, stretches, billows, reveals. Indeed, the veil performs the parting, the synecdochal substitution of the male body for the one part that must embody that body's significance and relevance as masculine.[15]

In *John the Baptist*, the figure confronts the viewer as if appearing from a dark mist, a prime example of Leonardo's *sfumato* technique. Lack of lighting notwithstanding, and with the improper part safely under wraps, the overall contours of the figure's body are nevertheless remarkably distinct and clear. The discreteness of the body's outline culminates in the precision rendering of the finger.

That situation is quite different in *The Angel in the Flesh*. While the crude penis is rendered with thick lines, the remainder of the body yields its contours through porous, fuzzy, and vague lines. The flesh dematerializes, loses its morphological integrity. That reverse effect culminates in the finger, too, with its outline nearly disappearing. Hence, the marked attention lavished on the representation of the penis disturbs the morphological relation between whole and part. In that way, the *Angel* forms Leonardo's own critique of the discreteness, symmetry, and proportionality of *Vitruvian Man*.

Masculinity depends on the distinction and the relationship between the whole and the parts of the bodily form in which it incarnates. Hence, that form revolves on the property and proportionality of the penis in relation to the whole. As the privileged *pars pro toto*, the penis must designate masculinity's complete and vertical form. Yet that same penis can also disturb, recalibrate, and reinflect the totality it must give figuration to. The synecdoche of desire that substitutes part for whole gives way to a supplementarity that disturbs the meaningful relation between the part and the whole. From a rhetorically privileged part, the penis becomes a haunting supplement, one capable of suspending the contours of bodily form. Ultimately, then, the evident blotting out and rubbing away of the contours of *The Angel in the Flesh* refer back to the morphological indeterminacy of the flat and seminal "that mark." "In the flesh," substantially, the same penis that signifies masculinity causes that gender's shape to be nearly smudged away.

PART THREE

PORNOGRAPHY

FIVE

SIGNIFICANT DISCHARGE

The Cum Shot and Narrativity

IN LACAN'S NARRATIVE OF THE CONCEPTION of meaning as bastard offspring, the moment and the image of ejaculation are precariously displaced. Hence, the phallus remains untouched by the temporality, visibility, and materiality that ejaculation brings to bear on masculinity and meaning. However, in contrast, popular culture offers an example where male orgasm seems spectacularly visible, temporal, and material, and where it is pivotal with respect to meaning and gender rather than marginal. Contemporary feature-length hard-core video and film pornography, both straight and gay, calibrates and celebrates masculinity in terms of the narrative temporality and visibility of male orgasm. The genre presents the so-called cum, pop, or money shot, the simultaneous visualization and narration of ejaculation, as its height of signification, the irresistible juncture where significance, pleasure, and masculinity are united.[1]

The cum shot forms hard core's pinnacle convention. It depicts ejaculation in close-up, always occurring outside of the body of the sexual partner.[2] Semen spurts, trickles, or gushes from the penis, and lands on the female or male skin of the buttocks, chest, belly, backside, or face. The cum shot nearly always forms the conclusion and culmination of the sexual encounters in the genre. The mandatory visibility of ejaculation as well as its specific function as narrative climax in the cum shot cannot but bear on the formation of masculinity that the genre puts forth. Indeed, those conventions appear to be intrinsic to the representation of masculinity, constituting elements, rather than attendant gimmicks or empty codes.

In "Male Gay Porn: Coming to Terms," Richard Dyer stresses the importance of visuality and narrativity for masculine sexuality. As Dyer argues, the visibility of ejaculation in hard-core pornography conforms to the general "importance of the visual in the way male sexuality is constructed/conceptualized."[3] In order to convince, masculinity must be foregrounded, produced into visibility, exposed. Thus, the cum shot may partake of the endeavor to make masculinity real, to realize or to authenticate it in the eyes of the viewer.

In addition, the function of ejaculation as narrative climax in the genre, Dyer continues, agrees with another aspect of the construction of masculinity at large. "It seems to me," he writes, "that male sexuality, homo or hetero, is socially constructed, at the level of representation anyway, in terms of narrative; that is, as it were, male sexuality is itself understood narratively" (28). The "sense of an ending" delivered by the cum shot, then, may likewise implicate the establishment of masculinity as a putative triumph, accomplishment, or goal.[4] Thus, visibility, narrativity, and masculinity join together most felicitously in the cum shot. "The emphasis on seeing orgasm," Dyer concludes, "is then part of the way porn (re)produces the construction of male sexuality" (28).

Specifically the male viewer of the cum shot does not so much merely observe the (re)production of the construction of masculinity along the lines of visuality and narrative, but rather (inter)actively participates in it. The cum shot, Dyer claims, enables the spectator "to see [the male performer] come (and, more often than not, probably, to come at the same time as him)" (28). Hence, the shot allows for a homosocial identification, a joint assumption of the image as inscribed in and through the body, through the agency of visual narrative.[5]

The privileged status of the cum shot in hard-core pornography mirrors the terms of the general understanding of narrativity that Peter Brooks proposes in *Reading for the Plot: Design and Intention in Narrative.* In Brooks's account, the friction of narrative pushes forward toward a moment of climax and resolution that he, with an apt choice of words, characterizes as the "significant discharge." Hence, the saturation of the bodily discharge of ejaculation with relevance and meaning through narrative in pornography finds its fitting theoretical counterpart in Brooks's narratology.

This chapter proposes a reading of the cum shot in terms of Brooks, and a rereading of Brooks in terms of the cum shot. My primary case will be the heterosexual porn film *Justine 2: Nothing to Hide.* Not only does that movie offer several conventional cum shots or pornographically significant discharges, but it also thematically elaborates on the production or performance of the cum shot itself. Its plot revolves on the male protagonist's initial inability to ejaculate in the right manner, and *Justine* thus makes clear the conditions under which the discharge of ejaculation may become either significant or meaningless, privileged or discarded, in the genre.

INTRODUCING THE CUM SHOT

I begin with specifying the conventions of the cum shot. In feature porn, ejaculation achieves its prominence under several precise conditions. Hard core does not restrict itself to a haphazard registration of more-or-less spontaneously occurring instances of male orgasmic pleasure on its sets. Three ubiquitous conventions are obvious. The first simply demands that ejaculation be visible. It is shown in the closest of possible close-ups. As the camera zooms in, the male performer withdraws from the body of his co-star, proceeds to masturbate, and ejaculates over her or his face, chest, belly, back, or buttocks.[6] Sometimes the camera will trace the trajectory of semen over the co-performer's body, as if to track its reach. Usually, another close-up of the ejaculating performer's contorted face accompanies or precedes the imagery of ejaculation.[7]

The second aspect concerns the importance of timing. Generally, the cum shot concludes the hard-core scenes. Thus, it must arrive after extended play and variation. A more-or-less obligatory kiss follows, and then the camera moves away, transfixing a detail of the scenery—for example, a window or lamp. Quite often a cut or fade terminates the scene. In sharp contrast, no female pleasure, *nor any male pleasure other than ejaculation*, is able to signal the culmination of the sexual encounter, because they lack the power to organize its narrative temporality. In this respect, two indices attest to the problematic of timing. The male performer frequently announces that he is on the brink of coming, presumably to alert his co-performers and the camera crew. Just as commonly, the transition from copulation to ejaculation is elided with a cut.[8] In that way, crew and cast may be carefully repositioned for the execution of the cum shot. If need be, moreover, a stand-in can be called in.[9]

Displacement of motivation is the third convention that regulates the cum shot. The male or female co-performers invite or coax their male partners to ejaculate outside of them. Thus visible and timed ejaculation is not so much presented as something that men desire, nor as something the camera or viewer demands, but rather as a specific, character-bound request. In effect, the co-performer's utterance prompts the appearance of ejaculation. As such, the request functions as a shunt or cog in the pornographic narrative. It performs the switch from the sexual encounter, which shows various modes of oral, genital, and anal sex in an alternation of wide-shots and close-ups, to the cum shot.

Hence, porn establishes distinguishable narrative levels. The most obvious level is that of the overall story line, progressing from title and opening shot toward the final credits. This story line frames various hard-core sequences or "numbers."[10] In turn, the level of the cum shot is embedded doubly, both in the story line and in the number, and serves as the switch between the two, concluding the latter and relegating narration back to the former. Each of these three levels presents their agents in a different way. If the story line presents characters, who are involved in a plot of sorts, then the number displays not quite characters but rather acrobatic bodies engaged in sex, and the cum shot presents neither characters nor bodies, but a body part and a bodily fluid—perhaps only rescued from an uncanny fragmentation by the image of the male face that looms over them.

Each of these discernible levels plays, so to speak, on a different stage. The transition from story to number, for instance, requires a series of marked adaptations. Often the lighting will be adjusted, since the number requires more extensive illumination than the story. If the story is set in a context that requires it to be dimly lit, say, a nightclub or a bar, then that setting will brighten up considerably as soon as the number commences. Moreover, extra-diegetic music sets in once the number initiates. While the dialogues of the story line usually offer synchronous sound, the soundtrack that accompanies the number is dubbed in postproduction.[11]

Finally, the camera will behave very differently during the sexual number. Though it largely observes basic Hollywood conventions during the story, the camera moves in from any vantage point, and gets as close to action as it possibly can during the number, selecting angles that ensure maximum visibility.[12] In turn, triggers such as the co-performer's request, the male performer's announcement of his ejaculation, or the elision-cut between the number and the moment of ejaculation prompt the careful repositioning of performers and other equipment for the cum shot.

Hard core's tiered and differentiating narrativity cannot but bear on the masculinity that the male performer embodies or enacts. The male actor and his body function in distinct capacities or roles within the genre's progressing narrativity: as a character in the story line, as a visible and acrobatic body in the sexual number, and as a set of organs and substantial traces in the cum shot. As a result, each level recounts a different modality of narrativity as well. Indeed, feature porn proceeds from act, to event, to effect.

The framing story line recounts the acts of the male character, who bears a name, and whose psychology is motivated in relation to the plot. But the number presents a sexual event that happens *to* him as much as it is caused *by* him. Finally, the cum shot displays the material and visible effect of that event in the traces of semen. At the level of the story, then, the male body operates as the carrier or vehicle for character identity, for subjectivity. At the level of the number, it functions as a flexible and plastic instance that is amenable to the image, to visuality. And, at the level of the cum shot, the male body serves as the site where affect and effect, the pleasure of ejaculation and the substantial ejaculate, are registered.[13]

All this suggests that in feature porn the male body is internally differentiated, told apart, into various modalities or aspects. In other words, hard core tells the difference, the differentiality, that inheres in masculinity. On the one hand, the cum shot can be seen as the furthest reach to the disintegration of masculine subjectivity—from coherent character to assorted images and pieces, from subject to bodily matter, and from agency to effect—and finishes the progressive slide, or drop, away from realistically motivated character action. On the other hand, the cum shot also shunts the narration back to the story level, so that its constituting elements or pieces are recuperated, redomesticated, through the character's subjective face, his name, and his agency. In that sense, the cum shot works to save male subjectivity from the pornographic lapse into a fragmented, pleasurable, amorphous, and bodily condition.

Hence, the shot can be seen to entertain the same question that, according to Serge Doubrovsky, animates the Proustian narrator's insistent scrutiny of traces of semen and ink: "how is *that* (by, from) *me?*"[14] How does *that*, the visible and material traces of semen, relate to the male subject? Hard core resolves the question by giving ejaculation a face, the countenance of the male performer as he comes. However, that does not change the fact that the cum shot visualizes ejaculation when the male character is partially suspended: first, as overruled by a functional and exhibitionist body; next, as fragmented into parts; and finally, as reduced to matter. Therefore, a potential gap or breach opens up between character and occurrence, between who does and what happens, between subject and coming, into which masculinity might well tumble.

JUSTINE: "I CAN'T BELIEVE YOU JUST CAME"

"I can't believe you just came," says Julie, the female protagonist of Paul Thomas's *Justine 2: Nothing to Hide*, with palpable disappointment and outrage, when the preceding orgasm of her male counterpart Simon fails to hit the mark.[15] The casual remark suggests a precise epistemology, performativity, and temporality of male orgasm in feature pornography. Knowing when and how to come is paramount. In Julie's eyes, "just coming" is an incredible and improbable misdemeanor.

What she specifically objects to, it seems, is the meaninglessness of her partner's ejaculation. Just coming implies merely coming; indeed, it scarcely denotes any coming at all. Hence, Simon's discharge is insignificant. *Justine*'s plot turns on the sentimental education of a male character, initially impotent within the regimented terms of the genre (he just comes), into the successful performance of the cum shot (he comes meaningfully). Thus, self-reflexively, the movie turns the construction and execution of hard core's decisive figure into an integral element of its plot line, starting off with the spectacle of the main hero's miserable failure to perform.

For, as Peter Brooks writes in *Reading for the Plot*, the suspense of narrative entails a particularly grave hazard: "the danger of short-circuit: the danger of reaching the end too quickly."[16] "It is characteristic of textual energy in narrative," Brooks continues, "that it should always be on the verge of premature discharge [*sic*], of short-circuit" (109).

Such was the blatant coincidence between the terms of male sexuality and narrativity in Brooks's critical language that Susan Winnett could effortlessly manufacture an entire description of the former from the book's pages. In the following passage from Winnett's article "Coming Unstrung: Women, Men, Narrative, and Principles of Pleasure," all quotes are appropriated from Brooks's book:

> We all know what male orgasm looks like. It is preceded by a visible "awakening, an arousal, the birth of an appetency, ambition, desire or intention." The male organ registers the intensity of this stimulation, rising to the occasion of its provocation, becoming at once the means of pleasure and culture's sign of power. This energy, "aroused into expectancy," takes its course toward "significant discharge" and shrinks into a state of quiescence (or satisfaction) that, minutes before, would have been a sign of impotence. The man must have this genital response before he can participate, which means that something in the time before intercourse must have aroused him. And his participation generally ceases with the ejaculation that signals the end of his arousal. The myth of the afterglow —so often a euphemism for sleep—seems a compensation for the finality he has reached.[17]

Winnett's description, à la Brooks, plays on the two axes of masculine sexuality that were suggested by Dyer: the visibility that runs from a "visible 'awakening'" to the ejaculation "that signals the end," and the narrative temporality, which proceeds from a trigger "in the time before" to a "finality . . . reached." These two axes should meet or cross at a specific instant to forge the significant discharge. However, that juncture is jeopardized by the specter of prematurity, of untimeliness, which turns power into impotence, the crucial distinction a matter of mere minutes.

Winnett's polemical "minutes" for the critical interval that distinguishes between meaningless prematurity and well-timed significance belittles the importance Brooks ascribes to postponement. Since the friction of narrative tension urges a pleasurable, yet untimely, and hence, meaningless, discharge, Brooks argues, the threatening release must be delayed, so that it can garner significance through a plotted course of action. In that way, Brooks continues, an incremented pleasure "can come from postponement in the knowledge that this . . . is a necessary approach to the true end" (103). Hence, immediate gratification must hold out for the approximation of a release that is truer and more meaningful.

The attribution of added meaning to the narrative discharge comes from formalization or binding. "Textual energy, all that is aroused into expectancy and possibility in a text," Brooks claims,

> can become usable by plot only when it is bound or formalized. It cannot otherwise be plotted in a course to a significant discharge, which is what the pleasure principle is charged with doing. (101)

Hence, just coming transmutates into a significant discharge due to a temporal delay, which enables the work of binding and formalization to take place, and which facilitates the eventual ending to be saturated with meaning. Mobile and libidinal energies are "bound," Brooks explains, through formal patterns of repetition.[18] This molding of energies into structured patterns is what permits "the emergency of mastery and the possibility of postponement" (101). Thus, the eventual discharge becomes charged, saturated, with meaning.

In Brooks's view, a story achieves meaning through the ordering it imposes on otherwise restless and formless energies. "Narrative demarcates, encloses, establishes, limits, orders," Brooks writes, adding that plot serves as its organizing principle, "demarcating and diagramming that which was previously undifferentiated" (4, 12). As both Winnett's perceptive parody and *Justine* indicate, gender is always already at stake in the proposed terms of such an ordering. Through the interplay of anticipation and retrospection, the ending of a story, a discharge as pleasurable as it is meaningful, must become the calibration point for the demarcation that the story as a whole performs. Leading up to that ending, the narrative trajectory in progress, in suspension, is designated by Brooks as the story's "dilatory space": "the movement, the slidings, the mistakes, and partial recognitions of the middle" (92).

It is in that dilatory space, presumably, that Simon, Julie's disappointing lover, becomes temporarily stuck. For his untimely and premature ejaculation short-circuits the flow of the narrative, preempting true meaning before it had the chance to be properly instantiated and finalized. The significance of the discharge is preempted; the story has come unstrung. So, does Simon manage to get unstuck in the remainder of the film?

Justine's opening scenes make clear that the inadequacies of Simon stem from his intense mourning over the death of his wife. When he jogs on a beach with his son Davey, the latter urges him to resume his love life. In the first hard-core sequence of the film, Simon's pathetic attempts to heed his son's advice are ironically, cruelly, parallel-edited with the son's successful efforts with his girlfriend; the same Julie, incidentally, who is to become his father's lover and educator.

The difference between father and son is underscored through their respective social positions. Simon is well-off but impotent, Davey is virile but, as a struggling musician, poor. Davey functions adequately in the sequence, ultimately producing a standard cum shot. Meanwhile, his father fails to copulate with a date due to his lack of erection. "I'm sorry, I can't," Simon explains. "It's psychic," the date offers. "It's my past," he adds. A lingering shot of his tormented face, the polar opposite of the facial shot that accompanies a successful cum shot, concludes the scene. Thus, the failed and insignificant discharge is given a face that expresses subjective frustration and disappointment.

When Davey then leaves town for a gig, Simon runs into Julie, whom he has not met before, in a sex shop where she is researching an article on the adult industry. For no apparent reason, Julie introduces herself as "Justine." They decide on a date, and in the second number of the movie, they have sex in an empty restaurant. This time around Simon is able to achieve an erection, but within moments comes inside Julie/Justine. Instantly turned off, she pushes him away and leaves, offering only "I can't believe you just came" by way of an explanation.

After a short while, Justine nevertheless contacts Simon and initiates the third number of the movie. Now, things look very different. At first she pleasures herself with the aid of a dildo, forcing Simon to do nothing but watch. They venture outside of Simon's house, where Julie chains him to a stairway. She proceeds to fellate him, and only then allows him to penetrate her. Finally, she asks, uttering the standard request ushering in the cum shot, "Do you want to come in my mouth?" A routine ejaculation shot follows, with Simon coming in her face and open mouth. "Was it worth the waiting?" she inquires. "Yes," Simon responds.

In terms of Brooks's narratology, Justine's question is redundant. For waiting decides value; postponement determines meaning. Only a controlled delay enables the requisite narrative binding to take place, and to recuperate Simon's later ejaculation from the fate of being just coming, an untrue ending. Predictably, Simon's masculinity is recovered in the process. In a later scene, the same date who was so sorely disappointed in the first scene explicitly compliments Simon on his regained manhood.

Brooks is careful not to specify what meanings are harvested at the totalizing, finalizing moment of the significant discharge or the true end, presumably because these vary considerably in different stories. His declared interest is formal rather than thematic.[19] Nevertheless, precisely because his view on narrativity is couched in terms of masculine sexuality, the object of Winnett's parody, his narratology cannot escape an excessive thematization of masculinity while remaining blind to its peculiarities. For instance, the emphasis on mastery, control, and postponement plays into the "delayed gratification" that is the hallmark of a mature, bourgeois, and virtuous virility.

As Simon's eventually successful education shows, the significant discharge of proper pornographic coming entangles worth with waiting, value with postponement, meaning with the sense of an ending, in close association with the establishment of masculinity as a form of control. In that specific sense, Brooks's narratology is indeed pornographic, or pornography is Brooksian in its narrative thrust. What is ultimately bound, demarcated, fixated, and quantified by and through the narrative at the juncture of the significant discharge is masculinity itself.

However, that dependency of masculinity on narrativity also allows for the possibility that, through narrative, masculinity may become *unbound*. For instance, the exteriorization of ejaculation in hard core, the way in which it tells and shows male orgasm as occurring outside the body, can also be taken to point to the similar way in which Brooks's narratology externalizes the significant discharge from a bodily reflex into a privileged narrative function, controlling the narrative as much as being controlled by it. Thus, the discharge of ejaculation figurates, becomes meaningful, only at some remove from the male body.

In *Justine*, it is not so much male pleasure itself that is turned into a "narratable" theme, but rather the wholly conventional representability of ejaculation in the cum shot. If Brooks is right, such a self-reflexive awareness implies a measure of recognition of the cum shot as a "divergence or deviance," something which requires narrative elaboration. Otherwise, there would be little to tell to begin with, no potential for storytelling. "For plot starts," Brooks explains, "from that moment at which [something] is stimulated into a state of narratability, into a tension, a kind of irritation, which demands narration."[20] Insofar as *Justine* thematizes the cum shot, then, it does not do so to make ejaculation its preferred figure of closure. Instead, the film seizes on its problematic and constructed nature. With *Justine*, the cum shot, the genre's significant discharge, becomes contestable, a pressing matter in need of further resolution.

THE CLIMAX OF INVOLUNTARY SPASM

The fact that *Justine* treats the cum shot as a narratable theme, as an irritant conducive to extensive and remedial plotting, may well be the logical next step in the historical development of the genre. For, as Linda Williams argues in her classic *Hard Core: Power, Pleasure, and the "Frenzy of the Visible,"* feature pornography came up with the cum shot as the paradoxical way to make *female* pleasure narratable and representable. In the wake of the problematization and politicization of sexuality in the 1970s, Williams claims, the genre turned to narrative in an attempt to come to terms with the problem of "*her* pleasure," thus articulating a long overdue "concern with the quantitative and qualitative difference of female sexuality."[21] The solution that the genre proposes turns out to be the cum shot, a figure absent in the film pornography of the years before.

According to Williams, that lasting mutation in hard core can be precisely dated. The year is 1972. The film is *Deep Throat* by director Gerald Damiano. As if the two should necessarily go together, *Deep Throat* both introduced narrativity in the genre *and* coined the cum shot as its defining figure. At its premiere, critics were quick to ridicule the film's plot, which centers on a woman unable to find gratification until she realizes that her clitoris is located in her throat, and thus best serviced by "deep throat" fellatio. But, as Williams argues, they

> missed the more important fact that the film had a plot at all, and a coherent one to boot, with the actions of characters more or less plausibly motivated. For the first time in hard-core cinematic pornography a feature-length film . . . managed to integrate a variety of sexual numbers . . . into a narrative that was shown in a legitimate theater. (99)

Marking the transition from the so-called stag movies of the 1950s and 1960s to the new genre of feature hard core still with us today, *Deep Throat* represents a landmark innovation in the genre. That becomes clear as Williams contrasts the film to the so-called stag movies that preceded it. Stags are relatively short and lack sound. No professional actors appear in them. They are illegally made and shown. There are no credits: authorship and copyright remain unclaimed.

Additionally, the films offer either a discontinuous narrative or no narrative at all. Usually, they revolve around a flimsy narrative theme, mostly voyeuristic in nature, but they do not expand or elaborate it. Stags restrict themselves to genital display, or, as Williams terms it, "monstration." Hence, stag movies present no characters, Williams argues, but bodies; no story, but fragmentation; no acts, but happenings; no closure, but "arbitrary cessation"; no ordered temporality, but "confused duration" (69).

Notably the cum shot is absent in stags; ejaculation is not shown in a particular or significant way. Instead, stag films offer a penetration or "meat" shot at their high point (72). Hence, the meat shot of stag oscillates between the attempt to signify "climax, culmination, possession," Williams writes, and the "undeniable fact that the 'scopic regime' of cinema cannot depict such climax, culmination, possession because the event of [*female*] climactic pleasure cannot be shown" (83). Attributing to the genre the masculine desire to show and know the female body and its pleasures, Williams concludes that stag, since female orgasm resists capture on celluloid, can only fail to arrive at a proper conclusion. Lacking a singular and undeniable sign, female orgasm cannot be shown adequately. Because female orgasm can be faked, it cannot securely be known, either. Thus, the progression of the stag film is forced to cease arbitrarily, somewhere in the middle, without being able to arrive at climax or closure.

However, that state of affairs became untenable, Williams continues, as societal pressure forged the narratability of female pleasure, urging "new, extended narrative treatments" (90–91). That broadening of the narratable and its subsequent fixation Williams allegorically reads in *Deep Throat*'s plot line. Initially, the film raises the problem of female pleasure in the shape of the dwelt-on inability of the female protagonist to find sexual satisfaction. Subsequently, it arrests the problem by putting forward the cum shot as the new standard of pleasure: the displaced clitoris of *Deep Throat*'s heroine facilitates the advent of visible ejaculation in her mouth and face. Hence, through obliquely considering the alterity of female pleasure, the genre settles on an extended and fixated figure of masculine sexuality, shifting in the process from stag to feature, from meat shot to cum shot, and from a deficient narrative to a completed narrative. Remarkably, this innovative calibration of narrative and the cum shot in the genre apparently also facilitated its newfound legitimacy ("a narrative that was shown in a legitimate theater").

Moreover, it is through the cum shot, Williams continues, that hard core finds what it had been seeking continuously, that is, the visual registration of pleasurable convulsions. In Williams's historical narrative, then, the imagery of ejaculation figures as the point of arrival or destiny for the male performer, for the sexual showpieces or numbers that make up the new genre of feature film, and for the quest of the genre at large:

> [W]ith the [cum] shot we appear to arrive at what the cinematic will-to-knowledge had relentlessly pursued . . . : the visual evidence of the mechanical "truth" of bodily pleasure caught in involuntary

> spasm; the ultimate and uncontrollable—ultimate *because* uncontrollable—confession of sexual pleasure in the climax of orgasm. (100–101)

However, according to Williams, that newfound visibility is internally divided. It may show the right kind of pleasure, mechanical, involuntary, spasmodic, but it does so with respect to the wrong gender. The image of ejaculation is inhabited by invisibility as much as it is by visibility. For the

> new visibility extends only to a knowledge of the hydraulics of male ejaculation, which, though certainly of interest, is a poor substitute for the knowledge of the female wonders that the genre as a whole still seeks. The gynecological sense of the speculum that penetrates the female interior here really does give way to that of a self-reflecting mirror. While undeniably spectacular, the [cum] shot is also hopelessly specular; it can only reflect back to the male gaze that purports to want knowledge of the woman's pleasure the man's own climax. (94)

Apparently, feature porn's new narrative success is forged at the cost of its visuality, replacing "female wonders" left unseen with mere male "hydraulics."

One objection to Williams's emphasis on the uncontrollability and mechanicity of the pleasure confessed in the cum shot is that it does not take into account the sense of purpose and deliberation that surrounds the performance and the precision editing of the shot. In addition, I object to the readily assumed familiarity of "man's own climax."[22] Because stag films did not display ejaculation in a specific manner, the cum shot of feature hard core can hardly be that instantly recognizable. If "we all know what male orgasm looks like," as Winnett states polemically, then that must be so precisely because of the cum shot's cultural dominance in rendering ejaculation, which, agreeably, resonates with the view of narrativity as turning on the climax of the significant discharge.

Hence, it is the cum shot that has, through narrativity, managed to *make* a specific representation of ejaculation familiar and well known. The "saming" of masculine pleasure and the "othering" of feminine pleasure, its continued mystification as a secret or wonder, are ultimately indistinguishable. Indeed, Williams's mirror only reflects back the self-sameness of ejaculation to the masculine viewer. Yet, that same reflecting specularity, when given a Lacanian twist, may usher in the alienation and exteriorization of masculine subjectivity.

Williams's historical interpretation can only proceed on the basis of a maintained set of interlinked binaries: familiarity and alterity, visibility and invisibility, masculinity and femininity. These may adequately describe the politics of the genre, its underlying ideology. But their continuance in Williams's reading also works to impede an analytic perspective moving beyond them. "[S]pectacular" yet "poor," in Williams's words, the cum shot apparently elicits a marked ambivalence, poised between visual excess and deficiency, showing both too much and too little. Moreover, Williams's terse admission that ejaculatory imagery may "certainly [be] of interest" begs the question, To whom? At the risk of stating the obvious, if the genre's criteria for representability are rendered moot, then a lot may turn out to be invisible and unfamiliar to male pleasures, and visible and familiar to female pleasures.

However, in Williams's reading, male visibility only forms an irrevocable feature of hard-core pornography insofar as it is overshadowed, and thus partially erased, by female invisibility. Such is the integral irony of the genre:

> while it is possible, in a certain limited and reductive way, to "represent" the physical pleasure of the male by showing erection and ejaculation, this maximum visibility proves elusive in the parallel confession of female sexual pleasure. (49)

Note the shift from a representation that is "limited and reductive" to "maximum visibility." Arguably, "[t]he physical pleasure of the male" is not quite the same thing as "erection and ejaculation." Partial and reductive, then, feature porn exhibits a generic and ideological preference for the visual evidence of male pleasure, for ejaculation. Thus, Williams's analysis restates the genre's own visual politics.

Consequently, Williams's interpretation does not reflect the genre's warped, biased, and thoroughly ambivalent investment in both gender and visuality. For, as Winnett argues, "patriarchy has a simultaneously blind and enlightened investment both in the forms of its pleasure and in its conscious valorization and less conscious mystification of them" ("Coming Unstrung," 507). On the one hand, straight hard-core pornography certainly participates in the ideological position that associates femininity with visibility, display, and exhibitionism. On the other hand, feature porn invests its touchstone of narrativity and visuality in the image of ejaculation, forging the display, the putting into the picture, of the male body, which is usually avoided at all cost in the culture.

As a result, Williams's argument also fails to acknowledge another stake patriarchy has in enforcing the ideology of female invisibility. Quite often the male visual presence in the genre is downplayed and glossed over, presumably lest it start to raise the specter of homosexuality. The men in heterosexual porn, a common argument goes, are negligible, ephemeral, inconsequential; somehow visually *there* and *not there* at the same time. In one gesture, it seems, the genre and its audience demand an image, to which they then turn a blind eye, professing ignorance or indifference. Paradoxically, Williams's analysis participates in the same attitude.

A typical case in point is offered by Joe Dolce, editor-in-chief of the men's magazine *Details*. Introducing an article on the adult industry's leading men in the September 1996 issue, Dolce easily owns up to the fantasy of being a male porn star. It should involve "being able to have sex with any number of beautiful, willing women and getting paid for it. Being adored. Even better, having it all immortalized on film *for other men to see*."[23] Before long, however, this visual immortalization is downplayed, as Dolce concludes that the men of straight porn are "considered [as] necessary equipment"; they serve as little more than "a tool of the trade" (44). In the article itself, "A Hard Man Is Good to Find," by Chris Heath, the stakes are raised: the men of straight porn are not so much things or instruments, mere props, but *women*. "Male porn stars are effectively substitute women, filling in the few roles women simply can't play."[24]

Ultimately, I contend, Williams's reading of the cum shot garners some of its credence from the age-old ontology that deems the image to be alluring, yet at the same time, necessarily illusory and deficient. Indeed, Williams discusses the genre's imagery of ejaculation in a chapter largely devoted to fetishism, titled "Fetishism and Hard Core: Marx, Freud, and the 'Money Shot'" (93–119). Driven by what she herself acknowledges as an iconophobic opprobrium for graven images, Marx and Freud expose the lie shaping the commodity or the eroticized accessory, pitting the "illusion of the fetish object's intrinsic value against their own greater knowledge of the social-economic or psychic conditions that construct that illusion" (104). In that vein, Williams considers porn viewing as "vicarious image-satisfaction." "We might compare the pleasure of viewing a contemporary porno film," she writes, "to the more straightforward exchange between prostitute and john, where the consumer does, at least momentarily, possess the 'goods.'"[25]

Rather than assuming the unproblematic familiarity and visibility of male pleasure, and the resulting understanding of the cum shot's imagery as vicarious and compensatory in relation to real sex and to the "wonders" of female pleasure, I view the cum shot as productive and constitutive of masculinity in its very ambivalence. I will track the possibilities for the alterity and alienation in and through the image of ejaculation in feature porn, between the happening of orgasm and subjectivity, and between material visibility and masculinity, in the remainder of this and the following two chapters. The next section continues my reading of *Justine*. For, as it transpires, neither the film nor the title character is quite done when Simon at last produces a successful cum shot.

"I WAS NOT FINISHED"

Justine offers an example that is in excess of the readings of the cum shot that Brooks and Williams allow for. Indeed, Simon's eventually reinforced control over his ejaculation and the recuperation of his virility do not form the finale, the happy ending, of the film. In fact, we are barely halfway through. Though the first part of the movie reinstates the proper cum shot as the genre's preferred figure of culmination, the second part sheds doubt on the shot's force in its continuing plot line. The simple fact that there is *more* narrative after Simon's triumph suggests that all is not said and done now that the cum shot is restored to its rightful place. The story continues, first bringing into play the theme of a female pleasure that resists and outlasts closure.

That theme is already hinted at in the beginning of the movie. Davey proposes marriage to Justine. She responds by asking him for time to think. But discord is apparent as she invites Davey to have sex in front of the windows. Feeling uncomfortable, he initially turns down the offer. Moreover, although Davey's subsequent performance comes across as satisfactory in comparison with the impotence of his father, Justine is not completely gratified when, after his cum shot, he leaves for the shower. In Davey's absence, she continues to masturbate with a dildo. "I was not finished," she explains to Davey as he returns from his shower. That same complement or coda returns even after she has initiated Simon into the proper dynamic of the cum shot. Once again, she is seen to masturbate on her own, this time in the shower with the water jet. Belatedly, Simon joins her.

More disappointment follows when Justine and Simon travel to a resort to meet up with a group of swingers. There, the fourth hard-core sequence of the film takes place, an extensive orgy scene. Justine initiates sex with two of the women; the men watch. One of the men asks Simon whether he "does [points to himself and Simon], too," but Simon gasps "no" in horror. Afterwards he expresses his doubts. Though he appreciates watching Justine having sex with other people, Simon cannot cope with his jealousy. Exasperated, Justine breaks up with him.

In the final unraveling of the plot, the three main characters come to realize the truth of the matter. Justine explains to Simon that Davey makes her feel safe and secure, while Simon makes her feel "alive." Seeing no solution, she decides to leave both men and to skip town, her unceremonious departure literalizing the elusiveness of her character and her pleasure.

Justine may well be a masculine fantasy figure, as her chosen alias indicates, conforming to the common pornogenic trope of female "insatiability." Moreover, as a journalist investigating the adult industry, and hence, cognizant of its codes and conventions, Justine serves as the epistemological authority that lays down the "law" (*ius*) for Simon, who just comes. Alternately, she might need to leave simply because a sequel, part three of the series that carries her name, lies ahead. Nevertheless, her actions repudiate and void the conclusive, exhaustive, logic of the narrative figure she initially appeared to endorse. Just coming is certainly not good enough for her, but *neither* is the proper implementation of the cum shot. Hence, *Justine* turns the generic convention of the cum shot into its own plot matter, simultaneously reendorsing and negating it.

In doing so, the film offers three perspectives on the alignment of visuality and narrativity in and through the cum shot. Pivoting on Simon's initial inability to produce the significant discharge, the first perspective supplies no image of ejaculation. Simon's orgasm is shown as a failure, triggering a theme of frustration and disappointment owing to his protracted mourning over his wife's death. In the second perspective, Simon manages to implement the cum shot, so that his masculinity and his psychic health are regained. In Brooks's vein, Simon's ultimately significant discharge brings about the culmination of this line of the narrative.

Hard-core narrativity saturates ejaculation with meaning, ascribes truth to the ending, and confers value on postponement, because that allows it to calibrate masculine power, granting the male performer leverage over his own body and those of others. The success of that endeavor is visualized to offer proof to the viewer, and narrativized to serve as the object for a relevant quest or passage. At the crossing or juncture between story and image in the cum shot, masculinity is recuperated from the troubles and challenges that were negotiated in the story's middle or dilatory space. Hence, if Simon's masculinity is initially revoked in the first perspective, then that is merely done to allow for its unequivocal reestablishment in the second one. Indeed, to the extent that pornography sticks to the sense of an ending that the cum shot affords, the genre remains singularly masculinist. As Frank Kermode suggests, there exists "a correlation between subtlety and variety in our fictions and the remoteness and doubtfulness about ends and origins."[26]

However, in the third perspective that *Justine* offers, that recuperation of manhood through the significant discharge is ultimately rendered moot. Though ejaculation is now properly timed and shown, the narrative does not culminate, but moves on, swerving to admit to other possibilities, such as feminine pleasure, homosexuality, however hesitantly, and the swinger's orgy. Thus, the cum shot cannot but become significantly less significant. The sense of an ending and the sense of masculinity are ultimately divorced from each other. Masculinity becomes unbound; it loses its visual anchorage in the image of ejaculation.

Therefore, the unfinished nature of Justine's sexuality pertains not only to her alone, to her "unfinishability" or her insatiability, but also applies to the cum shot. The shot can no longer be seen to deliver the sense of an ending to the hard-core narrative. That predicament is already attested to by the genre's tiered narrativity. For the cum shot does not form the finale of the plot line, it merely concludes the embedded sexual numbers. Hence, the significant discharge of ejaculation does not bring the whole film to a close, but finalizes each respective sexual encounter. This requires it to be repeated time and again throughout the course of each and any movie. This repetitiveness to the cum shot, I want to suggest, alludes to a perceived lack in the finalizing power of ejaculation.

In this respect, the last number of a film achieves additional significance. Not only should it manage to end that specific number, but it must also bring the framing story line to a successful closure. Yet it cannot do so. In hard core, the last cum shots are usually as routine, as conventional, as the previous ones. Apparently, then, there is little space left to expand on the established image of climax, no grande finale surpassing the routine cum shot. Instead, most features offer either an abundant orgy scene or a sexual encounter more romantic in mood than the previous ones. Hence, concluding numbers such as these attempt to arrest the narrative through a quantitative or a qualitative incrementation that arrives as the necessary supplement to the cum shot, which is thus revealed to be quantitatively and qualitatively insufficient for the narrative to cease. In the end, the cum shot cannot end; it can only repeat itself.

RETURN AND REPETITION

The flaunted instantaneity and singularity of the moment of ejaculation in feature porn is attenuated by the repetition and multiplication of cum shots in the sequence of hard-core scenes, both in each particular film and in the genre as a whole. Again and again, the genre returns to the same fixture, the same image, the same spectacle. In her characterization of the figure as offering "the visual evidence of the mechanical 'truth' of bodily pleasure," Williams alludes to a compulsive mechanicity at the core of the cum shot (100–101). In his interpretation of the shot, which I discuss at length in the next chapter, Paul Smith articulates a poignant "boredom" in response to the genre's incessant replaying of ejaculation.[27] What sense of an ending does ejaculation bring to porn, if it must be repeated at such an excruciating length?

The sense of repetitiveness of the cum shot is both signaled and countered by the request, spoken by the male or female co-performer, that immediately precedes it. Seeing the shot as the failed attempt to make an elusive female pleasure representable, Williams's reading can well explain the "genre's frequent insistence that this visual confession of a solitary male 'truth' coincides with the orgasmic bliss of the female" (101). The vocal request may also function as the way to make the cum shot narratively plausible, imparting a sense of *vraisemblance* or verisimilitude to the image of ejaculation, which would otherwise depart from the demands of realism. Without the request, visible ejaculation would appear unmotivated (at least since retraction of the penis before orgasm went out of style as a mode of birth control). With it, realism is saved: the other character likes it like that. In that way, moreover, each respective repetition of the cum shot is supplied with the incentive for its existence.

The dreary impression of repetition may be put down to hard core's lack of creativity or the assumed monotony of sexuality. Yet in an article dedicated to the works of actor-turned-director John Leslie, Joseph Slade suggests another possibility in passing. Disappointingly, Slade initially merely notes that the cum shot serves as "an inherently dramatic signal of closure," and as proof for the fact "that the sex is real."[28] But then he cites a retired porn actress, who brings up a different way of looking at the cum shot. In the actress's view, Slade writes,

> cum-shots are merely one rhythmic element in the structure of a sex scene.... In theory, ... anal intercourse ought to represent the ultimate climax, in a sort of dead-end ..., since there is no place left to stick the dick. (128)

Understood in that vein, pornographic narration seems split at its root, oscillating between a linear, climactic, and genital sequentiality, and a rhythmic and anal throbbing, which courses toward an entropy that, however flippantly, connotes death. Hence, the cum shot can be seen both as the genre's figure of climax *and* as its dead end, implicating both genitality and anality, culmination and voidance, accomplishment and entropy.

In *Reading for the Plot*, Brooks discusses three ways of thinking about repetition in narrative. In the precise manner of Brooks's own narratology, the third and last one overrules the previous two, which are nevertheless brought up in some detail. To begin, Brooks views repetition in accordance with the *fort/da* children's game as analyzed by Freud. The game involves the repetitively enacted disappearance and subsequent retrieval of a cherished object by the child. "The essential experience involved," as Brooks explains, "is the movement from a passive to an active role in regard to [the] mother's disappearance, claiming mastery in a situation to which [the child] has been compelled to submit" (98). Such a movement seems well suited to the pornographic cum shot, where the involuntary reflex of ejaculation is turned into an exercise in self-control.

Then Brooks suggests a second interpretation of recurrences in narrative. These perform the binding of otherwise mobile energies in the text, he claims. Bound by regular and returning patterns, narrative permits the postponement and ultimately well-timed occurrence of the significant discharge (101). Hence, the steady and potentially endless alternation between presence and absence, disappearance and retrieval, of the *fort/da* game makes way for the demarcation, fixation, and quantification of meaning.

Finally, Brooks's third argument is that the course toward the significant discharge in narrative is not only propelled by the Freudian pleasure principle, but also grounded in the death instinct. That latter instinct seeks to abolish the tension that pushes the plot forward, regardless of the need to calibrate meaning and pleasure together. In that sense, the repetition of the cum shot articulates a desire for the entropy, fading, or cessation of the narrative. Through iteration, meaning exhausts or voids itself in a dynamic that is recessive and regressive rather than forward-moving.

However, Brooks prevents that possibility from fully emerging. Pitting the pleasure principle and the death instinct against each other in a careful balance, the narrative approximation of the true end is recuperated:

> What operates in the text through repetition is the death instinct, the drive toward the end. Beyond and under the domination of the pleasure principle is this baseline of plot, its basic "pulsation," sensible or audible through repetitions that take us back in the text. Yet repetition also retards the pleasure principle's search for the gratification of discharge, which is another forward-moving drive of the text. We have a curious situation in which two principles of forward movement operate upon one another so as to create a retard, a dilatory space in which pleasure can come from postponement in the knowledge that this . . . is a necessary approach to the true end. (103)

Forged at the imbrication of pleasure and death, climax and pulse, meaning and entropy, the true end overcomes the two previous modes of repetition that Brooks considers: the pathetic and infantile claim to mastery through compulsive reenactment, and the death instinct's throbbing course toward fading out.

However, the intimate and intricate entanglement of those three modalities of iteration allows for the possibility that all three, to some extent, may inform porn's repetitive cum shots. Thus, the climax of the significant discharge, binding masculinity and meaning, is accompanied by the endlessly renewable and never quite established claim to mastery over the body, as well as by the entropic pulsation that wants to make subjectivity and meaning fade away. The latter two unbind what the first one binds. Shot-through with alternation and entropy, then, the linear and discrete point of climax, which the significant discharge of ejaculation brings to porn, becomes tangled and dense. Locally, the image of ejaculation becomes thick and blurry, overdetermined. Serially, the meaning of ejaculation is displaced and deferred over its numerous repetitions.

Ultimately, then, Brooks allows for the possibility of a thickening or coagulation in the narrative at exactly the joint where it seems to culminate. The forward-moving drive, search, or approach is doubled back on itself by the baseline, the retard, the momentum that "take[s] us back." Indeed, as Brooks concludes, "It may finally be in the logic of our argument that repetition speaks in the text of a return which ultimately subverts the very notion of beginning and end" (109).[29] The next chapter explores that notion of the significant discharge of ejaculation as a densely visible "return" rather than as a happy ending. Can the cum shot form the place where pornography gets stuck rather than where it culminates?

SIX

LEVERING EJACULATION

BRUCE LABRUCE AND RICK CASTRO'S campy and controversial gay porn comedy *Hustler White* offers few regular cum shots. The majority of the cum shots, which usually conclude the sexual sequences or numbers embedded in hard core's plot lines, are here all replaced by *literal* money shots; that is, by slow-motion images of dollar bills dwindling through the air and landing on bed sheets. Although these peculiar money shots are obliquely linked to the movie's theme of hustling or male prostitution, they largely arrive out of the blue. Spatially and temporally, the shots are unconnected to what happens in the various sexual encounters that precede them. If, for instance, a particular bed is part of the setting of a sexual number, then the dollars come to rest not on that bed, but on another in the literal money shot that ensues and that finishes the scene.

Moreover, no human figure appears in these money shots. One observes the fluttering descent of dollar bills on a bed, but no face, body, or hand in the frame to accompany and motivate the transaction in evidence. The shots of money that follow the various sex scenes are all virtually the same, and hence, wholly interchangeable. Utterly similar, the images come to relate to each other serially rather than to the specific junctures in the narrative at which they are presented. Additionally, the interchangeability of the shots is underscored through what makes up the images: sheets of worthless paper, which only derive their value from the conventional and iterable graphic designs imprinted on them. In a mise-en-abyme, then, the money notes reiterate the money shots of which they are part. Consequently, both the money shots and the dollar bills in them are transferable and repeatable. Finally, the paper-thin dollars make these shots come across as remarkably non-sticky and immaterial. While actual sperm would immediately cling to either skin or bed sheets, the bills of money may be easily levitated, rustling and fluttering through the air in slow motion.

Hence, *Hustler White*'s peculiar money shots form an astute interpretative comment on hard core's cum shots. Indeed, they expose the currency and value of the conventional cum shot as entirely dependent on the nonhumanness, exteriority, interchangeability, and iterability of the image of ejaculation. Because the repetitive money shots are nearly indistinguishable, they also attest to the sense of return and repetition that the cum shot in feature porn brings up. Rather than serving as felicitous climaxes or significant discharges, these money shots establish a persistent and compulsive fixture in the film. Returning time and again, they may trigger affects of interest or boredom, enchantment or annoyance, but in no case the triumph of closure.

In addition, the series of money shots in *Hustler White* work to displace the narrative that frames them. The film's main story line consists of the developing romance between the two main characters, which eventually culminates in a highly improbable happy ending. That comprehensive plot line embeds the succession of unrelated sexual encounters between other characters who set up the movie's numbers. But the ongoing chain of literal money shots is connected neither to the romance, nor to the numbers that fail to motivate and encapsulate them.

Thus, *Hustler White*'s money shots do not form the climactic juncture between story and number, but interrupt and disturb the measured alternation between the two that characterizes pornographic narration. In that sense, the shots remain untethered to the narrative. While the precise crossing or alignment of narrativity and visuality in the cum shot decides its functionality as the significant discharge (Brooks), or the homosocial instantiation of masculinity between performer and viewer (Dyer), these money shots impose an excess of visuality, which looms *over* the narrative rather than culminating it. This potential of the cum shot's imagery of ejaculation to sidetrack pornographic narrativity will be at stake in this chapter.

The chapter title, "Levering Ejaculation," condenses three different aspects of the shot. First, the fact that ejaculation organizes the genre's narrativity, delivering the sense of an ending to the number, grants the ejaculating performer leverage, the advantage or precedence, over both his own and other bodies. This leverage depends on the manual control over the lever, the knob or switch, that manipulates the narrative. Second, that same lever may start to act as a pivot or fulcrum on which the gendered ordering and differentiation that the narrative performs starts to turn, moving this way and that way, charging and discharging the meaning of ejaculation, binding and unbinding masculinity. In that sense, the repetitive motionality suggested by the levering points to the turns and returns of the cum shot in the genre.

Third, levering and leverage bring into play the working-class identity that is affixed to the men of porn and that is highly relevant for the two gay porn movies I will discuss in this chapter. This identity is relevant in two contradictory ways. As Susan Faludi's reporting on the adult business has shown, the male performers of straight hard-core porn pride themselves on their instrumental and utilitarian self-control in an industry that is dominated both by visuality and by female stars:

> [T]he men of porn cast themselves as the last workingmen of America. They are traditional men affirming traditional utility by showing that the one irrefutable proof of genetic maleness is up and running. "We're the last bastion of masculinity," [one male performer] said. "The one thing a woman cannot do is ejaculate in the face of her partner. We have that power."[1]

The power of ejaculation gives the male performers leverage, perhaps solace, over their female colleagues, who make considerably more money. However, in gay pornography, the image of blue-collar manhood is often sexualized and made desirable.[2] Both *Lunch Hour*, a movie I will discuss, and the portrayal of the male hustlers in *Hustler White* show such a sexualization of working-class virility. Thus, the leverage or power of men in the genre is levered, doubled back, to their function as objects of desire, there to be looked at. The "last bastion" of manly productivity gives way to the production of the image.[3] That image may haunt the narrative rather than participating in it. In the next section, therefore, I inquire into the (dis)alignment of narrative and visuality in hard-core porn.

PORN AS OPERA OR MUSICAL

Commonplace criticism of pornography often finds fault with the genre's tenuous integration of story and image, narrative and sexual showpiece. In fact, porn is discredited as easily for being too narrative as it is for being narratively deficient. On the one hand, "low" genres are generally understood to indulge in plot, action, and adventure. "[I]ndeed, plot [would be] that which especially characterizes popular mass-consumption literature," Peter Brooks writes, "plot is why we read *Jaws*, but not Henry James" (*Reading for the Plot*, 4).

On the other hand, the mass-consumption and "low" genre of hard-core porn is frequently disdained for its apparent lack of sophisticated plot lines. The genre's narratives, the argument goes, are threadbare, a feeble excuse to get people together in a room so that they can proceed to have sex (Williams, *Hard Core*, 99). "It is often said," Richard Dyer concedes, voicing a notion he wants to dispel, "that porn movies as a genre are characterized by their absence of narrative. The typical porn movie, hard-core anyway, is held to be an endless series of people fucking" ("Male Gay Porn," 28).

An additional critical motive judges the sexual displays of the genre, minimally narrative or unconvincingly motivated and visually overindulgent, as unrealistic, exaggerated, and farfetched. Such criticism, then, attests to a perceived unease about the interrelation between image and story in hard core. Ideally, showing and telling should be placed in a careful balance, a mutually motivating dependency. Porn, it would seem, experiences some trouble in achieving that end.

Attuned to the tension, Roberta Findlay argues that hard core is surprisingly similar to an unsuspectedly "high" genre: opera. "You have the opera story, but then everything stops when the soprano has to sing. It's the same thing in sex films. The story goes on, then it stops, then they have to screw," Findlay writes (quoted in Slade, "Flesh Need Not Be Mute," 115). In a similar vein, Linda Williams takes the Hollywood musical as porn's relevant intergenre. The song-and-dance routines in the musical, received wisdom has it, are actually all about sex. Turning the tables, Williams argues that feature hard core's numbers are all about "dance," the meticulously choreographed performance of turns and figures on a make-believe stage (*Hard Core*, 270).

However, the observed mismatch between the narrative and the visual in the genre may also be taken to fulfill an ideological burden with respect to the masculinity that operates in both. First, discrediting the narrativity of feature porn veils the fact that it is precisely and only on the basis of the narrative positionality of the cum shot as climax that ejaculation can get its accolade or privilege in the genre. Without the specific and regimented narrativity of the genre, the significant discharge and the male body that performs it would no doubt become considerably less significant.

Second, the critical disrepute heaped on hard core's hyperbolic sexual showpieces, which seem insufficiently motivated by the story line, lends more credence to the notion that the irrevocably present male bodies in the numbers are ephemeral, insubstantial, not really there. Therefore, the suspicion rises that the ostensibly sophisticated critiques of porn are not so much delivered on the grounds of formal, aesthetic, or compositional criteria, but rather signal the enduring difficulty of the genre's audience and critics in coming to terms with the hard-core visibility of the male body and ejaculation in the genre. If feature porn's visibility and narrativity, and especially their inadequate integration, are troublesome, then that must be so because of the extraordinary and explicit investment of masculinity in both. Centering on masculinity's vacillation in relation to ejaculation rather than unequivocally positing ejaculation's establishment of narrative climax and closure, the interpretation of the cum shot proposed by Paul Smith will help bring this ambivalence into focus.

VA(S)CILLATION

In his article "Vas," Paul Smith presents an alternative reading of the cum shot. Whereas Williams discusses the narration of male orgasm as the genre's figure of culmination, which should make good for an elusive female bliss, Smith's concern is with ejaculation as a visible and material event: he favors the visualization of ejaculation over the narration of orgasm. Consequently, Smith's analysis offers a different understanding of the masculinity that operates in film pornography. To him, this masculinity articulates a penchant for flight rather than arrival, for evanescence rather than closure. This view begs the question of whether the male subject is actually "present" at the moment of his own advent, his own materialization.

Deploring the dominance of the phallus in critical thought, Smith proposes an alternative notion to explore the articulation of masculinity and the male body in representation. That concept is the Latin noun *vas* (90). It means "vase," "jug," "can," in general "container."[4] The plural *vasa* refers to "plates and dishes," "household goods," "tools," "baggage," "equipment," and "outfit."

The new term avoids the reduction of sexuality to the body, Smith claims, since it does "not figure or suggest any specific organ in the way the word 'phallus' ultimately does" (90). But it does, too. *Vasa* also means "testicles," as would seem apparent from terms such as "vasectomy" and the "vas deferens" of the male genitalia, terms Smith alludes to throughout his article. Hence, Smith's argument is better taken as an attempt to supplement the account of masculinity and meaning on the basis of the image of the erect penis, with one taking the testicles as its vantage point, working to bring ejaculation to the fore. Indeed, "Vas marks the flexible and movable container," Smith writes, "where accumulations of imaginary 'substance' are built up and from which they can be lost" (100). Consequently, the condition of masculinity is "va(s)cillation" rather than stability (91).

Smith's emphasis on male substantiality seeks to counter a shift within the history of psychoanalysis. Early in his career, Smith argues, Freud predominantly concerned himself with masculine neuroses, revolving on anxieties about masturbation, contraception, venereal disease, and homosexuality. That path led him toward a substantialist theory of the male psychosexual economy, based on fluids, secretions, tensions, and discharges (92). Gradually, however, the problematic of the male body gave way to the topics of hysteria and femininity, which served to make Freud's reputation. The preceding substantialist theory of the male body was replaced with a symbolic theory of the female mind, a theory of fantasy, wishes, and repression (93). This shift Smith characterizes as a displacement, a replacement, ultimately as a loss of the male body from the emerging tenets of psychoanalysis (95).

The subsequent step, Smith continues, has been to transfix physicality and sexuality on the side of femininity altogether, in accordance with

> a veritable substantialist ideology of sexuality, where the woman's body contains substance, or "stuff." Within this substantialist ideology masculine sexuality is perceived inversely: it has been taken only as an action—or more precisely a reaction—and is nonsubstantial, being nearly an array of behavioral epiphenomena. (102)

Smith's aim, then, is to reintroduce a somatics of maleness in the analytical semiotics of the phallus in order to counter that substantialist gender ideology (102).

For that purpose, he appropriates the concept of *appareillage* from the work of Michèle Montrelay. As Smith explains, Montrelay uses the term to circumscribe the working of the male sexual imaginary. *Appareillage* condenses four meanings, some of which prefigure Smith's own *vas*. First, *appareil* means "appearance," suggesting the (dis)appearance and (de)formation of the male genitalia, their insecure and unstable posture within the field of vision, bringing to mind Lacan's play with the veil and with anamorphosis.

Second, its alternative meanings of "gear," "(military) equipment," "device," or "machine" point to the perception of the penis as a tool, apparatus, or weapon. Third, the complete noun, *appareillage*, denotes the work of "preparation" in its meaning of "making a ship or vessel ready for departure." Fourth, *appareillage* signifies the "departure" of a vehicle, suggesting notions such as take-off, launch, jumping off, and floating. The verb *appareiller* means "to cast off," "to set sail" (97).

Montrelay, Smith goes on, specifically connects the fourth meaning of *appareillage* (as "launch," "liftoff," "setting sail," or "departure") with the experience of orgasm and ejaculation. Observing in her male analysands associated feelings of loss and anxiety, Montrelay concludes that the imaginary scheme of *appareillage* serves "the function of deploying and marking out of a possible space to prevent ejaculation from leading to a destruction of the subject" (quoted in Smith, "Vas," 98–99). At the moment when the male body comes or arrives, masculine subjectivity needs to take leave from the body and seek out imaginary shelter elsewhere.

That flight is necessary, according to Montrelay and Smith, because the symbolization of subjectivity in the Oedipal phase is never complete. A residual amount of pre-Oedipal, unrepressed, and unsymbolizable material persists (97). At the moment that masculine subjectivity is threatened, that material returns into play, opening up the "abyss . . . of non-meaning" (99). In terms of Brooks, then, ejaculation threatens the possibility of the short-circuit, of the insignificant discharge, where and when the energies that sustain meaning and subjectivity become unbound.

Here, however, Smith's own interpretation moves away from that of Montrelay. The latter's view of the male imaginary of *appareillage* enables the masculine subject to flee the body once his control over it becomes tenuous. But in Smith's alternative of *vas*, the subject comes to terms with and celebrates surrender and loss. Noting that the loss inherent in ejaculation is only "a loss of subjectivity in relation to the phallus," a term too dominant in Montrelay's thinking for his comfort, Smith urges a consideration of the evanescent effect, "less [as] an aberrant or irrational moment of male sexuality and its defense, but more as something profoundly constructive" (99). Hence, Smith suggests a masculinity that oscillates between significance and insignificance, between subjectivity and its obliteration:

> Vas: that which men carry around in the real and which at the same time contains the unsymbolisable; it represents that which we consist in *and* that which we don't symbolise; that which we both carry and lose; or, to use an older vocabulary, that which we both accumulate and spend. (101)

In that way, Smith allows for an ejaculation that can be, albeit partially, devoid of meaning and privilege, a possibility that is difficult to pursue within the frames of Brooks's and Williams's readings. In Brooks's narratology, a meaningless discharge can only register as failure, as short-circuit, as significance escaping from its constitutive binding. For Williams, the cum shot *necessarily* fails in its address of feminine pleasure, but that is exactly what decides its meaning. However, Smith's *vas* seems to make way for the possibility that ejaculation may not mean much at all, or anything in particular. Or rather, Smith locates the significance of ejaculation exactly in its vacillation between meaning and nonmeaning. Arguably, the insistence of *vas* on a physical *gravitas*, on the male body as weighed down by its own baggage or stuff, troubles the quest for its *Aufhebung* to meaning. Preempting the upward movements of elevation and sublimation, Smith's new concept seems to keep the male body firmly to the ground, irreducibly material and visible.

Yet Smith's actual interpretation of the cum shot is phrased in a vocabulary that is much more suggestive of Montrelay's *appareillage* in its meaning of "floating" or "take-off" than of his own *vas*. Feature film pornography, Smith writes, continually replays and refigures a resonant "release," "*flottement*," or "launching":

> [S]o often repeating the image of cum scattered across a woman's body, [cum shots] speak to a masculinity for which the hysterical desire for somatic loss, the death of the body in an efflux of bodily substance, is a paramount element in its constitutive reality. Perhaps porn video figures in some measure an overcoming, around and on the bodies of women, of the terrible finality of the male orgasm of which Wilhelm Reich spoke. (107)[5]

Here, Smith seems to empty out the significance of the moment of orgasm due to a perceived iterability, a constant and compulsive replay, possibly compelling boredom rather than feelings of excitement or triumph (160, 107). The teleological curve of both the number and the genre that, to Williams, arrives at a cum shot that signals culmination and possession is substituted by a masculinity predicated upon flux, which emphasizes departure over arrival, evanescence over finalization. Because masculinity is not unequivocally present in ejaculation, the cum shot cannot instantiate masculine subjectivity.

Resisting a semiotic hastening to assign meaning to the image of ejaculation within a phallic economy, and countering the substantialist gender ideology that disavows male physicality, Smith's somatic reading of the cum shot, on the one hand, highlights the substantiality of the traces of sperm in the image, the "efflux of bodily substance." Because the cum shot pivots on a bodily substance, it does not correspond to the ideological view of masculinity, which decrees it to be an idealized arrangement of activity and agency, to what Smith describes as "nearly an array of behavioral epiphenomena" (102).

On the other hand, that predicament is largely compensated for because of Smith's invocation of an imaginary flight or launch. Ultimately, this shift prevents the recognition of masculinity in what is visible and material. As the masculine subject projects himself into thin air, the scattered traces of bodily matter remain stuck to the female bodies down below—not unlike a hot air balloon throwing excess luggage overboard to secure its position. Thus, masculinity comes to hover *above* the horizontal domain of both image and matter. Indeed, Smith's reading of the cum shot suggests a tableau in which woman takes on the horizontal register of image and matter, while man floats *over* the scene rather than materializing *in* it. Nevertheless, such a levitation, for Smith, does not signal the elevation and sublimation of meaning, culminating in the significant discharge of climax, but the anxious flight away from what ejaculation might bring to bear on both meaning and masculinity.

For Brooks, Dyer, and Williams, as I have indicated, the narrative ending supplied by ejaculation in the genre implicates both meaning and masculinity. For Smith, however, the repetitive imagery of ejaculation and semen in hard core articulates masculinity's flight from, or evanescence in relation to, meaning. In the first set of readings, masculinity becomes implicitly enshrined; in the second, it is partially voided. Yet in both readings ejaculation remains crucial with respect to masculinity, and in both cases the troubling materiality is left behind. With Brooks, matter is bound and formalized to yield narrative meaning. In Smith's reading, a viscous substantiality is deposited on female skin, with masculinity fearfully floating above and around it.

ABJECTION

If heterosexual porn films show images of sperm strewn over female skin, then it seems more probable that these serve as a convenient way to eject or project the substantiality of the body onto the sexual other, rather than as a way to allow for a masculine coming to terms with its own substantiality. Dumping the excess fluids in its *vasa*, a materiality necessarily excessive within the terms of an ideological masculinity, male subjectivity recuperates itself as it flees the scene, itself escaping unscathed.[6]

Not always, but often enough to be disturbing, the male performers of porn ejaculate their wads of semen in the faces of their female co-performers with apparent aggressiveness, hostility, and contempt. The "abject," a term entered into critical vocabulary by Julia Kristeva, enables further scrutiny of that feature of hard core. In *Powers of Horror: An Essay on Abjection*, Kristeva employs the term to designate the troubled relationship of the subject to its leaking and oozing body. Secretions such as feces, pus, mucus, blood, urine, sweat, and sperm may become repellent to the subject's perception, Kristeva argues, because these mess up the clarity or discreteness of the boundary between subject and object, identity and body. The abject, Kristeva writes, is something that is "[n]ot me. Not that. But not nothing, either. A 'something' that I do not recognize as a thing" (2).

The abject, Kristeva argues, returns the subject to the body, and ultimately to the body's place of origin in the disavowed maternal body, thus invoking the remembrance of the fact that subjectivity is "based merely on the inaugural *loss* that laid the foundation of its own being."[7] Hence, to Kristeva, what was once the maternal body for the subject is turned into the subject's abjection of his or her own body as soon as its contours become blurry (13). Yet the discredited and forgotten body persists through its leakage of secretions, which need to be forcefully dejected or abjected in order "to reassure a subject that is lacking its 'own and clean' [*propre*] self" (52).

In this respect, semen occupies a thoroughly ambivalent place. Kristeva lists it as one possibly abject substance among others (2, 53); but she also observes that sperm, notably unlike menstrual blood, is not considered to be "unclean" within most religious hygiene rules (71). Thus sperm may become both dirty and pure. Furthermore, Kristeva writes, it is only through and in an orgasmic *jouissance* that the abject "as such" can be experienced: "One does not know it, one does not desire it, one joys in it [*on en jouit*]" (9).

According to Kristeva, then, ejaculation and semen solicit a sense of the unclean, of the pure, and of an immanent rapture. When taken together, these three considerations suggest a dense ambivalence. Immanent and unknowable, the rapture of orgasm poses a problem for signification. When the ejaculatory abject is experienced as such, "in-joyed," it prompts the need for the renewed categorization of opposites. Consequently, the semen that is the material effect and remainder of *jouissance* is divided, split up, into an exalted substance that is good and clean, and an abjected substance that is bad and dirty.

Taken in this vein, the cum shot can be seen to perform a series of switches. The immanent enjoyment of ejaculation leads to the defensive and apprehensive abjection of the ejaculate, forked over to the sexual other who becomes burdened with it. In that way, the ejaculating masculine subject, threatened both by the immanence of "his" *jouissance*, which may be enjoyed but cannot be owned or known, and by the possibly abject effect of the viscous semen that blurs the body's outline, is reassured in his sense of an "own and clean [*propre*] self" at the cost of the abjection of the sexual partner.

This ejection or projection of the troubling substantiality for the proper establishment of masculinity onto the sexual other is what Smith's interpretation fails to recognize. As a result, his own analysis of the cum shot comes to feature in the same substantialist gender ideology that he wants to dispel. Only because it is projected onto the sexual other can the sticky substance be safely voided and avoided by the male subject. For the materially and visibly produced traces cling to the other, and not to the ejaculating performer, who can thus remain immaculate.

Following up on the dense return in the narrative (not so much culminating in the significant discharge but rather repeating itself, doubling back on itself, a possibility that Brooks ultimately admits); *Hustler White*'s literal and iterative money shots; and the hovering between enjoyment and fear that Smith sees as characteristic of masculinity's relation to ejaculation, the remainder of this chapter inquires into the cum shot in porn as a haunting or enchanting image.[8] In that sense, the cum shot poses as an excess of visuality within the narrative, obsessively turning and returning to masculinity. Each time, the shot posits Doubrovsky's question: how does *that* relate to *me?* Or, how does the seminal trace relate to masculine subjectivity? This question can be addressed through two case studies, starting with the gay hard-core film *Lunch Hour.*

STAINING THE IMAGE

Staging gay sex on an industrial work floor, the movie *Lunch Hour* makes explicit the working-class identity that is frequently affixed to the male performers in porn. To the actor quoted above by Faludi, this identity defines the men's status as the last workingmen of America, the last and irrefutable bastion of masculinity in the culture. Hence, utilitarian and manual control over ejaculation should give the men leverage over the women in straight porn. At the same time, the gay *Lunch Hour* participates in making the appearance of working-class masculinity especially desirable to the viewer, thus levering that identity the other way around, so that it becomes a spectacle, a gratifying showpiece.

Indeed, the film seizes on both those possibilities. On the one hand, *Lunch Hour* revels in the fierce differentiation between the men who ejaculate and the men who are ejaculated on, a strict demarcation that the film elaborates in terms of labor relations on the work floor. On the other hand, the movie also expands on the imagery of ejaculation, thickening, extending, and looping it. This imagery begins to loom over the sharp differentiation between characters that the story line establishes, blurring it out of focus. Insofar as *Lunch Hour*, even in its title, tells of a temporary "break" in the hierarchical relation between the workers and bosses who take part in the action, it can also be said to break the motile lever that forms the juncture between gender, power, narrative, and visuality in the genre. The film uses four strategies through which the image of ejaculation thickens or coagulates to such an extent that it comes to overbear, even prevent, the establishment of a conventional masculine subjectivity through the narrative of ejaculatory climax.

The opening scenes of *Lunch Hour* show the film's protagonist, a factory foreman named Spinelli, sleeping on a sofa with a document titled "First Quarter Production Goals" lying in his lap. A dream sequence follows, in which Spinelli finds himself on the job. He is confronted by three managers who inform him that the production goals have not been met, and that people will be fired as a result. Spinelli protests, complaining that the goals are "totally unrealistic"; the response of the bosses is to fire him on the spot.

Then, Spinelli smashes the computer that printed out the disappointing results, the high-tech symbol of managerial power; his coworkers join the revolution; together they overpower the arrogant managers and force them to dispense with their formal suits. Subsequently, the revolution takes the shape of an orgy scene that runs for most of the movie's duration. The factory men take their time to humiliate and rape their bosses, though it must be said that the latter get into their treatment rather quickly and voice only a modicum of complaint. In the reversed, yet strict, hierarchy of Spinelli's dream, the sex is continuously antagonistic and aggressive. None of the bosses is allowed to fuck a worker. After all, they do quite enough of that in real life. As one of the workers cries out, "Treat 'em like shit, like they've treated us. Put them in their place."

The reversed but fixed hierarchy of the workers' revolution, or rather, the hierarchy that is reaffirmed by its very reversal, requires that the managers be forced into passive roles, while the workers are granted sexual agency and control. The bosses are literally and figuratively put in their place at the "bottom" of the hierarchy, with the workers occupying its "top." In this way, *Lunch Hour* exposes what, in most gay and straight pornography, usually remains implicit: the socially differentiating agenda of sexual representation, which is itself made narratable and pornogenic here. Hence, the film partially plays out a socio-sexual hierarchization as germane to feature pornography, whether it takes place between the genders or, here, between men, workers and bosses.

The dream orgy, however, does not continue until the movie's finale. At last Spinelli awakes from his dream, prompted by a ringing telephone. It is Spinelli's boss, who calls to let him know that the factory's production results are up by no less than 15 percent. Terminations and pay cuts are entirely uncalled for. A relieved Spinelli celebrates the good news together with his boyfriend in the last hard-core number of the film. In sharp contrast to the preceding scenes in the dream, the sex is now romantic, consensual, and collaborative in nature. Spinelli even reciprocates fellatio, a favor he certainly did not bestow on his bosses in the dream. This resolution may form something of a convenient cop-out, but it does relieve the rigidity, antagonism, and aggression of the dream with images that present an alternative view on sexuality. As is usual for the genre, the final number attempts to resolve the conflict that propels the story line through a qualitative incrementation or additional emphasis.

However, there is another and more far-reaching way in which *Lunch Hour* counteracts the differentiating function of the narration of ejaculation in the cum shot that pertains even to the dream sequences in which the discrimination between workers and bosses is at its fiercest and most uncompromising. This thwarting or canceling mode of representation consists of the film's extension of the image of ejaculation in such a way that its specifically narrative significance as climax becomes equivocal.

The first strategy of expanding on the image of ejaculation simply entails the multiplication of cum shots. That may seem readily obvious, because a gay porn film involves more than one male performer, and more than two in its orgy scenes; hence, there will simply be more cum shots to go around. However, the mere presence of more than one cum shot per hard-core number reduces its status of being the narrative high point and end point, the significant discharge. Even in *Lunch Hour*'s lengthy dream sequence, the humiliated bosses produce ejaculation shots of their own. Another director, Kristen Bjorn, raises the stakes. His films increase the number of cum shots to such an extent that the point of their functionality as narrative climaxes becomes entirely moot. A rave review of Bjorn's *Manwatcher* in *Adult Video News* tallies up the count to a "grand total of sixty-three. That averages one every two minutes." Consequently, the singular significance of the cum shot becomes diffused by repetition and multiplication.

This multiplication of ejaculation concerns not only the number of shots, but also the viewpoints from which each ejaculation is shown. *Lunch Hour* presents cum shots that are made up from footage shot from several camera positions: from below, from above, and from the side.[9] The same ejaculation is visualized from different perspectives, further serving to fracture the supposed singularity and instantaneity of narrative climax.

Next to the multiplication of quantity and perspectives, the second strategy through which ejaculation becomes visually thickened, arresting the course of the narrative rather than precipitating it, is called *looping* in the industry. One of *Lunch Hour*'s cum shots takes no less than 44 seconds to complete: the ejaculation is first shown from below, interrupted by a facial close-up; then the same ejaculation is shown once again, now filmed from the side, also followed by a facial shot; the camera is then moved back to its original position, pretending to continue to show the ejaculation in process from below. That last shot is actually a rerun of the first one, a loop.

Another cum shot from *Lunch Hour* pulls off the same trick, and also forms an example of the third strategy that I want to highlight. In gay porn, the performers sometimes ejaculate into the camera itself, staining the lens. One performer ejaculates straight into the camera, positioned low, and blemishes the lens with semen. Another high-positioned camera registers the same ejaculation. The edited sequence then cuts back to the initial camera position, where a still-transparent camera lens is stained once more, in the same way as before. Again, the last shot is actually a loop, a rerun of the first take. Such a staining of the glass of the lens divorces the image of ejaculation from the narrative in which it is embedded. It emphasizes a viscous and enduring visuality that temporally halts the trajectory of the story rather than forming its instantaneous and discrete point of culmination. Indeed, the stains of semen on the lens turn ejaculation into something that is materially and visually compelling rather than narratively climactic.

The fourth and final strategy, the staging of self-reflexivity, *Lunch Hour* only establishes indirectly. As Dyer argues in "Idol Thoughts," the cum shot's laborious staging and editing breaks the rules of classical realism. Ejaculation is not shown as if happening in reality, but instead is presented as a self-consciously staged performance, "drawing attention to the process of video making itself" (53). For Dyer, such a self-reflexivity does not diminish the thrill that the shot offers, but adds to it. That extra excitement follows from the realization "that you are watching some people making a porn video, some performers doing it in front of a camera, and you."[10] Hence, the constructedness apparent in the cum shot enhances its effect, but does so by exposing that constructedness rather than by obfuscating it. Again, this self-reflexivity thwarts the climactic narrative of hard core. Instead of functioning as the sense of an ending that naturally and inherently follows from the sexual sequence, and that is narratively motivated by what precedes it, the cum shot becomes a separate, self-conscious, and highly staged performance.

Kristen Bjorn's *The Caracas Adventure* offers a scene that is self-reflexive to the extreme. One performer is sprawled against a car window; another sits inside the car in the driver's seat. When the former ejaculates against the windowpane, which doubles for the camera lens, the latter stares at the viscous and mottled traces of semen that slowly descend on the glass. One side of the window functions as the camera lens, the other as the produced image, the cum shot. Consequently, performer and viewer, substance and vision, flatten themselves against the transparent but impenetrable screen that connects, yet separates, the two. Here the narrative trajectory in progress does not culminate, but stops short at the imagery of semen that slowly traces the glass of the window.

In these four ways—multiplication, looping, staining, and self-reflexivity—these cum shots extend the image of ejaculation far beyond the necessity of delivering the culmination and authentication that is in accordance with the formation of masculinity. Instead, they seize on the produced, constructed, material, and visible image rather than performing the ideological reproduction of masculinity. For if ejaculation is exposed as a performance and a construction that is entirely conducive to the image, to a material visuality, then the gendered subjectivity that the execution of the cum shot should prove cannot but become less important.

Against the background of *Lunch Hour*'s dense play with ejaculatory imagery, it becomes possible to appreciate the sharp edge on which their counterparts in straight porn are poised. Heterosexual pornography must show external orgasms, since these serve as the visual foregrounding of a utilitarian and powerful masculinity, a subjectivity with leverage. However, straight hard core cannot indulge in such imagery beyond the strict narrative and visual necessity of delivering a sense of culmination and authenticity without raising the specter of the possibility that images of ejaculation and sperm might be pleasurable, entertaining, or compelling to look at in their own right.

A gay film, *Lunch Hour* does not need to observe such a critical constraint. On the one hand, the movie makes the socially differentiating function of the narration of ejaculation explicit and narratable: telling the difference between the bodies of men and women as well as the bodies of managers and workers. In the reversed hierarchy of factory politics, the workers shoot their semen in the faces of their bosses with apparent contempt.

On the other hand, the extended visual play with ejaculation starts to outweigh the story line that revolves around making these crucial distinctions. Images of ejaculation become alluring showpieces in their own right, looming over the narrative, suspending it rather than participating in it, and rendering the differentiating agenda of the story line equivocal. Indeed, the differences imposed on the narrative characters dissolve and become unfocused through the play of and with the imagery of semen. Crucially, these cum shots no longer matter much in establishing the masculine distinction of the performer, the actor. Instead, they are deliberately and self-reflexively veered toward a viewer, who may welcome them.

HAND

The pornographic formation of masculinity largely depends on the manual, instrumental, utilitarian, and quasi-technical control over the male body. Indeed, as Susie Bright remarks, "Pornographic Man" first and foremost embodies "competence."[11] The idea that the male sexual body should serve as a controllable instrument is commonplace, and already attested to by Dolce's characterization of the men of porn as the genre's "props" or "tools of the trade"; by Smith's *vasa* in its sense of "tools" or "equipment"; and by Montrelay's *appareil* in its meaning of "gear, "device," or "apparatus." These readings presume manual control over the body and its pleasures. Indeed, as Leo Bersani writes, the hand "is the subject's principal tool for manipulating the environment."[12] Apparently the male subject's body is to some extent a part of this "environment" rather than the unequivocal agency operating in it.

Habitually, the male performers back away from the body of the costar, continuing to masturbate themselves in order to be able to execute ejaculation with some measure of precision. Thus, ejaculation is shown as an exercise in manual self-control. In accordance with utilitarian masculinity, then, it is the masturbating *hand*, and not so much the penis, ejaculation, semen, or the body at large, that functions as the juncture or lever between the subject's agency, the event of ejaculation that is pushed into motion, and the material effect that is its result.

The simple fact that the male performers usually masturbate themselves to climax is easily missed, passing nearly unnoticed due to its conventionality, its practical self-evidence. Yet one immediately notices this elementary feature of the cum shot once it is lacking. Intriguingly, the gay porn director Kristen Bjorn has made hands-*off* ejaculations his trademark. In his oeuvre, virtually all the cum shots portray male orgasms as unassisted by manual control. As a result, the shots in his *Caracas Adventure*, for example, suggest more of a surrender to a paroxysmal pleasure, showing male bodies shivering and shuddering with the effects of pleasure rather than a precision control over ejaculation, if only because the trajectory of semen cannot be securely aimed in that way.

The companionship between the hand and the penis in the cum shot poses a crucial question: Does porn show hands-on ejaculations because, once visible, they require the assistance of the male performer's hand, or because porn wants or needs to portray instrumentalized and controlled ejaculations to begin with, so that these cannot but be external and visible as a result? The ideological and commonplace stress on masculinity as an instrumental performance and the deliberation and purpose surrounding the execution and editing of the cum shot strongly suggest the latter possibility.

In Aristotle's treatise, the masturbatory hand is not considered, because his approach is determined by reproduction. Nevertheless, Aristotle's close scrutiny of the visible and concrete qualities of sperm suggest that the substance he observed was in fact produced through masturbation; for in reproduction these material qualities would not be observable as such at all. Serrano's images cut the hand from the frame, so that the trajectory of semen can appear as an autonomous and quasi-celestial occurrence. Yet the "masturbation kit" from *Van Gogh's Ear*, which supplies a rubber glove, attests to the relevance of the hand in the conception of the images. In Lacan's account, the agency of the narrator's hand is both obfuscated and stressed by the veil, which is drawn and withdrawn with deliberation.

Presumably, the hand and the penis should appear in the cum shot as aligned together under the heading of a voluntary agency, which substantiates conventional masculinity. However, the fact that the body appears here as the hand and the penis can also be taken to betray an inner dehiscence. In the shot, the male body is split into, or doubled between, two of its parts.

These may well come to mirror, counter, or overrule each other. For example, does the hand confer the value of instrumentality on the penis, or does the penis turn the hand into its instrument? "In masturbation," Bersani claims, "the . . . body, more specifically the penis, disciplines the hand that would rule it" (*Homos*, 103).

Also, both the hand and the penis are internally divided between two aspects. Each can serve as an instrumental extremity or limb *and* as a sense organ, its tactile and sensitive skin registering motion, touch, friction, and warmth. The same hand that operates as the masculine trope, the lever, for instrumentality and control, ushers in a series of redoublings and exchanges that continues the fracturing of masculinity. In the final analysis, the instrumental hand cannot function as the lever between the masculine character and the event of ejaculation in pornographic narration.

Rather, masturbation stages a sensory motionality through which the distinctions between the hand and the penis, between agency and effect, and between instrumentality and tactility are rendered equivocal. Pressed and rubbed together, pressing and rubbing each other, the two become nearly indistinguishable, establishing an excitable zone of contact, friction, and exchange. That zone becomes palpable and visible once the discharged sperm flattens itself against the co-performer's skin, tracing it and clinging to it.

Instead of penetrating an opaque interiority where it could fulfill its mythopoetic and ideological destiny, saturating the body of the sexual other with its presence and transforming that body from within, the semen visibly attaches itself to skin, externally and superficially. In that way, the opalescent substance, the textured skin, and the resulting image consisting of both become material and tangible. In other words, the image becomes a *stain*. In the cum shot, image, semen, and skin are layered together, superimposed on each other. Hence they mirror and reiterate the tactile, sensory, and responsive dermatic surfaces of the hand and the penis, of the male body, that an instrumental masculinity must disavow, yet cannot but bring into play as it attempts to instrumentalize ejaculation. Thus the causal and linear narrativity of porn becomes condensed, flattened, or entangled in and through the two-dimensional and layered image of ejaculation in the cum shot.

The pornographic hand functions doubly. It serves first as the motile lever that joins the body to the narrative. Narrative supplies the causal linearity that connects the male body, the penis, the ejaculation, and the semen with one another, all manipulated and timed by the male subject's hand. Through the hand, the male body's hypothetically polymorphous or amorphous potential for pleasure and signification is wedded to the climactic, linear, and causal narrative, which arrives at closure in the cum shot. Yet that narrative calibration also allows for a metonymic slippage between the different aspects that set up the course toward the culmination of the narrative through ejaculation.

Such a metonymic association ultimately makes it difficult to decide where the male body exerts its power. The hand may instrumentalize the penis, or the body may turn the hand into its instrument, as Bersani argues. The hand aims the semen away from the male body, or that body itself becomes viscous and material because of the sticky substance that is presented as contiguous to it. The controlled ejaculation may either become the discrete point of climax or invoke a flat immanence where opposites are reinscribed and entangled with each other.

In *Hustler White*, the second film I want to discuss, the pornographic hand is rendered moot. This movie cuts not only the hand, but also the face and the body of the male performer entirely out of the frame of its literal money shots; it also has one sexual number that revolves around the literal amputation of a limb, and its ultimate appeal is to let go of all manual control. Thus, its central imperative is to let go: "*Lass es gehen.*"

"LASS ES GEHEN"

In *Hustler White*, Tony Ward stars as the male prostitute Monty. Co-director LaBruce plays the part of Jürgen Anger, a nerdy German with an anthropologic interest in the cruising and hustling around Santa Monica Boulevard, Los Angeles, an aesthetic fascination with Hollywood suicides, and above all a libidinal infatuation with Monty. The two meet at the beginning of the film; they get each other at the end, although by then Monty will be dead.

Toward the movie's conclusion, Jürgen takes Monty home. The latter unceremoniously slips on a piece of soap, hits his head, and drowns in a jacuzzi before their budding romance has a chance to be consummated. Jürgen takes Monty's corpse to the beach to ponder the transience of life and beauty there. In a reference to Visconti's *Death in Venice*, Jürgen's black hair dye starts to run. As Jürgen confesses his love to the lifeless body, Monty miraculously rises from death, and they kiss and caress. In what seems a deliberate and ironic appropriation of the Hollywood-style happy ending, the two frolic on the beach under the orange glow of the sunset. Jürgen throws in a one-handed handstand out of pure joy. As the final credits start to roll, it appears that *Hustler White*, however ironically and improbably, augments narrative closure rather than offering a new perspective on it.

But this romantic ending arrives only in the wake of a series of semi-pornographic numbers that show no routine cum shots at their conclusions, but instead offer the shots of money bills dwindling down on bed sheets in slow motion. The affair of Monty and Jürgen frames several other unlikely encounters: between a born-again country singer and an escort, a fetishist and an amputee, a boy and a transvestite mortician, a blond porn star and a gang of black men, and an aging soap star and a dominator. Playing up both a romantic tenderness and an extreme violence, these numbers scandalized audiences and reviewers alike.[13] The mortician ultimately kills the boy, the soap star is stroked with a razor blade, and the fetishist revels in the amputation of his object of desire.

Crucially, all these encounters do not end with exalted ejaculations to signal completion. Some close with a kind of suspended bliss, others simply abort halfway through. For instance, the gang rape of the blond porn star by a group of black men, a number that revels in racist imagery, suddenly halts when a pager goes off and the men frantically search through their garments to figure out whose attention is called for. When Jürgen attends the shooting of a porn scene, the performance is discontinued at first when one of the actors fails to "live up to his contractual obligations," as Jürgen puts it. Monty serves as "fluffer" on the set: his job is to bring back the failing performer's erection. While reading a book, he distractedly jerks the actor's member back to life. But as soon as the shooting resumes, the performance halts for a second time when the actors crash from the bed onto the floor. Thus, *Hustler White*'s numbers are either interrupted or aborted, while the literal money shots merely signal the financial consummation of the encounters, and the non-humanness, exteriority, interchangeability, and iterability of the cum shot, as I have argued.

The contrast between the physically and sexually clumsy performances and the repeated shots of the dollar bills is related to the two "cum shots" that *Hustler White* does deliver. They form the outer frame of the movie; outer, because the first precedes the film's proper beginning with the opening credits, and the other follows its closing with the end credits. Hence, the plot's curve or trajectory from beginning to end is densely literalized and problematized.

Hustler White opens with a scene that shows Monty floating facedown in a jacuzzi. His voice-over, explaining his untimely death, sets up a flashback to two months before, when the plane carrying Jürgen lands at the airport. Images of the descending airplane and the sounds of its engines are crosscut with images of Monty turning a trick with a client and the soundtrack of his moaning. Alternately, the shots of Monty show him masturbating on his own and being taken from behind by the client. As the plane descends closer to the ground, Monty moves closer to orgasm. The images and sounds reach a crescendo, and Monty ejaculates. His sperm sprays into the air with a faint popping sound and then travels down again. The title credit appears on the screen. Only then does the plane touch the ground. Monty's satisfied face concludes the sequence. Since this cum shot is split between showing Monty on his own and with a client, and is interrupted by Jürgen's arrival by plane, it triggers the story line that will relieve Monty's solitude with the romance that, albeit after his death, culminates on the beach.

The rolling end credits that follow that last, happy scene make way for another supplementary scene and another "cum shot." A man wearing only a pair of jeans sits in a chair. His face is not in the frame. "Let it go, man. *Lass es gehen*," an off-camera voice directs. Moaning as though he comes, the seated man urinates in his jeans. Whereas Monty's first cum shot opens up the narrative of romance, this last one is largely divorced from that narrative. As an encore, it disrupts the preceding story of a romance in retrospect. Moreover, it stresses the passivity, substantiality, and abjectivity of the male body. Hence, this supplementary "cum shot" forms the exact opposite of the conventional cum shot. The man does not perform, he lets go; the discharged substance is not semen but urine; and the substantiality of the urine is not projected onto the body of someone else, but soaks and darkens the man's pants.

In this sense, this extra "cum shot" relates back to the other encounters that did not end in the full consummation of romance or sexuality through narrativity. Instead, they zoomed in on the vulnerabilities and eccentricities of the body, of desire, and of pleasure: the porn star's difficulty in maintaining his erection, Monty's accidental slip in the jacuzzi, the amputation of a foot to the delight of the fetishist, the masochistic bliss of the aging soap star who is gently stroked with a razor blade. Thus, *Hustler White* proposes a hard-core pornography that does not center on the reified and instrumentalized agency of masculine subjectivity over the body, but puts forth the vulnerability and awkwardness of that body with pornographic effect.

Admittedly, the extreme violence of the movie makes that potential seem not only pleasurable, but also disturbing and threatening. However, the violence can also be taken to signal the sheer force that is necessary to make space for the representation of masculine pleasure beyond the ideological conventions that enshrine and anchor it. For, through and next to the violence done to male bodies, the movie articulates those bodies' potential for a sexual bliss that leaves behind the rigorously maintained image of ejaculation that hard core delivers in the cum shot. To let it go, then, is *Hustler White*'s enduring and pertinent appeal to the genre.

As a comment on hard-core pornography and the cum shot's privileged place in its universe, the film offers two equally impossible alternatives. The supplementary "cum shot" of the male figure urinating in his pants, and the sex scenes that are as clumsy as they are painful and/or pleasurable, point to a physical liability that runs from hilarious slapstick to extreme masochism. Releasing the substances of the male body forges the release, the letting go, of a conventional masculinity. The body fluids shed—blood, semen, and urine—are shown as nearly indiscriminate and contagious. Because the fluids are not projected onto the sexual other, this contagion also applies to the male body. The viscous liquids cling to the body that releases them. Hence, *Hustler White*'s elaboration of a slapstick masochism, of sexuality as physical comedy, makes way for the recognition of a masculinity that is irrevokably substantial rather than predicated on agency.

In contrast, the literal money shots cut the body entirely out of the frame. Hence, the alternative to the physical masochism and slapstick that the movie entertains is commodification: the serial production of the image that sells hard-core porn. This image, the cum shot, however, is revealed to be wholly immaterial, iterable, external, and non-human. In entering into pornographic representation, *Hustler White* seems to propose, masculinity finds itself suspended between these two options: *either* the liability of the body in its substantiality and its awkwardness *or* the commodification of the image that erases the body altogether.

Eclipsed in that stark opposition is the conventional cum shot, which can now be read as a compromise between these two extremes. The yielding of the substance of semen in ejaculation is transformed into the narrative high point that instantiates the masculinity of a voluntary and instrumental agency. Apparently this masculinity is threatened by, and may be alienated through, the two tendencies that ground it in the cum shot: the substantiality and clumsiness of the male body, of ejaculating and sperm, which remains ideologically cumbersome with respect to masculinity, on the one hand, and the endless iterability of the commodified image, which works to reiterate and displace masculinity, on the other.

Insofar as the image of ejaculation fits porn's regimented narrativity, it endures as the signal for a specifically masculine performative competence. Doubrovsky's question, How does *that* relate to *me*?, is then answered: ejaculation and semen serve as the sign of masculine leverage or precedence in the genre. But as soon as the image of ejaculation starts to turn on the narrative, haunting or arresting it, or endlessly reduplicating itself, other possibilities become palpable: masculinity as entranced or burdened by a material visibility and a bodily performativity that it cannot quite account for, either because of its irreducible substantiality as physical comedy or masochism, or because of its endless reproducibility. Hence, the image of semen becomes either an inert and arresting stain or an apparition so fleeting that it flutters away, much like the dollar bills in *Hustler White*'s money shots. In both cases, the image of ejaculation escapes from the masculine subjectivity that wants or needs to claim it as its own instantiation, as the sign that proves its reality. Doubrovsky's *that*, then, becomes the trace of masculinity's levering, its suspension, between the male body's awkwardly material physicality and the adult industry's reproduction of the image of ejaculation.

CODA: FEMALE EJACULATION

So, what about female ejaculation?[14] Under the generic heading of "squirting," some hard-core porn does indeed include imagery of female ejaculation. What is extraordinary about these scenes is the sense of exhilaration and jubilation that surrounds them, something conspicuously missing in the case of the terse, constrained, and deliberate performances of male ejaculation in the standard cum shot. In one clip, I saw a woman on a couch in the throes of a lengthy orgasm, emitting gush after gush of fluid on a series of plastic bags that were laid out on the floor in front of her, while the men and women in attendance applauded and cheered her on.

In the previous chapter, I have shown that the narrative functioning of hard core binds and disciplines male ejaculation into the climax of the number, which makes orgasm an exercise in masculine self-control. As a result, the paroxysms, substantiality, and carnality of ejaculation—in a word, its pleasure—are largely withdrawn from sight: the genre does not so much show male orgasm as a bodily pleasure, but rather as a masculine accomplishment. In this chapter, I have tried to show that imagery of ejaculation can nevertheless also vacillate in relation to the narrativity that enjoins it, so that it returns to the story line as an arresting, haunting, or enchanting image. If it is true that, as Linda Williams has famously argued, the cum shot partly serves as the surrogate stand-in for the female orgasm that cinema or video would not be able to capture, then perhaps the images of squirting women in straight porn may articulate precisely what men have lost because of ejaculation's function as a narrative and masculine trope in the genre.[15] Within the restricted but specific terms set up by Williams's reading of the genre, the surprise, wonder, and delight that accompany female ejaculation can be taken to betray how tersely and flatly, how devoid of fun, the male ejaculations in porn are shown. Hence, the images of squirting women can become the displaced reminder of the male body's awkward but pleasurable physicality that hard core is at pains to erase; they show the exhilaration of "letting go."

SEVEN

"NOW TAKE ONE OF ME AS I COME"

Pornographic Realities

IN A POIGNANT SCENE FROM Pedro Almodóvar's film *Kika*, the titular heroine and her lover Ramón retreat to the bedroom to make love. Quickly, Ramón produces a Polaroid camera to register the couple's passion. He takes pictures of Kika, who dutifully indulges her partner by overacting the throes of her pleasure, and of himself as he penetrates her. But then, handing over the camera, Ramón requests of Kika, "Now take one of *me* as I come."

Kika obliges, but Ramón remains dissatisfied. "Again, maybe you've moved," he orders. Unfazed, she replies, "Of course, you're not exactly lying still." Once more Ramón attempts to wrest a credible performance from his body, but now Kika remains unconvinced. "Oh no, that is too artificial," she judges. Ramón gives it another try, his third, but Kika is fast losing patience. "Aren't *you* coming?" he pleads. A fed-up Kika moves away from him and exits the room, leaving Ramón to mull over the series of Polaroids in bed. As Kika, both the character and the film, move on, the Polaroids, material images within the film, remain lying on the couple's bed, summarily discarded by the ongoing narrative.

This particular attempt to capture the motions of bodily pleasure in the visual medium of photography remains infelicitous, in vain. Between authenticity and artificiality, between Ramón's frantic motions and the freeze-frame of the camera shutter, and between Ramón's determination and Kika's apparent disinterest, the transitory moment is irrevocably lost, and no proper cum shot is produced. Specifically, Kika's lack of enthusiasm in the face of Ramón's efforts, so different from the jubilant attitude with which the co-performers of hard-core porn normally salute the advent of visual ejaculation, adds to the failure of the project. If this cum shot misfires, it is mainly because there is no response to motivate or to affirm it, no expression of facial delight or vocal support to enjoin it.

Ramón's utterance is characteristic for the genre of hard-core porn at large. "Now take one of *me* as I come" redirects attention away from the usual pornographic spectacles of femininity toward the visual authentication of masculine sexuality, a switch literally figured here by Ramón's handing over of the camera to Kika. Apparently, what is now desired or demanded is an image of masculine pleasure, and no longer the masquerades, wonders, or secrets of an elusive and mystified feminine bliss. Indeed, Ramón's gesture embodies the heuristic move I have been advocating in the two previous chapters.

Significantly, the discarded Polaroid images form the material remainder of an attempt to integrate and privilege ejaculation in and through narrativity. As this remainder, ejaculation becomes the instance where the story gets stuck, where it restlessly vacillates between the oppositions that should determine its meaning, rather than serving as the juncture where the movie's story line comes to a closure. Consequently, the story must embark on a new and different course. Since Kika's noted disinterest fails to motivate the produced cum shot, adding to its failure, it remains to be seen where the now-lacking motivation will eventually turn up. For the moment, the burden seems squarely reinvested in Ramón. In this way, the movie counters the conventional displacement of the motivation for the cum shot in the genre. So, why does Ramón want or need to capture an image of his own ejaculation?

From its opening scenes, *Kika* makes the shift from feminine spectacle to the visual authentication of masculine sexuality explicit. The film opens on the image of a keyhole. The camera moves in front of the lock, and through it one observes a female model who slowly undresses. This scene is accompanied by the sounds of a feverishly clicking camera shutter. Subsequently, the lock makes way for the image of a rose, its petals receding into an opaque interiority. When the rose disappears, the former scene comes back into focus. Ramón, a professional photographer, is shooting pictures of the model, whom he directs to position herself in exaggerated postures of relaxation, arrogance, pleasure, and so on. The loud clicking of his camera accelerates as the scene progresses.

Next to his professional work, it later appears, Ramón also creates artistic collages made from feminine pin-ups, tableaux of saints and starlets in stereotypical postures. That these various attempts to capture and to get to know the intricacies of feminine spectacle are intimately related both to Ramón's mother, an aging diva of the stage who excels in a melodramatic style of acting and singing, and to an implicit mortality becomes clear as the opening sequence segues to Ramón at his mother's villa, where she has just taken her own life.

The established association of femininity, visibility, and death is followed through in the next scene, situated three years later.[1] It shows Kika teaching a class of would-be cosmeticians. Her usual working practice, she explains, includes female models as well as the recently deceased. Kika's lesson triggers an anecdote she shares with her pupils, shown in flashback. After meeting Nicholas Pierce, an American writer and the lover of Ramón's mother, and hence, his stepfather, behind the scenes of a television show, Kika is requested by Nicholas to do the make-up for his stepson's corpse. To all intents and purposes, Ramón, lying rigid on a bed, appears to be dead. But just as Kika cautiously starts to apply rouge on his pallid cheeks, Ramón awakes. As it turns out, he suffers from narcolepsy and is occasionally given to catatonic, near-dead lapses. Having thus met, the two become a couple.

As a narcoleptic, Ramón is poised on the boundary of life and death. This also applies when he seems to be alive. Kika repeatedly expresses her exasperation over his emotional coldness or "deadness," his unwillingness to discuss the psychic matters in which she, an ardent pop-psychologist, revels. Ramón's not-quite-alive existence also makes him enter into the nexus of spectacle and mortality that is normally reserved for femininity. Hence, his move from the subject to the object of the photographic gaze, his handing over of the camera to Kika, and the attempt to have his ejaculation captured on photographic film all participate in Ramón's wish to reconvince himself of the fact that he is, indeed, alive, that his existence as a man is real.

Thus, *Kika* makes clear that, if the cum shot of hard core serves to deliver evidence of the fact "that the sex is real," a common notion argued, for example, by Joseph Slade, then the salient question to ask is why this mediated confirmation is necessary to begin with, and for whom ("Flesh Need Not Be Mute," 129). What is the underlying rationale for the demand for the visual authentication of male pleasure? The case of Ramón suggests a masculine need to have one's ejaculation be caught on camera in order to authenticate one's own existence as a man for oneself, a goal that can only be accredited in the eyes of someone else, a viewer. Generally and generically, similar burdens may well apply.

Having shifted gears from its opening sequence centering on femininity (the lock, the female model, the rose) to Ramón's unsuccessful cum shot, *Kika* continuously inquires into what can make masculinity real, what may realize it in the eyes of an onlooker. That investigation takes the film from the reality-TV show *The Worst of the Day*, sponsored by Le Real milk, which is obsessed with capturing footage of male-committed crimes such as murder, rape, and incest, to the debatable significance of moustaches, to the hidden and incomprehensible motivations of a male serial killer, and to the "professional" rapist and porn performer Paul Bazzo, who will eventually produce a cum shot of his own to rival and supplement Ramón's.

Through these trajectories the movie becomes an illuminating essay on the senses of reality and realness that hard-core pornography and the cum shot prepare for their audiences. To bring out these trajectories, I will compare and contrast Ramón's failed cum shot with the shot in its typical guise in porn, as well as with the second cum shot of Paul Bazzo that *Kika* delivers in course. I will also inquire into the relationship between the banal and stereotypical vagaries of the pornographic story line and the excessively staged nature of the sexual numbers, especially with respect to their contrasting but related modes of establishing realistic credibility or *vraisemblance*. In this respect, the psychological motivation for the cum shot that *Kika* discloses gains further weight. Moreover, as will become clear, *Kika* considers gendered realities in close relation to different modes of representation: the theater, the realistic novel, and the documentary. Finally, the second cum shot of *Kika*, next to Ramón's, is a way to reconceive of the realness or reality of the cum shot in the genre. In the next section, I begin by discussing the "hard core" of ejaculation in porn as the irreducibly somatic and material instance that is allegedly before or beyond representation and semiosis.

HARD CORE

The representation of ejaculation is easily seen as the pinnacle of realism, as argued by Slade, among others. The causal, temporal, and physical proximities between the cum shot and the occurrence of ejaculation seem irresistible. For if ejaculation is understood to proceed involuntarily and uncontrollably, an aspect stressed by Linda Williams, it does not hold the capacity to pretend, fake, or lie; it can only confess to its own physical truth.[2] As a piece of the real, ejaculation comes to operate at some remove from semiosis. At most, pornographic representation and narration serve as the unnecessary packaging of this irreducible bit of somatic realness. Indeed, the generic nomen "hard core" promises precisely such a kernel of unsymbolizable material—even when the putative solidity at the heart of the genre paradoxically consists of a fleeting instance and a bodily matter that is substantially fluid and unstable.

Though it conflates the "significant discharge" and the "true end," the terms of male sexuality and narrative truth, Peter Brooks's view on narrativity, discussed in chapter 5, makes clear that the true discharge requires the extensive binding of narrative in order to become intelligible as such. Both "just coming," as *Justine*'s Simon learns the hard way, and coming too determinedly, as Ramón's failed efforts show, can short-circuit the narrative machinery that is able to make something emerge as the culmination of meaning. Thus feature porn does not so much package a slice of the real that could well be real on its own, but rather puts forth an image that the genre, through its particular narration, represents as authentic.

Julia Kristeva's emphasis on the immanence of orgasm—which cannot be known or owned, only "in-joyed"—and the possible abjection of the ejaculated semen shows that the "hard core" of porn may be internally riven. At the least, the cum shot comes apart between orgasm, as a series of spasms that radiate and course through the entire body, and ejaculation, as a singular, local, externalizing, visible, and material production. The fact that the two usually, but not always, go together seems insufficient for establishing that the latter proves the reality of the former. Rather, orgasm and ejaculation, differently placed with respect to visibility, point to and suggest each other without quite being one and the same thing.

Once expulsed, furthermore, the semen vacillates between being perceived as pure and as dirty, and is dependent for its significance on whether the sperm is deployed to share in the viscous substantiality it brings to two or more participants, or whether it deposits the burden of substantiality onto the sexual other with apparent contempt. Even the rudimentary materiality of the fluid shown in the cum shot, then, does not necessarily make the semen one and the same thing.

Next to the vacillation between Ramón's determination and Kika's indifference, what is striking about the cum shot that *Kika* presents is the elaborated precariousness of ejaculatory timing, so much at odds with the secured narration of ejaculation as climax in most porn. This acknowledged precariousness, too, makes the "hard core" of porn considerably less solid and singular. In the scene, this temporal liability results both from Ramón's movements and the freeze-frame of the used Polaroid camera, and from the singular occurrence of ejaculation and its iterative displacement that results in its eventual loss. It remains unclear whether or not Ramón did in fact ejaculate, and, if so, at what try, the first, second, or third. This kind of temporal trouble is also readable in some of the possible interpretations of the cum shot I have been discussing.

Linda Williams rhetorically questions, "[D]oes feature-length hard-core pornography simply reflect the sexual activities performed in American bedrooms in the wake of the sexual revolution? Is the money-shot a realist reflection of these activities?" (*Hard Core*, 128). Yet at the same time Williams attributes a strong sense of reality to the cum shot as "the visual evidence of the mechanical 'truth' of bodily pleasure caught in involuntary spasm; the ultimate and uncontrollable—ultimate *because* uncontrollable—confession of sexual pleasure in the climax of orgasm" (101). Apparently, the noted lack of realism in porn, the genre's indifference toward or failure to reflect real-life sexual practices, does not prevent the evidentiary status of the male orgasms shown.

The realness, rather than realism, of the cum shot in Williams's reading emerges from the simultaneity between the occurrence of ejaculation and its capture on film or video. The figure presents the body as "caught," as grasped *both* by uncontrollable pleasure *and* by the camera in a single instant. But whereas the former may indeed be uncontrollable to some extent, the latter is certainly not, as the precious performance, registration, and subsequent editing of the shot shows. Hence, the putative simultaneity of the instant of the body being caught by the spasm and by the camera elides the subsequent steps taken to ensure that the cum shot looks real. Perhaps Ramón could have been saved by a savvy director and editor. The temporal differentiality that the efforts of capturing adds to the instantaneity of ejaculation is signaled in *Kika* by the loud, repetitive, and accelerating snapping of the camera shutter on the film's soundtrack. However frantic its pacing, it never succeeds in obtaining the right image.

Such a mock simultaneity also applies to the separate temporality of viewing the cum shot. In the interpretation of Richard Dyer, the shot satisfies a masculine desire for proof or literalness and enables a viewer "to see [the male performer] come (and, more often than not, probably, to come at the same time as him.)" ("Male Gay Porn," 28). This view suggests that the sense of proof or literalness is in fact only realized when and if the viewer and actor ejaculate simultaneously. Hence, the effect of realness is produced in and by the body of the spectator as it responds to the interpellation by the image.

Paul Smith gives the lie to such a temporal *approchement* in his reading when he stresses "a sensation akin to Roland Barthes's recognition that in photography the thing shown was *once* really there" as relevant for viewing cum shots ("Vas," 106; emphasis added). True, a motion picture may seem more lively than still photography, yet the temporal gap that this "once" introduces is as imperative for the cum shot in film porn. The ejaculation joined by the male viewer is long over and done with.

All this suggests that the cum shot becomes most real or authentic when and if three instances of "shooting" appear to happen simultaneously: the actor ejaculating on the set, the camera capturing this ejaculation as it happens, and the viewer coming at home. The proximity, not collapse, of these temporally different moments must appear as close to each other, as smoothly superimposed on each other, as possible. But as a relational category, dependent on the situatedness of the body with respect to scale and distance, proximity is profoundly relative: the three simultaneities that decide the realness of the shot are only approximate, merely more-or-less established. This relativity opens up the possibility of temporal and spatial gaps between what happens and what the image shows, between the occurrences of ejaculation and orgasm, and the cum shot, and between the production and the reception of the ejaculation.

Indeed, if Ramón's cum shot fails, it is because the performances of his body, of the camera wielded by Kika, of Kika as his female costar, and of Kika as viewer do not succeed in bridging the gaps between the series of oppositions at play here: between distance and closeness (as a participant in the sex she shoots as well as observes, Kika is too close to or too involved in the action), authenticity and artificiality, interest and indifference, instantaneous capture and iteration, happening and registration, and life and death. As a result, Ramón's near-death existence continues. As I will show, *Kika* offers another cum shot that takes the spatial and temporal gaps between the pleasurable event, its capture, and its reception to the extreme, stretching these out to an extraordinary extent.

No wonder, then, that hard-core porn relies heavily on additional measures to grant the status of reality to the sexuality and cum shots it presents. The genre makes considerable effort to ensure that its imagery comes across as real for its viewers; feature porn emphatically does not show "just" sex, but choreographs, stages, and frames the action on display in such a way that its reality status can be taken for granted. This alone implies that the ejaculations hard core trades in are not a priori or automatically real or authentic—not "hard." As it happens, *Kika* thematizes many of the ways in which the genre achieves its effects of reality.

MUNDANE DETAILS: REALITY-EFFECT

Overdetermined as the dimension of the subject that is bare, rudimentary, and authentic in Western culture, sexuality forms the domain where the subject is understood to be most truthful to the self and to others in confessing and living out his or her deepest desires. Hence, one would expect hard core's most persistent reality-effect to be located in the graphic display of sexual acts. Once a movie shows actual and nonsimulated sex acts, then it would follow that these hold the capacity to make that movie offer an unadulterated sense of reality to the viewer. The fact that "realist" and "pornographic" have often served as near-synonyms—the first serving as a euphemism for the latter, and the latter serving as the idealist charge leveled against the former—is a case in point here.

Umberto Eco's short essay on the genre is provocatively titled "How to Recognize a Porn Movie." Thus, Eco suggests that the identification of a film as belonging to the genre may not lie exactly in the obvious visibility of real sex, and consequently, that hard core's basic establishment of a recognizable reality has to be found elsewhere. Eco's reading focuses on the narrative bits *between* the sexual numbers that many commentators neglect or write off as being banal, minimal, or merely functional:

> Pornographic movies are full of people who climb into cars and drive for miles and miles, couples who waste incredible amounts of time signing in at hotel desks, gentlemen who spend many minutes in elevators before reaching their rooms, girls who sip various drinks and who fiddle interminably with laces and blouses before confessing to each other that they prefer Sappho to Don Juan. To put it simply, crudely, in porn movies, before you can see a healthy screw you have to put up with a documentary that could be sponsored by the Traffic Bureau.[3]

The thematic that Eco suggests (gentlemen, girls, laces and blouses) admittedly seems rather quaint with respect to the genre and somewhat at odds with the "Traffic Bureau documentary" that consists of cars and hotels. The point is that Eco considers the scenes between the numbers not as mere filler but as integral to the genre's recognizability as well as its effects.

At first he attributes to such temporizing and spatializing scenes—driving for miles and miles, wasting huge amounts of time at hotel desks, sipping a variety of drinks, endless fiddling with pieces of clothing—the function of delay for reasons of physical (for the performers) or psychological (for the viewers) economy. But then he concludes that these scenes serve to establish "a background of reality." A "pornographic movie," Eco specifies, "must present normality—essential if the transgression is to have any interest—in the way that every spectator conceives it" (207).

Hence, the seemingly redundant story scenes ground the sexual numbers they anticipate and embed in reality, or rather, in realism. This cannot but suggest that the numbers, though showing actual sex, are neither real nor realist on their own. The "transgression" that the "healthy screw," according to Eco, brings to the genre is wholly dependent on the background of normality that the story line sets up. This implies that the screw only becomes healthy, and hence no longer much of a transgression, once that level of normality is already safeguarded. Consequently, Eco's formulation also implicitly articulates the possibility that the sex can become less healthy, genuinely transgressive, only if the realism of the story line is put under strain, and not necessarily when a number includes alternative sexual acts generally taken to be more transgressive than the healthy screw.

What counts, then, is not so much the content of the sexual scenes, but the way in which these scenes are related to and framed in the normalizing background. More precisely, neither the content of the sexual numbers, nor the content of the reality of the story line that links them in a series, matters much in making either of them real or realist. What matters are the separation of and the interrelation between the two, the precise maintenance of the switch between story and number.

Furthermore, that this realism of the story is as normative as it is normal is clearly betrayed in Eco's fragment by the juxtaposition of the thematic of gentlemen and girls, and the documentary-style registration of their comings and goings. The realism of the narrative scenes also entails stereotypically recognizable characters who inhabit a world that to some extent matches the reality as most people think they know it. The fact that Eco's description suggests adultery as well as lesbianism adds to this effect of verisimilitude. The presence of well-established pornographic themes and the documentary-style registration of the mundane facts of life work together to produce the realism of the story line.

Eco's reading of porn shows some similarity to the elements of narrative that Roland Barthes, in his famous piece on "The Reality-Effect," proposes as figuring "concrete reality," namely, "casual movements, transitory attitudes, insignificant objects, redundant words."[4] Devoid of symbolic significance and narrative function, such features, Barthes argues, have often been excluded from analysis or treated as mere filler or padding (135). Yet, precisely because they lack further meaning or function, these ostensibly insignificant or redundant movements, attitudes, objects, and words manage to create the impression of a rudimentary reality in or against which the story plays out. The fact that they *seem* banal or meaningless is exactly what allows these features—Eco's cars and drives, hotels and check-ins—to produce the effect of realism.

Once this basic but elusive sense of realism is set up, the story can then trust other forms of plausibility to take hold. Mainly, Barthes points to aesthetic and doxic plausibilities, based respectively on alluring images or descriptions, and on convention and a majority-led consensus (139). Moreover, Barthes suggests, these different modalities of plausibility, redundant, visual, and ideological, work most surreptitiously and effectively when they are woven together, as in Eco's description (139). Hence, exactly the uninteresting and stereotypical banalities of pornographic storytelling serve to make the genre realist. Hard core's narratives are not so much nonrealist because they are threadbare, fickle, or vague. Rather, it is *because* they are that the genre produces its reality-effect. In this way, the genre sets the stage for the aesthetic, visual, and doxic plausibilities of the sexual numbers—one of which entails their mandatory culmination in the cum shot.

SEXUAL THEATRICS

As I have indicated, the sexual number generally breaks with the realism that the typical pornographic story line observes. Eco's cars, drives, and hotel check-in counters make way for the improbably theatrical and acrobatic renditions of sex in the numbers. Continuity montage, for example, is substituted for by the spatial and temporal gaps produced by the selection of angles that ensures maximum visibility. In due course, characters are replaced by acrobatically sexual bodies.

Indeed, many numbers, like Spinelli's revolutionary dream in *Lunch Hour*, explicitly and literally take place outside of recognized reality: they are (day)dreamed, fantasized, remembered, or hallucinated. In feature porn, one finds many of the cinematic devices used to shunt a story line from reality into nonreality, such as fades, dissolves, dreamy music, and close-ups of intensely watching or closed eyes. Just as typically, a barrage of ringing phones, alarm clocks, and similar rude awakenings pull characters back into the real life of the story.

In addition, the imperative of visibility makes many numbers and cum shots come across as excessively staged. At a minimum, the lighting and setting will be adjusted when the number commences. Several other indices point to the staging of a number and shot. For instance, when being orally pleasured, female and male performers take care to fold and keep the hair of their partner behind his or her head. Female stars sometimes, typically after the cum shot, look straight into the camera, acknowledging the viewer with a look or a smile. Specifically in gay porn, the performers sometimes ejaculate on the camera lens, staining its surface with semen. Both gay and straight porn show a marked avoidance of horizontal or missionary positions, as these would restrict camera access. Finally, the progression from the sexual sequence to the cum shot is often interrupted by a cutaway shot that concentrates on the face of the male performer.

The question, then, is how do story and number relate to each other in their establishment of reality, realness, or realism? The answer boils down to an odd chiasmus of opposite values: the story, though uninteresting or redundant, produces the necessary background of normality or reality; the number may be exciting and alluring in that it shows nonsimulated sex, but it presents that sex as fantastic and staged, hence as unreal. In *Hard Core*, Williams proposes an explanation for the genre's particularly phantasmic and staged representation of sex. Inferring the Hollywood musical as porn's relevant inter-genre, she points out a structural similarity between two genres that are seemingly further apart than any.

If the lavish production numbers of the musical are actually all about sublimated sex, then the sexual numbers of hard core may be about "dance": the meticulously choreographed performance of rhetorical figures on a make-believe stage (*Hard Core*, 270). Arguing that mass entertainment generally has an escapist or utopian function, Williams claims that both the musical and feature porn cautiously bring up sociopolitical tensions and inequalities in their narratives. *Lunch Hour*'s sexualized labor politics are a case in point, as are the adultery and female homosexuality hinted at in Eco's description. Since the scenes Eco brings up implicitly contrast monogamy and promiscuity, and heterosexuality and lesbianism, they are not as inconsequential as they may seem. Next to the representation of mundane facts of life and the use of stereotypes, then, this negotiation with thorny sociopolitical issues adds a third way in which porn's narratives become realist.

The embodied rhetoric or dance of the numbers, Williams goes on, must offer imaginative resolutions to punctuate and relieve the tension triggering the narratability of the story. Porn locates this placatory potential in specific sexual practices that, because of their intensity or abundance, should be able to resolve the tension that pushes the story forward (145). Alternatively lesbian, oral, incestuous, orgy, and anal numbers are put forth to do the job, Williams concludes. The realist preoccupations of the embedding story line, tentatively acknowledging real political and social tensions, are ultimately resolved by the "musical" numbers that deliver imaginary resolutions.

Since it is liable to the quick inflation of the effects of its imagery, the genre's privileged number now seems to be the "double penetration" of female stars. Such an inflation of rhetorically effective sexual showpieces partially explains the dissatisfaction the genre currently shows with what Williams describes as its "musical" aspect. While feature porn seems determined to increase the production values of its numbers, delivering ever more grand, sophisticated, and technically accomplished sex scenes, other subgenres that take different routes to remedy the lack of reality in the genre's numbers are proliferating.

For instance, "amateur" films show supposedly real people, not professional performers, having sex in their own homes (even though their performances seem intent on acting out the numbers of feature porn rather than replacing them with real-life sexuality). "Gonzo" porn includes the camera and its operator/director as participants in the action (although it largely maintains the separation between this alternate level of reality and the sexual numbers performed). Popular "blooper" tapes present allegedly failed performances by the cast, and "reality-TV" sex films claim to register spontaneously occurring encounters on closed sets. So-called "nasties" or "extreme" films, inimical to the "politically correct" or "pretty" sexuality that their directors decry, add the degradation and humiliation of the female stars to the pornographic menu, often centering on scenes of abuse and rape.[5]

Such supplementary realities attest to the apparently shared recognition that the usual numbers of feature porn are not sufficiently real or realist, even when the proposed alternatives seem scarcely more so. If Eco and Barthes are right, then the most effective sense of reality that the genre produces lies not in what is shown, but in how what is shown is framed.

Hence, it ultimately makes little difference whether a number is set up by a narrative of cars, hotels, and blouses (feature porn according to Eco), the porn crew's arrival in a real home (amateur), the exploits of the cameraman (gonzo), accidents on the set (blooper), television conventions (reality porn), or the spitting, slapping, and cursing of "forbidden" sexuality (extreme films or nasties). All of these different frames paradoxically serve as redundancies—if the sex is already so real, why bother?—that are required to ensure that the sexuality looks real precisely insofar as it diverges from reality. This paradoxical dynamic is nicely summed up by "extreme" producer and director Jeff Steward, who describes his films as "hard hardcore."[6]

Something similar happens for the pornographic materials now available through the Internet. In her introduction to *Porn Studies*, Linda Williams coins the term "on/scenity" to account for the insistent presence of what used to be deemed *obscene*, in its meaning of "off-stage," "in the new public/private realms" of home video, DVD, and the Internet.[7] "On/scenity marks both the controversy and scandal of the increasingly public representations of diverse forms of sexuality *and* the fact that they have become increasingly available to the public at large," she writes (3).

In his contribution to the same volume, Eric Schaefer argues that hard core's newfound "on/scenity" also allows the genre to shed the narrativity that characterizes the pornographic feature film.[8] According to Schaefer, narrative was only necessary for a time to entrain the attention of the viewer in a public theater and ward off boredom (381), to ascribe to the films the social or artistic merit that legitimized their showing in public theaters (384), and to serve as a flexible frame for including variegated sexual encounters (393). However, the new technologies of porn viewing, such as video, DVD, and the Internet, have now rendered this narrative elaboration obsolete, so that the genre could revert to what Schaefer calls "plotless ruttings" (371).

Part of the porn offered on the Internet does indeed flaunt the immediacy and realness that make it similar to gonzo's supposedly "plotless ruttings." Nevertheless, a large part of what the Internet offers consists of numbers from feature-length films that can be viewed "on demand." Some Internet porn may do away with the elaborate plot line or anecdote that characterizes fully narrative hard core. But the scenes on view by and large maintain the secondary narrativity of the sexual number, including their requisite finalization in the cum shot. Hence, it seems that the—necessarily narrativizing—cum shot of feature porn has so far survived the technological, social, and generic changes that have touched the genre since the 1970s. Still mandatory, the shot supplies each scene or clip with a mini-narrative, which culminates in ejaculation. For as long as the cum shot remains dominant in hard-core representation, the genre cannot be "plotless." Hence, the interactivity that the remote control and the computer are supposed to deliver ultimately cannot supply an alternate "sense of an ending" to the sexual number. In her contribution to *Porn Studies*, Zabet Patterson employs Slavoj Žižek's notion of "interpassivity" to indicate the digital porn viewer's restricted, embedded, and disciplined agency.[9] Consequently, the cum shot's reality-effects remain in place. The heightened reality that some Internet porn promises is merely a setup for the recalibration of the trope of ejaculation as the generic real thing.

Indeed, the stylized numbers of feature hard core do not diminish the genre's original claim to realism, because the fantastically staged sex scenes are narrated as a diversion from or a transgression of the background of reality and normality, which is established by the banalities and plausibilities of the embedding story line. The numbers are precisely realist to the extent that they do look unreal, fake, or exaggerated in relation to the story line. And this applies even more when it appears that the subgenres mentioned, including the porn that is on offer on the Internet, though introducing different types of normalizing backgrounds, still observe the visual and doxic imperative to end most, if not all, sexual encounters with the cum shot. Thus, the subgenres mentioned bring in supplementary objects, movements, and attitudes that garner reality-effects in order to continue to pass off ejaculation as the genre's "hard core," its touchstone, its preferred piece of reality.

Hence, the realism of porn does not entail the actual sex shown in the hard-core sequences, but the specific manner with which the genre separates, and alternates between, story and number, between dreary realism and theatricalized sex. The genre holds that the sociopolitical tensions and inequalities it touches on can only be resolved sexually, while at the same time it situates sexuality at some remove from real life, on a make-believe stage. The phantasmically offered resolutions cannot seep back into reality; neither can the prohibitions and problems of social existence decisively inform the staging of sexuality in the numbers, serving merely as their occasion. As a result, the aesthetic, visual, and doxic plausibilities of the genre's exposition of sex can remain in place, notably and especially the unchallenged privilege accorded to ejaculation in the cum shot.

Yet, it is precisely the maintenance of the boundary between story and number, realism and theatricality, life and sex, that *Kika* undoes when it allows Ramón's tortuous psychology to percolate not only into the sex scene but also into the cum shot. Ramón does not switch from (realist) character to (theatrical) performer once the sex begins; no, he stays "in character" throughout. Paradoxically, this makes the failed cum shot all the more realist, yet all the less real in terms of the visual politics of the genre. For now, the realness of Ramón's ejaculation cannot be conclusively proven. The simple fact that Ramón's desire for the cum shot is in fact fully psychologically motivated abducts the figure from its supposed narrative and visual inevitability, its formal necessity. One is tempted to infer that this entry of a particular and gendered psychology into the figure of the cum shot is in itself already sufficient to make it inevitably fail.

Given these psychological bearings, the cum shot according to *Kika* is no longer the requisite significant discharge or a matter of narrative and generic form; the shot is weighed down by its own content, its motivation. It forgoes the realness routinely attributed to the representation of ejaculation while simultaneously becoming more realist. This shift suggests that the usual cum shot can only become real and authentic on the condition that realism is kept at bay. This requirement, however, isolates the realization of the proof of masculinity through ejaculation, cordoning it off from the realistic male character, who is replaced by the "musical" performer who carries out the cum shot in his place. This isolation makes the latter's masculinity a theatrical and phantasmic accomplishment, neither real nor realist. For all its realness, the cum shot belongs not so much to the genre's realism but rather to the nonrealism and rhetoricalness of its "musical" aspect.

As the privileged figure in what Williams describes as an embodied and choreographed ballet, the cum shot must resolve, relieve, and bring to closure the stresses and strains triggering narratability. The rhetorical effect of the cum shot must overrule its reality; hence, it must stand apart from the reality that embeds it. Yet *Kika* allows the temporizing and spatializing correlates of the story line to stretch into, to contaminate, the performance of sex, so that the cum shot becomes dislocated from its privileged position. Indeed, *Kika*'s failed cum shot takes place in the reality of its characters' existence, and not on some make-believe stage.

In sum, Almodóvar's film takes up several conventionally gendered oppositions, in order to then displace and reverse them. At first, the narrative is marked by the conflict between feminine theatricality and masquerade, and a masculine genuineness that has little at stake in self-display; in other words, between feminine representation and masculine presence. This conflict triggers Ramón's quest to fathom feminine appearances, his photographic attempts to capture the postures of femininity, linked to the theatrical melodrama that characterizes both his mother's life and her job. But then that initial opposition is recoded as an opposition between the emotional expressivity and transparency of the female characters and Ramón's impassivity, coldness, or deadness. This opposition in turn propels Ramón's attempt to visibly authenticate his own pleasure and his existence in the eyes of Kika, who refuses the invitation. While the thrust of hard core is that visible and timed ejaculation should precisely not be motivated, or alternatively be displaced onto the co-performer, *Kika* inquires into the psychology of its existence. And once realistically motivated, the cum shot cannot but fail.

THE MEANING OF MOUSTACHES: VERISIMILITUDE

Not motivated at all, or with its motivation displaced onto the costar, the conventional cum shot becomes the privileged figure of reality in feature hard core. In itself a merely arbitrary or conventional fixture of the genre, it becomes the naturalized and necessary way to conclude the sex scenes. Hence, the cum shot can be seen as an instance of the generic verisimilitude or *vraisemblance* that Gérard Genette, in an article titled "*Vraisemblance* and Motivation," describes as an "amalgamation" of narrative probability and propriety or decorum, in a word, as ideology.[10]

Because of its general acceptance, the motivation for the shot can remain implicit or be gratuitously displaced, so that the genre comes to function, Genette continues, "as a system of natural forces and constraints, which the narrative follows as if without perceiving and, *a fortiori*, without naming" (242). Appointing a forceful *because* to make one forget the *why*, implicit vraisemblance serves, Genette writes, "to naturalize, or to realize (in the sense of: to make pass for real) fiction while dissimulating what has been 'prearranged' in it" (253). The fiction that feature hard core passes off for real is the privilege of ejaculation, and hence, of masculinity, while dissimulating its precious construction and maintenance.

Such a tacit servility to ideology Genette mainly associates with popular genres; his example here is the western (240). On the opposite extreme, he places radical, modernist, or avant-gardist works that flatly refuse or flout the platitudes of public opinion and ideology (242). But this is not what *Kika*, in its dealings with the rules of *vraisemblance*, does. For that film neither obeys the generic plausibilities of porn in its renditions of sex, nor simply refuses realism.

Instead, it forges a new rule or maxim of probability to realistically account for the cum shot: "Men need to have their ejaculations captured on film because, emotionally near-dead, they want to reconvince themselves of their being alive." The implicit motivation for the cum shot is thus replaced by a new and explicit one. What is singular, particular, material, or individual to Ramón's case does not so much corrupt the generally plausible; no, it simply sets a new rule of plausibility. This fresh rule stems from the contemporary discourse of pop-psychology, to which Kika repeatedly pledges her allegiance.

This surprising, perhaps postmodern, strategy partakes of the film's specific handling of *vraisemblance*. The probable according to *Kika* does not so much serve as the crucial but implicit means through which the movie becomes able to narrate a credible story, but rather as the subject matter of the story itself, making it steadily more and more incredible and extravagant. That is to say, probability becomes the explicit and contested stake of the narrative itself. Indeed, no matter how farfetched or contradictory, the film's characters repeatedly resort to readily available platitudes, maxims, and non sequiturs in order to make sense of each other's behaviors.

Consider the case of Nicholas Pierce, the American writer who was the lover of Ramón's late mother and hence, his stepfather. As Nicholas visits the television talk show *Reading Makes Wise* to promote his novel *I Married a Comedienne*, in which said comedienne is murdered by her husband, the show's host points out the striking similarities between the book's plot and Nicholas's own life, briefly bringing up his implication in the police investigation following his wife's suicide. Nicholas retorts by referring to the established convention of wife killings by male writers; his examples include Louis Althusser and William Burroughs.

When discussing his second novel, *A Lesbian Killer*, in a later scene, Nicholas volunteers the information that that book had been inspired by newspaper reports of murders that only had their apparent lack of motive in common. To account for the senseless serial murders by the title's character, Nicholas has phrased the following comparison: "Murder is like clipping toenails. The idea tires you at first, but once you do it, you quickly discover the result. Then you think it'll take long before you'll have to start over again. But when you least expect it, they've suddenly grown back." When his friend Andrea Caracortada reviews the manuscript, she initially compliments this analogy's realism: "Wonderful! The urge to kill could not be described any better." But then Andrea launches a critique of the passage's *vraisemblance*. "Then again, it is voiced by a woman," she argues, "and as a lesbian, I know that no woman will ever tire of any form of physical maintenance." Nicholas concedes the argument.

However, this little piece of established truth is immediately countered by Kika's lesbian maid, Juana. When Kika encourages her to remove her prominent moustache in another scene, Juana replies: "Moustaches are not the privilege of men. Men with moustaches are either fascists or faggots, or both." Kika concurs.

Thus, *Kika*'s proliferation of contradictory maxims of probability effectively disturbs the movie's *vraisemblance*. According to Andrea and Juana, both lesbians, women may either take pride in their moustaches or eschew any lack of physical maintenance. Meanwhile, the fact that the protagonist of Nicholas's book is a lesbian rather than a heterosexual killer lends credence to that story's probability, since the lesbian vampire or psychopath is a familiar trope. Yet even that received notion does not go uncontested as the narrative suspense of the film starts to turn on the question of whether either Ramón or Nicholas, similarly unforthcoming in sharing their inner emotions and motivations, is the actual and real-life serial killer whose murders are detailed in the book's pages.

Of course, the murderer turns out to be Nicholas. One should have expected as much, since no man can be bothered with clipping his toenails at regular intervals. In authoring the dubious comparison, then, Nicholas has effectively pointed the finger at himself. The simile makes sense only when spoken by a man. But the established association of Ramón and Nicholas, equally inscrutable and both suspected of the murders, also supplies the missing motivation for the latter's murders. Nicholas's killings are made probable by his referring to the newspaper reports of senseless murders that formed his inspiration, the convention of wife-killings by writers, the analogy of the growing toenails suggesting a returning and increasing necessity, and finally by Ramón's comparable psychology. If Ramón is a voyeur obsessed with capturing the postures of femininity as well as the ejaculatory proof of his own existence as a man, then Nicholas does much the same by killing women. To this pathetic and pathological pair of men, *Kika* adds a third male character: the convicted rapist and professional porn star Paul Bazzo.

BAZZO'S ESCAPE

The switches of *Kika*'s meandering and tangled narrative involve different genders as well as related modes of representation. Initially the movie follows Ramón on his quest for the truth behind alluring feminine appearances. As Ramón's mother, the melodramatic actress, Kika's job as a cosmetician, and Ramón's careful posing of the models, saints, and starlets all suggest, the master genre in which femininity makes its appearance is the theater, as it refers to the staging and enacting of gender with the help of stereotypical costumes, postures, and gestures. As a result, the reality of femininity turns out to be elusive; it can only materialize as a symbolic convention.

This first and inconclusive mission finds its counterpoint in the search for the hidden and inner motivations of the masculine characters, the psychology that drives Ramón's attempt to capture photographically his ejaculation and Nicholas's dissimulated recounting of his own murders in his novels. The enigma or mystery that the movie now tries to fathom is no longer feminine exteriority and spectacularity, but the intimate emotions that the male characters so hesitantly express and share.

In accordance with that second project, the movie also changes its guiding genre. With Nicholas's career as a writer of literary novels as the pertinent clue here, masculine character psychology is entertained in the mode of the realistic and narrative novel, which prompts the lengthy and contradictory excursions on relevant maxims of *vraisemblance*. Hence, femininity is theatrical and performative, masculinity is realistic and novelistic, the film seems to suggest. The former depends on established stereotypes and conventions; the latter claims to offer a semblance to real life. However, the second narrative line ends as inconclusively as the first one: the proliferation and preemption of rules of plausibility ultimately cannot sufficiently account for the inscrutable and disturbed behaviors of the male characters.

Hence, *Kika* changes course once more. A third line of inquiry punctures the deadlock of masculine realism and feminine theatricality. Its object is the male body itself, especially its capacity for pleasure and violence. The alternative generic model that the film now turns to is the reality-TV documentary. This shift is prepared for by the TV show *The Worst of the Day*, which presents real footage of male-committed crimes such as murder, incest, and rape; Ramón and Kika are frequent watchers.

As the couple watches an episode of the show together with Juana, Andrea Caracortada, the program's host, introduces video images shot at a religious ritual in which the participants flagellate and puncture the skin of their shoulders and backsides in honor of the Virgin Mary. Its grainy imagery, pale coloring, and shaky and uncertain camera movements show the male worshippers, masked and robed but for their exposed backs, inflicting bloody wounds on themselves and one another in a spiritual frenzy.

Andrea's voice-over recounts that the prisoner Pablo Méndez, a.k.a. Paul Bazzo, ex-legionnaire, ex-boxer, and ex-porn star, is among the worshippers. Having been granted a day off to attend the ceremony in his hometown, the felon convicted for rape and indecency has taken advantage of the situation to flee. Paul escapes the law through his participation in a ritual that ordains that his face be masked and his body be wounded and scarred. He has effectively disguised himself in his own body, a gendered body that is now not so much theatrical or realistic, but rather substantial and material.

Watching the images, Juana seems more perturbed than strictly necessary. The reason for that becomes clear when, in a later scene, Paul makes a visit to the apartment. Juana and Paul turn out to be siblings. Juana scolds her brother for his insatiable lust and his imbecility; Paul, it turns out, is retarded. Together, the siblings hatch a plot to steal the costly photographic equipment lying around the house. To conceal Juana's complicity in the theft, Paul ties her to a chair and knocks her unconscious. Free to peruse the apartment, Paul enters the bedroom where Kika lies asleep. Instantly aroused, he takes off his shirt, so that the wounds and scars on his back sustained in his escape become visible. He decides to leave and then returns to the bedroom.

Paul gazes intently at the painting that hangs above Kika's bed. It shows a female nude in a reclining posture, ornamented with pieces of fruit. His eyes travel to the nightstand next to Kika's bed, where a partially peeled orange attracts his attention, and then to Kika's sleeping body. He undresses and starts raping Kika, threatening her with the fruit knife. Unfazed, Kika engages her assailant in conversation, starting with proper introductions. "You are not doing such a good job," she judges. "They say I'm the best in the movies," Paul responds. "This is not a movie, but a real rape," Kika fires back, to then usher in her trusted discourse of pop-psychology, "I think you have a lot of problems. Paul, stop this and tell me about your problems." Paul declines the invitation.

The viewer witnesses part of this rape scene as focalized by an anonymous voyeur, who inhabits the house across the street and who observes Kika's bedroom through a telescope. His line of vision is frequently and regularly interrupted by a block and tackle that moves up and down against the apartment building's façade, carrying furniture and groceries. The voyeur calls the police. Meanwhile, Juana has regained consciousness and barges into the bedroom. "It's Paul Bazzo, the escaped porn star," Kika informs her. "Aha, a professional!" she responds. As she tries to remove Paul from her mistress, she is joined by two policemen who arrive at the scene. But, having come only twice, Paul perseveres in order to reach his third ejaculation.

Paul's third and last orgasm coincides with his escape. He jumps on the balcony and continues to masturbate. The balcony, windowsills, and curtains behind him frame his posture as if on a theatrical stage. Eventually, drops of his sperm travel several stories downward, following the trajectory of the tackle rope. Below waits the face of Andrea Caracortada, the host of *The Worst of the Day*, apparently tipped off as to the whereabouts of the escapee. In slow motion, Bazzo's sperm lands on her face.[11] However, the event fails to present her with adequate footage for her TV show, since her camera, mounted on a helmet on top of her head, is positioned too close to capture the moment. Paul then makes his getaway with the help of the tackle rope. Andrea is quick to propose an exclusive interview, but Paul steals her motorcycle and flees.

Flatly refusing Kika's attempt to psychologize his behavior, Paul is not touched by the *vraisemblance* that burdens Ramón and Nicholas. Apparently, the generic rules of the realistic novel do not apply to him. Both an imbecile and a professional porn star, Paul is neither a fully fledged character nor a proper masculine subject. He stands at some remove from the reality that the other male characters inhabit; that is why he is able to escape their world.

This marginal position is specified by his inability to differentiate between representation and presence. Paul's rape of Kika is prompted by what can be described as an iconic way of looking, conflating the reclining nude on the painting, connoting passivity and availability, with Kika lying fast asleep on the bed on the ground of the partial similarity between the two.[12] Furthermore, he is also unable to distinguish between his performances on the porn set and the rape that he is committing. *Mutatis mutandis*, this inability to separate performance from action, representation from real life, must also bear on the cum shot that he produces. Conflating the cum shot and reality, the scene suggests, is a retarded way of looking at the figure.

In the second and bizarre cum shot that *Kika* presents, two visual apparati are juxtaposed. Whereas Ramón attempts to capture his own ejaculation with the help of the photographic camera, this scene has a telescope as well as a television camera. However, just like Ramón's Polaroid camera, both these instruments fail to grasp Paul's cum shot. Andrea's helmet camera is too close to the action. Surprised by Paul's semen, Andrea fails to direct and zoom her camera in time to capture the cum shot. Across the street, the voyeur's telescope suffers the same fate by being too far off. Neither of these devices succeeds in registering the piece of reality offered up to them; the movie supplies no focalized imagery of Paul's ejaculation through either the television camera or the telescope.

Nevertheless, the viewer does see Paul's ejaculation. It takes place in a way that suggests a particularly staged performance. The balcony, windowsills, and curtains that form the backdrop of this cum shot transport Paul's body into the theater, onstage. Hence, both the reality-construction of the realistic novel and the documentary-style registration of reality by the visual apparati fail, while the theater succeeds in finally rendering the sought-after ejaculation. Previously associated with the exteriority and spectacularity of feminine appearances, *Kika* ultimately re-renders masculinity as theatrical, as a symbolic and conventional performance, akin to femininity. Hence, the reality of masculinity, specifically of ejaculation, cannot be realistically and narratively accounted for, and neither can it be just grasped by a camera or other visual device; it can only be staged.

That, in fact, was Ramón's earlier mistake: placing too much trust in the camera to capture his living reality. The contrast between the two ejaculating men, Ramón and Paul, is underscored when it appears that Ramón is in fact the anonymous voyeur, spying on his wife with the telescope from across the street. What he ironically ends up witnessing is the adequate performance of visible ejaculation, exactly the thing he himself failed to produce earlier. Thus, when ejaculation takes place in relation to a realistically motivated character, the cum shot fails; when it is performed as divorced from realism and self-consciously staged, it succeeds. Paul, the imbecile but professional porn star, jumps onstage to temporally replace Ramón, compensating for the cum shot that the latter can neither produce nor capture, and in the process reduces Ramón to its spectator rather than its performer.

Thus these two characters in *Kika* concretely take up the two masculine positions in the cum shot: the character of the story line and the physical performer of the shot, respectively. The incommensurability between the two is literalized in *Kika* through the two characters exactly pinpointing the deficit of reality in the genre. Ramón lacks the ability to execute ejaculation in the requisite manner so that it can serve as the mandated proof of reality and masculinity; Paul, as an imbecile, lacks the relevant psychology that should work to make it realistic. This contrast implies that the conventional cum shot of the genre functions precisely as the quasi-musical figure or embodied rhetoric that should ultimately resolve the glaring contradiction between these two separate masculine realities, between the acting character and the performing body, between masculinity as realism and masculinity as theater.

Unlike the genre of film, theater requires that the bodies of the actors be physically present in the same space as the viewer. In accordance with that aspect of the stage, Paul's body is initially introduced in an indexical manner, dependent on a close contiguity between the sign and its object; this is specified by the grainy, pale, and shaky documentary footage in which he makes his first appearance, and by the scars emphasized on his body just before the rape scene. Yet the ejaculation that he produces is not captured by either Ramón's telescope or Andrea's television camera.

Hence, there is no established simultaneity between the occurrence of ejaculation and its registered image: Paul's pleasure is not "caught" in Williams's sense. Neither is there any simultaneity between the production and the reception of the ejaculation, as the drops of sperm travel several stories downward in slow motion before they hit Andrea's face. As indexes, then, the ejaculation and the semen are stretched out, spatialized and temporized, to an extraordinary measure—to such an extent, in fact, that there is sufficient space and time for the ejaculation to entertain three different views: the telescopic and the televisual look, both equally infelicitous, and both framed in the theatrical look of the viewer, which works. Indeed, the interval between the production and the qualified reception of the ejaculation gives Paul sufficient opportunity to escape the law once again.

Paul's bodily indexicality is ultimately reframed in the symbolic theatricality that was previously associated with the feminine characters. Ejaculation thus becomes a symbol based on little more than convention. The iterability that this implies is highlighted by the triple repetition of orgasm in the scene, and by Paul's apparent "citation" of the figure from his previous experiences as a professional porn star. *Kika* does show a "real," in the sense of indexically proximate, ejaculation. Yet it can only become intelligible by its reliance on a symbolic convention, through reiterating and citing a generically established figure. Paul jumps onstage to physically quote the cum shot as he ejaculates for the third time.

As a film burdened with the residue of iconic realism that also marks the novel, *Kika* takes up the privileged figure of reality from the genre of hardcore porn to displace and criticize it. With the verisimilitude of realistic narrative rendered moot, the movie first links ejaculation to the indexical documentary that suggests its heightened reality, and then ultimately reframes it as symbolic theater, the least real of the modes of representation considered. Semiotically, then, the cum shot as theatrical symbol overrules its status as realist icon and as real, contiguous index. Indeed, the latter two are problematized and reconceived in terms of the former. To perform and to see the cum shot as unquestionably real, then, is a feat only an idiot like Paul can get away with.

PART FOUR

THEORY

EIGHT

THE SUSPENSE AND SUSPENSION OF BLISS

Barthes

IN THE PREVIOUS THREE CHAPTERS, I have attended to the imagery of ejaculation that hard-core feature pornography presents; in the next chapters, I will discuss three theoretical concepts that are highly and densely informed by considerations of orgasm, ejaculation, and semen. Roland Barthes's *bliss* [*jouissance*], Jacques Derrida's *dissemination* [*dissemination*], and Georges Bataille's *expenditure* [*dépense*], all three staples of contemporary theory, become intelligible anew and in surprising ways when read as notions that bear concretely on masculine sexuality at least as much as they do on signification. Indeed, in continuously reconsidering signification in terms of ejaculation and semen, these three concepts cannot but problematize masculinity and the male body in the process. Thus bliss, dissemination, and expenditure all stage the question of how the male body and its pleasures may relate to significance and signification.

Though these male authors are often headed together under the generic title of poststructuralism, my aim is not to trace the historical development of the notion of ejaculation in their works, with Bataille serving as poststructuralism's *avant la lettre* existence or pre-history, Barthes as the hinge between structuralism and poststructuralism, and Derrida as the latter's full realization. Instead, I take each concept separately as an invitation to (re)think ejaculation in relation to the male body and to masculinity. As I will show, bliss, dissemination, and expenditure envision different (but conceptually related) accounts of how ejaculation might matter to signification and masculinity. Although I thus stage a contemporary and anachronistic dialogue among the three authors, whose texts are now equally and simultaneously available for analytical usage, this discussion does not imply the erasure of historicity and temporality altogether.

For the concepts coined by the three thinkers all react against historical, patriarchal tradition while taking up one of its privileged terms: the supposedly "seminal" aspect of relevance and meaning, the imagination that treats ejaculation and sperm—in a mixture of speaking literally and figuratively, the precise balance of which is ever difficult to ascertain—as the privileged tropes for an account of signification. Furthermore, the three concepts also allude to temporalities *other* than the linear and teleological development toward full realization, completion, or totalization that ejaculation as climax so easily accommodates. Such alternative temporalities include breaks, ruptures, and gaps; stoppages, intermittences, and entropy; thrusts, blows, and triggerings; a multifaceted fracturing; and a convulsive, iterative motionality adequately comparable to "hiccups." Hence, ejaculation and orgasm are not so much entertained as the discrete high points and end points of making meaning and making masculinity, but rather as the dense instances that prevent or convolute both.

Co-opting the voyeuristic pleasure of the aesthete and the connoisseur, Barthes makes way for another pleasure that suspends masculine individuality rather than enshrining it. The monumental *semina aeternitatis* of classical thinking are cannily replaced by unpredictably motile "seeds" that wander through the text, and that can be traced by an embodied, sensorially vulnerable, and ecstatic reader. Derrida comments on the ideal of autoinsemination, homoinsemination, or reinsemination of the "good son" by the father-teacher as crucial for Platonic philosophy and pedagogy, and disrupts that Platonism's economy through a disseminative diaspora that makes the cherished seed always-already lost. What Derrida terms the seminal nostalgia, *logos spermatikos*, and mythological panspermism of philosophy must be undone by deconstructive readings attuned to the "de-seeding" and dispersion of meaning and semen, he argues. Bataille, indebted to Hegel, is ever haunted by the hierarchies between the high and the low, semen and urine, spirit and matter, and concept and image, that he wants to turn on their heads, while simultaneously championing the masculine glory to be reaped from intense intermale rivalries, including the one between himself and Hegel.

Neither should these chapters be understood to take away anything from ongoing attempts to revisage the nexus of meaning and gender, signification and corporeality, with the help of alternative tropes and concepts that are either non-male or, perhaps even more critically, non-sexual. Though I admit that inquiring into ejaculation and semen runs the serious risk of merely continuing or reiterating their privilege in patriarchy, I am convinced that treading the fine line between tradition and critique that the notions afford can be highly productive, for both understanding and criticizing masculinity's fraught relation to ejaculation and semen. That fine line, moreover, remains to be followed through to its ultimate consequences.

True, replacing the phallus for ejaculation as an organizing principle, heuristic searchlight, or reading guide in itself does not change the maleness of the discourse. However, replacing the phallus with ejaculation may also imply the former term's displacement. Though the ejaculation of semen is undeniably male, it does not automatically follow that it is also unproblematically masculine, or that the masculinities conceived through ejaculation will necessarily always assume the same conventional shape. In this first chapter in the series on available concepts of ejaculation, I start with Roland Barthes's specific understanding of what he terms "bliss" [*jouissance*].[1]

CONNOISSEUR

According to some, the later Barthes should be seen as the exemplary connoisseur or man of taste. With equal conviction, Barthes is either reproached or complimented for the refined aesthetic sensibility and world-weary knowingness that characterizes his later work by authors such as Terry Eagleton, Frank Lentricchia, and Susan Sontag. In his *Literary Theory*, for example, Eagleton casts Barthes in the role of the hedonist who "luxuriates in the tantalizing glide of signs," the reader who delights "in the textures of the words," the intellectual who savors "the sumptuousness of the signifier."[2]

In a similar vein, Lentricchia argues in *After the New Criticism* that Barthes would enact the "ultimate gearing-up of the Kantian engine." "As a seeker of pleasure in isolation from social, cognitive, and ethical dimensions of selfhood," Lentricchia goes on, "[Barthes] reaffirms the fragmented personality upon which Kant erected his aesthetic system, while turning his back upon those ideologies in force which produce that fragmentation."[3] In a marked contrast, Sontag paints a favorable picture of Barthes as dandy, arbiter of the senses, man of elegance, taste, and pleasure, in her introduction to the anthology *A Barthes Reader*.

Barthes himself appears to have acted as the prompter or ventriloquist of the terms of his own critique or recuperation. In *The Pleasure of the Text*, he comments on the "entire minor mythology" decreeing that pleasure should be a "rightist notion," whereas all "knowledge, method, commitment, combat" would naturally belong to the Left. "On both sides," he notices "this peculiar idea that pleasure is *simple*, which is why it is championed or disdained."[4] For Barthes, one is to understand, pleasure is complicated, possibly complicating. Throughout the essay, Barthes continues his opposition to the disqualification of pleasure. For example, he complains that our culture is marked by two modalities, the one of platitude, the other of political or scientific rigor, both of which work equally well in obviating pleasure (46). Or, he gleefully foresees the reactions of two policemen who will rush to apprehend pleasure in the name of politics or psychoanalysis: "futility and/or guilt, pleasure is either idle or vain, a class notion or an illusion" (57).

Additionally, Barthes's diverse characterizations of pleasure admit, even tentatively endorse, poignant experiences of distress and anxiety to such an extent that these can hardly be written off either as mere masochistic intensifications of pleasure, or as the obligatory protestations of the guilty conscience of the bourgeois pleasure-seeker. In Barthes's eyes, pleasure does not necessarily imply having any fun. Barthes traces a sensory potential in the workings of readerly luxuriating, delighting, and savoring that does not anchor the subject. If that is true, then Barthesian pleasures cannot but have some bearing on the social, cognitive, and ethical dimensions of selfhood on which Lentricchia sees Barthes turning his back. Pleasure matters to politics.

Certainly, Barthes does write that the pleasurable text "is (should be) that uninhibited person who shows his behind to the *Political Father*" (53). However, obviously, showing one's behind to someone is not quite the same thing as turning one's back. Moreover, as it juxtaposes Father and behind, phallus and ass, high and low, Barthes's interrogation of pleasure specifically targets masculine and, hence, hierarchized figurations of gratification. If pleasure can be circumscribed as showing one's behind to the Father, then it is at the least not to be enjoyed in any shape *like* or *with* the Father. Unwilling to consider the ways in which pleasures are socioculturally (en)gendered, Lentricchia himself, rather than Barthes, reaffirms the Kantian fragmentation he decries.

Barthes's pursuit of a possibly subversive aptitude within sensory and bodily experiences does remain wedded to gratifications of a conventional kind: to petty, sexist, elitist, bourgeois, aestheticist, sadistic, and voyeuristic indulgences. For instance, the essay's language of erotic and sensuous appreciation; its avoidance of the conventions of society and regular politics; the appearance of a striptease (11); the program for a "*Society of the Friends of the Text*" (14); the description of the text as an "islet" beyond common social relations (16, 38); the imperative that bliss not yield to criticism or analysis (21); its embrace of delicacies, luxury, and extravagance; and especially the essay's characterization of a comfortable reading praxis ("house, countryside, near mealtime, the lamp, family where it should be, i.e., close but not too close [Proust in the lavatory that smelled of orrisroot], etc." [51])—all these features easily lend credence to the idea that Barthes uncritically promotes the "good life" for the mature and masculine members of the leisure classes.[5]

At other points, however, the text slyly changes the terms of the gratifications that such a lifestyle can well afford, and therefore criticizes the formation of masculinity it implies. The strategy at work is the one of "*subtle subversion*," as outlined by Barthes himself (55). Indeed, the connoisseur's, aesthetic's, or bourgeois's masculinity and its dominant pleasures are not directly opposed, since such a move, Barthes cautions, would remain caught up in what it contests "in an ultimately complicitous fashion," but instead are appealed to and accommodated to be undermined in due course (55). Other subjectivities, usually defined in contradistinction, are brought into a close and contagious contact with the well-established one, so that its vectors start to diffuse and give way. Pleasure, Barthes suggests, may well be childish, cowardly, or queer in nature.

In contrast to the idea that aesthetic pleasure is an adult function, a token of maturity, Barthes revels in oral figures that make it come across as childish, if not infantile. The pleasured reader tastes, sucks, and gobbles down the text. A masculinity based on vigor and agency, expressing a form of pleasure Barthes characterizes as muscled, phallic, and violent, finds its counterpoint in the numerous antimilitaristic references in the essay. In the text, Barthes writes, the war between various ideological languages and idiolects is not so much won or overcome, but made momentarily "tranquil" (29). In opposition to what he calls the "insidious heroism" of Bataille, the "pleasure of the text (the bliss of the text) is . . . like a sudden obliteration of the warrior's *value*, a momentary desquamation of the writer's hackles, a suspension of the 'heart' (of courage)" (30).[6] Only "defection . . . approaches bliss" (45). Finally, the heterosexual pursuits of the strip parlor are countered by cruising [*la drague*]: "I must seek out this reader (must 'cruise' him) *without knowing where he is*" (4). The cruise moves on to a bar, where Barthes enjoys its bustling sounds in a state of semisleep, and compares the experience to a Tangerine souk (49).[7]

This diversification of pleasures, masculine, childish, cowardly, and/or queer, is followed through by the critical pair of terms that Barthes introduces. Barthes's subject, with an image Platonic in origin, must keep "in his hands the reins of pleasure and bliss" (14). Whereas Plato's charioteer negotiates between the horses of reason and passion, beauty and lust, Barthes's driver must control and distinguish between two different modalities residing within Plato's second terms, namely, between "pleasure" [*plaisir*] and "bliss" [*jouissance*].[8]

In general terms, "pleasure" commands values like contentment, comfort, relaxation, ease, plenitude, satisfaction, and assurance, while "bliss" is characterized in terms of shock, ecstasy, tremor, loss, annulment, drift, and fading. Alternatively, the two terms characterize different historical periods (broadly, traditional versus modernist or avant-gardist books); different semiotic potentials residing within most texts, if not each text; different modes of reading; and, finally, different effects, or affects, in readerly reception. The sheer weight the two terms must carry already appears excessive, hyperbolic—somewhat like a parody of the scholarly urge to classify.

At the same time, the two notions are continuously relegated to the general and comprehensive term "pleasure," which encompasses both. Since a general notion of pleasure splits apart into a secondary pleasure and bliss, the conceptual clarity of the distinction is put under pressure. Hence, the catch may be that the reins of the two horses, the distinguishable modalities of enjoyment, easily and inevitably become entangled, twisted together.

As Michael Moriarty argues, moreover, even the ostensibly more radically flavored bliss may easily loop back into its opposite. On the one hand, Moriarty claims, bliss points to the eclipse of the subject, its fading or annihilation. On the other hand, he suggests, *jouissance* also implicates the specifically legal constitution of the subject, who "enjoys"—read: possesses—inalienable rights, properties, or good health [*jouir d'un droit, la jouissance d'un bien, jouir de la santé*].[9] Thus, the distinction between pleasure and bliss is coined and qualified in the same gesture.

Indeed, "a margin of indecision," Barthes writes, makes the whole distinction, the would-be controlled handling of the two horses, "precarious, revocable, reversible"; "*Pleasure/Bliss:* terminologically, there is always a vacillation—I stumble, I err," he adds (*The Pleasure of the Text*, 4). That last sentence poses the question of whether this vacillation or stumbling is merely terminological or, rather, indicative or constitutive of pleasure itself. The dash performs the vacillation that allows for both readings. Therefore, "I stumble, I err," directly following the mute but gear-switching dash, can be taken as a description that indicates the abrupt and largely unpredictable transition from pleasure to bliss, the reins getting twisted. Hence, the erring or stumbling between the two is more important than the distinction per se. Another pair of terms, discussed more fully below, takes up this same relation of connectedness and abrupt differentiation: *suspense* and *suspension*. The close association of the two is suggested by the similarity between the words, but, as I will show, Barthes gives the terms radically different inflections with respect to the temporality and narratability of male pleasure.

For the moment, the point is that pleasure is an internally differentiated category for Barthes; that it is complex and complicating; and, consequently, that it can make a (political) difference in relation to gender and sexuality. In what follows, I first pursue pleasure in its narrow sense [*plaisir*] before outlining its simultaneous synonym, counterpart, and opposite, bliss [*jouissance*]. I give special attention to the ways in which Barthes phrases both pleasure and bliss in connection to male orgasm and ejaculation, as well as to the ultimately undecidable relation between the two terms. Then, I discuss the relations that Barthes suggests between pleasure and the ordered temporality of narrative under the heading of climax or high point. Finally, I trace the alternate temporalities and appearances of masculine pleasure that Barthes fleetingly entertains. For Barthes not only pits the two terms against each other in an opposition that allows only for the choice either to come in a stereotypically masculine fashion or to come undone altogether, but also suggests different figurations of what male coming might possibly look like.

TAKING ONE'S PLEASURE

The erotic enjoyment of the reader may follow from certain pleasing textual qualities. Broadly, Barthes views two aspects as particularly pleasurable: excess and two-sidedness. *Cobra*, a work by Severo Sarduy, spoils its reader silly with an escalating quantity of words (*The Pleasure of the Text*, 8). A text pleases the reader, then, when and where it exceeds functionality and economy. Two-sidedness, in turn, entails the friction between two sides or edges of language, the one conformist and canonic, the other mobile and subversive. Neither aspect, Barthes cautions, is pleasing in itself. The gap between, or the collision of, the two is gratifying. In Sade's oeuvre, the friction between the exemplary grammatical sentences and their less than exemplary content is particularly pleasing (6). These two initial kinds of pleasures firmly reside within the text. There, they can be pointed at and identified.

However, congenial effects can also be produced by doing something to a text that may otherwise not please that much. Reversing a text is one way to achieve such an effect. "The more a story is told in a proper, well-spoken, straightforward way, in an even tone, the easier it is to reverse it, to blacken it, to read it inside out (Mme de Ségur read by Sade). This reversal, being a pure production, wonderfully develops the pleasure of the text," Barthes writes (26). A second strategy for the production of pleasure involves a kind of do-it-yourself editing or cutting: the reader skips some passages, "descriptions, explanations, analyses, conversations," to speed to the "warmer parts of the anecdote" (11). Barthes compares the operation to the behavior of a visitor to a strip parlor, who jumps on stage to accelerate the striptease by helping the dancer out of her clothes (11).

Excess, two-sidedness, reversing, cutting—these four modes of pleasure can only take place on the basis of the fundamental boundary between object and subject, text and reader. The first two specify inherently enjoyable qualities of the object; the last two entail the subject's imposition of the terms and conditions of his own gratification on the text. Simultaneously, the two distinguishable angles of operation are joined under the singular heading of the "pleasure of the text." Consequently, the sense of pleasure starts to float, move back and forth, between the object and the subject of reading. Apparently, the feeling cannot but be mutual.

The figure that enables this comprehensive and mutual pleasuring of text and reader is the ambiguity of the genitive in "the pleasure *of* the text." It vacillates between *genitivus subjectivus* and *genetivus objectivus*. The standard example for this figure is the Latin phrase *amor matris*, which can be translated as "the subject's love *for* the mother" (*objectivus*) as well as "the love *of* the mother for the subject" (*subjectivus*). One might speculate that this example is exemplary precisely because it promises a perfectly mutual, circular, and shared validation. In this sense, the alternate translations become virtually tautological. Thus, pleasure appears to denote a reciprocal sense of well-being that circulates between reader and text; what the reader *takes* and what the text *gives* are congruent, nearly one and the same thing. As a result, the possibility of textual resistance is foreclosed.

Symptomatic of this collapse of reader and text is the surprising ease with which Barthes shifts between the phrases "pleasure of the text" and "text of pleasure." As indicated, the former can well be achieved by manipulating the text, by reading it against the grain, or by cutting it up. The question, then, is whether the pleasure of the reader automatically renders the text as pleasurable, as out to please. Whose pleasure is it, anyway? "*Pleasure of the text, text of pleasure*," Barthes writes, "these expressions are ambiguous." He clarifies this ambiguity by differentiating the single noun *pleasure*: it "sometimes extends to bliss, sometimes is opposed to it." Additionally, he argues, the word refers both to a generality ("pleasure principle") and to "a miniaturization" ("minor pleasures") (19).

Yet the italicized phrase as a whole, consisting of two genitives that are linked and reversed, is also ambivalent in a different way. For, as two related, gender-specific French expressions make clear, the matter of gender, in sharp contrast to the exchange of the imaginary love of the *amor matris*, derails the smooth transition between the two. A *homme de plaisir* ("man of pleasure") is a "pleasure-seeker," the subject of pleasure. But a *fille de joie* ("girl of joy") is a "prostitute," pleasure's object. Hence, pleasure may boil down to the appropriation of the text by the reader. In this respect, even *jouissance* may insinuate a cynical financial transaction, as Moriarty suggests.

With regard to the fantasy that animates this dimension of wholesale and pleasurable appropriation of the text by the reader, it is relevant to note that an idiom of indiscriminate orality pervades Barthes's text. Next to the ambiguity of the genitive, this language of orality is the second way in which Barthes suspends the difference between reader and text. In the "oral-sadistic phase," Laplanche and Pontalis explain, libido and aggression are directed to the same object, and are expressed through notions such as sucking, licking, biting, and devouring (*The Language of Psychoanalysis*, 288–89).

In *The Pleasure of the Text*, the idiom of orality functions initially to denounce a boring, frigid, and "prattling" text (4–5). The language of this sort of text "foams," is "unweaned"; its phonemes "milky," it merely offers the motions of ungratified "sucking, of an undifferentiated orality" (5). Subsequently, however, Barthes notes that Sarduy's verbal excesses offer the reader distinct pleasures of the oral kind: "we are *gorged* with language, like children who are never refused anything or scolded for anything or, even worse, 'permitted' anything" (8, emphasis added). Additionally, the impatient voyeur visiting a strip club is compared to "a priest *gulping down* his Mass" (11).

This being "gorged" and "gulping" describe pleasure in its narrow sense, but orality features equally in the reading mode reserved for the modern, avant-gardist text susceptible to bliss: "not to devour, to gobble, but to *graze*, to browse scrupulously" (13, emphasis added). The writer's object, Barthes continues, is the "*mother tongue*," the maternal body to be "played with," "glorified," "embellished," "dismembered," and "disfigured" (37). Finally, the language of the political stereotype decrees that it be "*swallowed* without nausea" (44, emphasis added). The many references to the maternal body and to orality work to cancel the distinction between reader and text, and suggest a diffuse and mutual pleasuring that bypasses the import of gender.

Since the (pre)subject's experience in the oral stage is relatively undifferentiated, its idiom figures equally to characterize the text that does not please, the text that does please, and the text that brings about bliss. In accordance with that lack of distinction, the notion of pleasure both differentiates (in opposition to bliss) and un-differentiates (as the overriding term). This dynamic of making and un-making distinctions, then, also applies to the difference between text and reader, the smooth transition from the pleasure of the text to the text of pleasure. The predominant, oral urge seems to be to consume and ingest the text: to graze, devour, and to gobble it down. Consequently, it becomes difficult to imagine any textual resistance or opposition to this eager and demanding mouth in terms other than, say, indigestion or choking. So far, it appears that the text cannot be or do anything to resist the reader's consuming pleasure, to force him or her to switch gears. Then again, Barthes recodes this reading pleasure as specifically childish, perhaps regressive.

BEING TAKEN BY BLISS

In fact, the possibility of choking does appear in the text. Gorged with language by Sarduy's generosity—"*more, more, still more!*"—the pleasure of the reader suddenly tips over into something more sinister: "*Cobra* is the pledge of continuous jubilation, the moment when by its very excess verbal pleasure chokes and reels [*bascule*] into bliss [*jouissance*]" (8). This choking, then, is considered as the last and only obstacle to the wholesale oral appropriation of the text, the acute sensation of being overwhelmed or smothered by the breast, milk, or verbal abundance. "[M]*ore, more, still more!*" suddenly becomes "too much."

The sentence articulates a temporality that moves astray. The book promises a "jubilation" that should be "continuous." Nevertheless, that enjoyment is stopped short or punctured by the instantaneity of bliss. Tripping into bliss brings about a different temporality than the one that pleasure is seeking out. Reading promises an ongoing satisfaction, but one that might, instead of culminating in a pleasurable climax, be interrupted in its motions, and switch gears.

The notion of choking returns when Barthes describes the intense instantaneity of coming in terms of the impossible moment just before the last of possible moments, of nearly suffocating to death. "The pleasure of the text is that untenable, impossible, purely *novelistic* instant," he writes, "so relished by Sade's libertine when he manages to be hanged and then to cut the rope at the very moment of his orgasm, his bliss" (7). Switching gears from orality to genitality, this ecstatic choking is now related to orgasm, alternately described as reeling, falling, or tumbling [*basculer*]. This awkward and vulnerable motionality brings back to mind the phrase that I highlighted above: "I stumble, I err" (4). Apparently, riding the waves of joy, the subject falls through the plane of pleasure into another dimension. The temporality of that dimension is neither continuous nor climactic, but so instantaneous that it is nearly impossible.

The distinction between pleasure and bliss is played out somewhat differently in another passage from the text. In the space of a few lines, two expressions referring to orgasm are linked up as if they were virtual synonyms, as if the one unproblematically extends to the other, while their terms nevertheless subtly vary. Imagining a societal outcast, an antihero, Barthes specifies, "he is the reader of the text at the moment he takes his pleasure [*prends son plaisir*]. . . . [T]he subject gains access to bliss [*accède à la jouissance*]" (3–4). Like *jouir*, *prendre ses plaisir*, it turns out, is a standard French expression for "coming."

However, "taking one's pleasure" presupposes considerably more subjective agency and control than "gaining access to bliss" does, and certainly more so than "tumbling into bliss." In the course of Barthes's considerations of orgasmic reading pleasures, then, the agency of the masculine subject vis-à-vis his own gratification can be reified [*prendre son plaisir*], qualified [*acceder à la jouissance*], or interrupted [*basculer dans la jouissance*]. The next and final step is the renunciation and transfer of agency altogether. "[I]n the midst of bliss," Barthes writes, it is a "*dissolve* which seizes [*saisit*] the subject" (7). Ultimately, bliss takes the passive subject rather than the other way around.

In Barthes's text, two resonant words capture this interrupting and unsettling aptitude of bliss. The first is *perte*, "loss": "What pleasure wants is the site of a loss [*perte*], the seam, the cut, the deflation" (7; see also 14, 15, 19, 39, 41). Typically, the chosen term *perte* condenses morality, economy, and sexuality. *Perte* means "loss," "waste," and "leak," but also refers to "downfall," or "ruin"; its plural denotes "(financial) losses" (as opposed to gains). *Pertes séminales* stands for "involuntary ejaculation." Also, note the possibly penile and economic correlates of "deflation," the final term that Barthes gives.

This ideological entanglement connects *perte* with the second word, which makes but one appearance: *chute*, for "fall." The subject, Barthes writes, "simultaneously enjoys, through the text, the consistency of his selfhood and its collapse, its fall [*chute*]" (21). Again, the insidious concatenation of moral and economic meanings surfaces in the various meanings of the word: "ending," "ruin," "failure," "sudden (economic) devaluation," and "decrease in value." *Perte* and *chute*—indeed, "I stumble, I err" (4). Pleasure's vacillation or indeterminacy is at once moral, masculine, sexual, and economic. At stake in bliss is not only masculinity's sexual aspect, but also that gender's moral and economic correlates. Barthes suggests that orgasm, conceived as "fall" or "loss," features as the abrupt interruption of the mutual and imaginary sharing of pleasure between mother and child, text and reader, object and subject, which was implied by the ambiguous genitive and the idiom of orality he uses.

On the one hand Barthes deploys the notion of pleasure to suspend distinctions: between pleasure and bliss, between reader and text. On the other hand, pleasure equally turns on a crucial and abrupt differentiation, the agency of bliss, which heavily implicates the subject. Thus, in reading, in entering into textuality, the reader may trip over a surprise lying in wait there, and be returned to his own body, which has changed in the process. In a similar vein, the text figures as a malleable object that can be appropriated, swallowed, without reserve or remainder, and as the irreducible resistance that makes the reader gag, fall, come. What feature of textuality allows for such extremes?

THE CERTAIN BODY

So far, Barthes offers little clarification of the ways in which the text can make the subject come, in the sense of suffocating or tumbling. What force does the text exert in forging the reader's agency to become qualified, interrupted, or revoked? At what frictional instant does pleasure turn into bliss? An answer is suggested by two fragments from *The Pleasure of the Text* that ascribe contrasting but related materialities to the text. In the first, the text is described as a body; in the second, as a piece of wood; what connects the two is the presence of "veins," the fine, heterogeneous, dense, textured, and material markings that bodies and wood have in common.

"Apparently Arab scholars, when speaking of the text," Barthes observes, "use this admirable expression: *the certain body*" (16).[10] That certainty remains unclear. The textual body is not, Barthes hastily explains, the *corpus* of anatomists, physiologists, grammarians, or philologists. Yet,

> [W]e also have a body of bliss consisting solely of erotic relations, utterly distinct from the first body: it is another contour, another nomination; thus with the text . . . Does the text have human form, is it a figure, an anagram of the body? Yes, but of our erotic body. (16–17)

Relational in nature, this body cannot be securely classified or divided. "[T]here are no 'erogenous zones' (a foolish expression, besides)," Barthes adds (10). Hence, the erotic body, be it of the text or the reader, resists clear and easy classification when it is given over to bliss.

Later, Barthes explains that the reader may seek out the figuration, as opposed to direct representation, of the erotic body "in the profile of the text" (56). This body may be that of the (nonbiographical) author, of a character, or of the text itself: "a diagrammatic and not an imitative structure, [the text] can reveal itself in the form of a body, split into fetish objects, into erotic sites" (56). The difference is between a body conventionally divided into localizable and quantifiable zones, and a perverse body that yields unexpectedly arousing sites. These qualifications once again bring up the danger of the "profile" of the text and the erotic body of the reader collapsing, so that the text comes to function as a pliant and accommodating body.

But the idea of profile can also be taken up to suggest a stubborn material individuality, capable of resistance. Referring to the reader who cuts or edits the text, Barthes writes that he enjoys "the abrasions [he] impose[s] upon the fine surface" (11–12). Hence, this reader adds nicks and scrapings of his own to a surface that is itself already densely textured, fine. This potential is followed up in a passage that compares the text to a piece of wood, a material that, unlike, say, wax or clay, has little anthropomorphic makings:

> If you hammer a nail into a piece of wood, the wood has a different resistance according to the place you attack it: we say that wood is not isotropic. Neither is the text: the edges, the seam, are unpredictable. Just as (today's) physics must accommodate the non-isotropic character of certain environments, certain universes, so structural analysis (semiology) must recognize the slightest resistances of the text, the irregular patterns of its veins. (36–37)

Instead of willfully adding abrasions of his own, the reader must now acknowledge, feel out, the text's profile, its pattern of minute resistances.

Engrafted in wood, moreover, these slight features do not easily give (in). Hence, they do not necessarily, *a priori*, yield to our erotic or perverse body, anagrammatically or diagrammatically. Instead, they cause friction. Because these markings are described as quasi-physical veins, and because Barthes at several points suspends and abolishes the distinction between text and reader, the possibility of a reversal of the metaphor opens up as well: the resistant veins of the texts are able to etch or graft themselves into the reader's erotic body, which has become hypersensitive through the pleasures of reading. Thus, they may reinscribe, rewrite, the reader who trips or tumbles over them, rather than the other way around. However small, these veins are sufficient to interrupt the pleasure of reading and to make the subject tumble and choke, come. Consequently, the reading subject becomes "writable," "scriptible." Here in Barthes's essay, one finds a cautious and suggestive description of the material agency of the text.

The possible fits and misfits between pleasure, masculinity, and narrative, a concatenation that Barthes repeatedly invokes, bring out that potential more forcefully. On the one hand, narrativity brings about the ordering of the features of the text, as well as of the energetic pleasures of the reader, so that both, linearly, episodically, and progressively, gear up on a course toward resolution and climax—to what Barthes calls the "solution of the riddle, the revelation of fate" (11). In Peter Brooks's narratology, such a discrete point of resolution is described as the "significant discharge," the timely collapse of heightened meaning and pleasurable release (see chapter 5). Suggestively, Barthes approaches narrative climax as orgasmic pleasure in its narrow and conventional sense. Through the ordering that narrative produces, text and body, object and subject, become classifiable. Consequently, timely and untimely pleasures, privileged and disavowed satisfactions, fore- and endpleasure, as well as different incarnations of masculinity can be distinguished and judged.

On the other hand, according to Barthes, this narrative organization of the text does not entirely manage to "cover" or subsume the intricate profile of the non-isotopic veins of the text. As a result, the course of narrative processing and the calibration of signification in its terms may suddenly stumble over the edges and seams that remain stubbornly in place, prompting the reader to come blissfully; the veins of the text become trip wires. As I will argue, the difference between pleasure and bliss can best be appreciated in relation to narrativity as well as masculinity. Reveling erotically in the text, the reader may appropriate the text's flexible and malleable body without reserve or remainder. Or the reader may find his pleasure in the gratifying and painful frictions that the text performs, resisting its narrative ordering and making the reader gag, trip, come, rather than safely and ultimately arriving at the "solution of the riddle, the revelation of fate." So, to whom does the "certain body" of the text belong?

FROM SUSPENSE TO SUSPENSION: TUMBLING OR FREEZING NARRATIVE

In *The Pleasure of the Text*, masculinity is hardly brought up directly; gender is not an explicit topic of consideration. Nevertheless, Barthes repeatedly inquires into the concatenation of masculinity, narrativity, and textuality as he coins and articulates his pleasures. What does narrativity afford masculinity? How can textuality prevent the solidarity between narrative representation and gender norms that Barthes observes? And to what extent is the narrative pleasure of climax different from what Barthes calls bliss? Barthes proceeds by taking into account two closely related aspects of male coming. The first is its precision timing, the temporizing of pleasure so that it appears at the narratively "right" moment, and not prematurely or belatedly. The second aspect concerns the visual appearance of orgasm, the image of ejaculation that emerges. Mainly, Barthes's thoughts on narrativity, pleasure, and gender are developed with the help of two figures: a stripper and the father. The scandal is that, ultimately, these two figures get mixed up.

At two separate junctures, the essay seems intricately burdened with the question of masculinity. Both concern the visual form or appearance of orgasmic pleasure in relation to temporality and narrativity. In the first passage, Barthes refutes the necessity that pleasure arrive in a particularly masculine and powerful shape: "The pleasure of the text is not necessarily of a triumphant, heroic, muscular type. No need to throw out one's chest. [*Pas besoin de se cambrer*]" (18). The statement suggests a pleasure that emerges in another shape than a triumphant achievement, an arrived-at goal. Hence, pleasure may well arrive as a withheld accomplishment or prevented telos, as failure or embarrassment.[11]

The second passage goes further. Now Barthes considers bliss as the active deregulation of the progression toward culmination or climax:

> [Emotion] is a disturbance, a bordering on collapse: something perverse, under respectable appearances; emotion is even, perhaps, the slyest of losses, for it contradicts the general rule that would assign bliss a fixed form: strong, violent, crude: something inevitably muscular, strained, phallic. Against the general rule: *never allow oneself to be deluded by the* image *of bliss*: agree to recognize bliss wherever a disturbance occurs in amatory adjustment (premature, delayed, etc.) . . . (25)

Bliss can only appear in its regulated shape, strong, violent, crude, muscular, strained, and phallic, on the condition that it arrive in due time, with the "amatory adjustment" running smoothly. However, bliss can also take on a wholly different form, intimated here as "bordering on collapse," whenever it occurs at the "wrong" moment, when it arrives too soon or too late. This noted concern for timing and pacing closely connects male pleasure with narrativity.

Barthes then relates narrative to the Oedipal father. "Oedipus," Barthes surmises, is "at least good for something: to make good novels, to tell good stories" (47). The acclaimed

> Death of the Father would deprive literature of many of its pleasures. If there is no longer a Father, why tell stories? Doesn't every narrative lead back to Oedipus? Isn't storytelling always a way of searching for one's origin, speaking one's conflicts with the Law, entering into the dialectic of tenderness and hatred? (47)

The idea of the narrative quest for the origin, initially embodied by the father, is also brought up in another passage that, switching the genders, compares the suspense of narrative with "corporeal striptease" (10).

In turn, this analogy is only suggested *after* Barthes has argued that the body surfaces most erotically when the skin appears intermittently, flashing between two pieces of clothing or textile borders—for example, between trousers and sweater, glove and sleeve, or the open neck of a shirt. "It is this flash itself," Barthes explains, "which seduces, or rather: the staging of an appearance-as-disappearance" (9, 10). This intermittent temporality of the erotic flash does not coincide with the precision-paced temporality of narrative and striptease.

The flashing appearances of skin are, subsequently, favorably opposed to the principle of gradual unveiling that underpins narrative and striptease alike:

> The pleasure of the text is not the pleasure of the corporeal striptease or of narrative suspense. In these cases, there is no tear, no edges: a gradual unveiling: the entire excitation takes refuge in the *hope* of seeing the sexual organ (schoolboy's dream) or in knowing the end of the story (novclistic satisfaction). Paradoxically (since it is mass-consumed), this is a far more intellectual pleasure than the other: an Oedipal pleasure (to denude, to know, to learn the origin and the end) . . . (10)

Hence, narrative and striptease solicit the reading subject's expectation of or hope for a full disclosure, which they will eventually deliver, offering up the finalized appearance of the origin and the end, or the sexual organ of the stripper, rather than the much more erotic staging of an appearance-as-disappearance. But, then, that latter mode of staging is itself effectively upstaged as Barthes moves on to consider further the figure of the striptease. Meanwhile, both the erotic of the flash and the body of the father are temporarily bracketed.

Though classical narrative furnishes a gradual unveiling similar to the striptease rather than the erotic staging of the flash, it may nevertheless contain "a sort of diluted tmesis," Barthes argues. This tmesis is actualized by a reader who modulates the intensity of his reception rhythmically. Some passages are skipped in order to speed to those that promise to precipitate "the solution of the riddle, the revelation of fate" (10, 11). "[D]oing so," Barthes specifies, "we resemble a spectator in a nightclub who climbs onto the stage and speeds up the dancer's striptease, tearing off her clothing, *but in the same order*, that is: on the one hand respecting and on the other hastening the episodes of the ritual" (11). Such a procedure may prepare the pleasure of the reader. Yet this pleasure is also discredited as "diluted," merely following the "simple principle of functionality" or the "simple temporality" of reading (11, 12).

That this pleasure is simple and diluted becomes clear when Barthes describes bliss as the wholesale deregulation of the functional temporality of narrativity that this reader merely speeds up. Now, the reading mode is to "graze, to browse scrupulously," to cling to the text: it "skips nothing; it weighs, it sticks to the text" (12, 13). Only in that way, one learns, might the hole open up through which the subject tumbles to his bliss:

> It is not (logical) extension that captivates [this way of reading], the winnowing out [*l'effeuillement*] of truths, but the layering [*la feuilleté*] of significance; as in the children's game of topping hands, the ex-

> citement comes not from a processive haste but from a kind of vertical din [*charivari*] (the verticality of language and its destruction); it is at the moment when each (different) hand skips over the next (and not one *after* the other) that the hole [*trou*], the gap, is created and carries off the subject of the game—the subject of the text. (12)

Hence, a narrative pleasure that is gradual, extensive, and progressive is punctured, ruptured, by an anticlimactic bliss that is sudden and momentous.

The story that is "to be continued" to its ending and the striptease that cannot but culminate are stopped short, arrested without compromise. The word *l'effeuillement* plays on both registers. Implicitly referring to *feuilleton*, a "continuing story" or "soap," *effeuillement* means the "falling of leaves," while *effeuillage* denotes a "striptease," and *effeuilleuse* a "stripper." Rather than obeying the anticipated but deferred gratification of a full disclosure, be it narrative or voyeuristic, the reader gets caught up in the layering and shimmering of sensual possibilities, a simultaneous but heterogeneous "layering" [*feuilleté*]. The root word here is *feuille*, for "leaf" as well as "page"; *feuillage* means "foliage." Meaning is not disclosed page after page, leaf after leaf, but takes place instantly, as the rustling of leaves or pages. The shuddering, rippling, and shimmering of these "leaves"/"pages" as they catch the light or a gust of wind supply an image for male orgasm that replaces the phallic "image of bliss." It suggests temporality, but one that cannot be subsumed in a teleological approximation of climax. It suggests visibility, but cannot be said to look particularly masculine.

Indeed, "din" [*charivari*] (for "tumult," "tangle," or "disturbance") captures an orgasmic instantaneity that resists timing and calculation. It pinpoints the precise instant when the reins of the two horses of pleasure and bliss become entangled. Elsewhere, Barthes once more underscores the unruly temporality of bliss:

> The bliss of the text is not precarious, it is worse: *precocious*; it does not come in its own good time, it does not depend on any ripening [*mûrissement*]. Everything is wrought to a transport at one and the same time. . . . Everything comes about; indeed in every sense everything *comes—at first glance*. (52, 53; emphasis in the text)

This ejaculation is, precisely, premature; anticlimactic rather than climactic. The schoolboy who should await the eventual revelation of the sexual organ and the reader who must hold out for the final materialization of narrative truth come too soon.

In this respect, Barthes strategically contrasts *suspense* with *suspension*. The former characterizes the meager but conventional pleasures of narrative and striptease. The notion returns when Barthes aptly observes that pornography habitually represents not so much the erotic scene itself, but rather its anticipation or expectation (58). And, when the sex scene does finally arrive, there is often little more than "disappointment, deflation," he writes (58).

Suspension, however, is described as a force that actively prevents meaning: "it is a veritable *époché*, a stoppage which congeals all recognized [*signified*] values (recognized by oneself)" (65). So, where narrative suspense can only pledge erotically disappointing and canonic revelations of "the origin and the end," antinarrative suspension forecloses the import of what Barthes terms *doxa* (popular opinion) and ideology owing to a temporal and visual freeze, thickening, or fracturing. Hence, preempting climactic pleasure by way of the deregulation of bliss may be one way to prevent ideological formations from holding sway, from becoming enshrined in and through the narrative. Indeed, coming too soon, untimely bliss, preempts the reification of climax as well as the values calibrated at its timely arrival.

However, that explanation cannot entirely account for Barthes's reinscription of "proper" climaxes. What exactly is at stake in coming "in good time"? Generally, one could argue that Barthes subtly subverts a conventional masculinity predicated on a reified agency and control, to be exerted over one's own sensual pleasures. The most prevalent example of this tendency is perhaps delivered by hard-core pornography's maintenance of the phallic image of bliss, of ejaculation, as the requisite ending to each sexual encounter. Additionally, Barthes's stress on precocious or premature bliss can be understood to contest the so-called delayed gratification that is paramount to adulthood, and that is underwritten in Brooks's narratology. For "bliss," Barthes writes, "does not depend on any ripening [*mûrissement*, "maturation" or "coming of age"]" (52). However, I want to append another explanation, one that must surely short-circuit the Oedipal and narrative suspense that allows for the proper finalization of pleasure: the intrusion, flashing, or staging of a particular body that I have so far skipped.

UPSTAGING THE FATHER

I started this analysis of the concatenation of masculinity, narrative, and pleasure by noting that, for Barthes, narrative suspense prepares for the emergence of the origin, embodied by the figure of the Oedipal father (47). This father reappears at a surprising juncture in the text. His reentry is staged right in between the two other stagings that I have considered above.

The first staging entails the exposure of skin between two textile seams, deemed "most erotic" by Barthes: "it is this flash itself which seduces, or rather: the *staging* of an appearance-as-disappearance" (10, emphasis added). The second one concerns the simile which had a visitor to a nightclub jumping "onto the *stage*" to speed up the striptease (11, emphasis added). Hence, Barthes connects and differentiates between two theatrical frames, two stages, in which the body makes an appearance. The first one turns on intermittent and brief glances at pieces of skin, appearing and disappearing. The second one, in the mode of narrative suspense, anticipates and ultimately delivers the disclosure of the sexual organ. However, exactly at the seam or gap between these two erotic theaters, Barthes interjects an entirely different stage on which the body of the father returns to view.

Right in between the gaping pieces of clothing and the brouhaha of the nightclub, where the stripper scrupulously paces her disrobing, at the edge between these two forms of staged exposure, the paternal body itself flashes, intermittently appears, in the text. I cite the fragment, a separate paragraph in the text, in full:

> The pleasure of the text is not the pleasure of the corporeal striptease or of narrative suspense. In these cases, there is no tear, no edges: a gradual unveiling: the entire excitation takes refuge in the hope of seeing the sexual organ (schoolboy's dream) or in knowing the end of the story (novelistic satisfaction). Paradoxically (since it is mass-consumed), this is a far more intellectual pleasure than the other: an Oedipal pleasure (to denude, to know, to learn the origin and the end), if it is true that every narrative (every unveiling of the truth) is a *staging* of the (absent, hidden, or hypostatized) father—which would explain the solidarity of narrative forms, of family structures, and of prohibitions of nudity, all collected in our culture in the myth of Noah's sons covering his nakedness. (10, emphasis added)

Narrative seems to stage an absence, the absence of the father's body, the body not to be unveiled or denuded in narrative. The reference to the Noah myth arrives as a throwaway comment, an afterthought restating the obvious, what we already know. It summarizes an improbable range of phenomena ("narrative forms," "family structures," "prohibitions of nudity"). Additionally, it is twice removed from the main argument: "if it is true," "which would explain."

In the passage, Barthes stresses the covering of Noah's nakedness rather than the preceding episode of the story in which it is exposed, even though the immediate context of the reference, from the skin flashing between textile seams to the striptease, points to erotic exposures. All this works to make Noah's entry on the scene highly negligible, hardly noticeable. Surrounded by the schoolboy's dream and the setting of the nightclub, and set up by the Oedipal reference that makes one anticipate a denuding of the mother, the reader is manipulated to expect the ultimate disclosure of the *female* body. Yet, the arch father's nakedness is at issue here.

In "Géricault and 'Masculinity,'" art historian Norman Bryson discusses the biblical account of the relevant episode in the life of Noah (Genesis 9:21–29). Noah's youngest son, Ham, chances upon his father in a state of undress, sleeping off a wine-induced hangover in his tent. As soon as Ham's brothers learn of this, they take swift action. Walking backward into the tent, their eyes averted, they cover the dormant Noah with a robe. Once Noah awakes from his alcoholic stupor and hears about the incident, he curses Ham and condemns his offspring, eventually to form the people of Canaan, to the servitude of the tribes that his brothers Shem and Japheth will generate.

Bryson sheds light on the dynamic at work in the story with the help of a personal anecdote. Visiting a rehabilitation center for Vietnam veterans, he observes that, while the vets shower together with their superior, only the officer wears a pair of swimming trunks. Bryson concludes that the penis of a man with authority over other men, a father (Noah, the officer), may not be seen by his subordinates (the sons, the vets), because that would enable them to appropriate with their looks the powers and privileges that the parental penis embodies. This reading is accredited in rabbinical tradition, according to which Ham not only would have seen his father's naked body, but also would have taken advantage of the situation by castrating him. This subsequent castration would have been deliberately omitted from Genesis.[12]

In *Francis Bacon and the Loss of Self*, however, Ernst van Alphen takes issue with this analysis. Stressing not so much the possibly symbolic significance of the episode, he asks, simply, what Ham has actually seen. In any case, van Alphen argues, *not* "a proud penis, the iconic sign—motivated by resemblance—of patriarchal privilege, but . . . instead a shriveled shrimp—a sign of an altogether different kind. And such a sight would make it painfully clear that the privileges associated with the penis are arbitrary, imaginary" (179).

Seeing the penis, van Alphen concludes, can undo the belief "in a motivated relationship between penis and phallic power." In itself, the penis, once visible, fails to support a phallic, paternal, and powerful masculinity. Instead, it is its vulnerable "Achilles' heel" (180). Whereas Bryson's analysis pivots around the possible appropriation of phallic power, the son becoming father, van Alphen's reading deflates, undoes, the semiotics of fatherhood. For, having seen the "shriveled shrimp," the embarrassing sight of the father sleeping off a hangover, the son's access to an idealized fatherhood is now prevented, foreclosed. Rather than an icon of paternal power, the penis becomes an index for the vulnerability of the male body. Or, seeing the penis puts before the eye the (in)sight that the presumed icon of male power is a Peircean symbol, motivated merely by convention.

This analysis can be made more meaningful if one considers another perspective. To all intents and purposes, it seems, Ham was not out looking for "the origin and the end." He just happened to find himself in the wrong place at the wrong time, a wandering facilitated by Noah's own loss of control. Paradoxically, then, the crucial event of this story is itself untimely, accidental, incidental: insufficiently narrative. The story is strangely devoid of suspense. Because of that, it scarcely allows for the teleological structuring of delay and ultimate revelation. There is no buildup of expectation, no kindling of desire or hope by a temporarily withheld disclosure. Thus, the event functions as the suspension of narrative rather than as partaking of narrative suspense. Narrative, after all, does not unveil existing truths. Through its temporal ordering of anticipation and delay, rather, narrative *produces* the effect of "truth," the effect of added relevance and significance. Narrative compels excitation, desire, or hope, thus inducing the belief in what is finally given. The wait generates the meaning of the outcome. The story of Noah, however, opens up the possibility of a sudden glimpse at a paternal, yet nonphallic, nudity.

Hence, through Barthes's use of the Noah story, and through its strategic placing, the desire of the schoolboy and the voyeur to see the female sex is effectively replaced, upstaged, by the suspension caused by the introduction of the father's nakedness on the scene. As a result, the powers of narrative come unglued: "If there is no longer a Father [but just a father], why tell stories?" (47). If the parental body is allowed to flash within the narrative, but without forming its ultimate telos, then the drive or dynamo of narrativity cannot but hamper. Indeed, the deflation of the phallus also deflates the arched trajectory of narrative progression. For, "if it is true that every narrative (every unveiling of the truth) is a staging of the (absent, hidden, or hypostatized) father," as Barthes argues, then narrativity becomes sidetracked once the paternal body makes however brief an appearance before the footlights of the text (10). Thus, the Noah reference in Barthes's text, ostensibly negligible and insignificant, is precisely the juncture where the essay itself offers up a non-isotopic place of resistance, a glitch that derails its intelligibility.

For, if the father embodies the ground of narrativity, then that structural dependency also implies the possibility that the paternal body might momentarily, intermittently, surface into the narrative. As the Noah reference suggests, narrative serves to cover the paternal body on which it imposes itself, which supports it, while simultaneously promising the paternal body's disclosure. If that disclosure is ill timed, then that body may briefly emerge in a shape or form that does not substantiate the telos of paternal or masculine status and privilege. Rather, it insinuates a physicality that is vulnerable and embarrassed. Apparently, the extra layer of organization that narrativity adds to a text, like the robe that Noah's sons draw over his naked and dormant body, and like Lacan's veil that accompanies the phallus, is not entirely smooth: the profile of the shrouded body, described by Barthes as intricate "veins," persists. Hence, the "certain body" of the text belongs to this father, both hidden under and supporting the narrative. The orgasmic bliss that Barthes calls "din" occurs when the relation between the ground of the narrative, the paternal body, and the surface of the narrative that covers it becomes disturbed; when some aspect of that body crosses over or emerges into the story.

That body's eventual emergence in one shape or the other is unpredictable; it cannot be calculated or prepared with deliberation. For, as I have contended, Barthes does not argue for the crisp distinction between the effects of pleasured reading, for the maintenance of differences. Suspense and suspension, pleasure and bliss, narrative and text are intricately entangled, enfolded into each other. Hence, text and narrative, ground and surface, form fitting and ill-fitting folds that can be traced, felt out, tripped over.

Barthes's recourse to Noah ultimately implies the replacement of those other, foundational, and invariably murderous myths of patriarchy: Oedipus, the primal horde. Apparently, the father does not necessarily have to be killed in order for the son to become a father, thus inevitably resuscitating the ideal of fatherhood. It quite suffices that the paternal body be seen, enabling the son to see through the myth of masculinity. The suspense works as long as the sought-out paternal body remains present in its absence, its inaccessibility to the glance. However, this suspense itself becomes suspended when that body becomes the object of the look. Narrative tumbles or freezes, and the hold of myth with it. With narrative temporarily held in abeyance, other figurations of male pleasure than the requisite image of bliss can now be noticed and considered.

WANDERING SEEDS

Barthes's programmatic slogan to "*never allow oneself to be deluded by the image of bliss*" enables alternate forms of male pleasure to move into focus. These take place within the frame of narrative, yet work to sidetrack or bracket it. I have already considered several of them. Enjoyment must be recognized not only in the shape of climax, but also, perhaps rather, in its disturbances, the deregulation of the "amatory adjustment": pleasures arriving too soon or too late. Bliss may well appear in the shape of a sudden and awkward loss of control, as falling, stumbling, or reeling. Additionally, it might follow up on pulsating flashes of unexpected exposures in the text, or be experienced as the suspension of narrative suspense, congealing signification and the ongoing flow of the narrative.

Barthes considers three more specific figurations of pleasure. The reading mode that clings or sticks to the textual surface offers an entirely superficial contact with it, floating *over* the text rather than penetrating it: "like a cork on the waves, I remain motionless, pivoting to the *intractable* bliss that binds me to the text (to the world)" (18). On the last page of the essay, the pleasure of being penetrated appears: the reverberation of a voice, supple, lubricated, granular, in the hollow of the ear: "it granulates, it crackles, it caresses, it grates, it cuts, it comes: that is bliss" (67).

The final figuration of ejaculation returns to the profile of veins, the finely textured pattern of resistances graphed in the text, and prefigures the dispersal of semen and meaning indicative of Derridean dissemination, the concept under scrutiny in the next chapter. "The text," Barthes writes,

> is no more than the open list of fires of languages (those living fires, intermittent lights, wandering features strewn in the text like seeds and which for us advantageously replace the "*semina aeternitatis*," the "*zopyra*," the common notions, the fundamental assumptions of ancient philosophy). (16–17)

Here, ejaculation is accorded full semiotic relevance. The wandering seeds of bliss replace the eternal semina, the common assumptions of philosophy and ideology.

To conclude, bliss, conceived as orgasm and ejaculation, is the affect and effect of the reader, who has become embodied owing to his arousal or titillation while reading. Co-opted by narrative, this readerly pleasuring may largely ignore the materiality of the text and veer toward the culmination of satisfaction and significance when the story arrives at closure. The specific form of pleasure thus produced Barthes terms the image of bliss, an ejaculation that appears timely, as well as in a shape that Barthes describes as phallic, masculine, and muscled. However, the course of narrative cannot but negotiate the irregularly textured terrain of the text, where a body lies asleep, partially covered by, and partially supporting, the narrative in progress. The features this body brings into play—irregular veins, wandering seeds, and intricate folds—cause friction and can make the reader trip, fall, stumble, thereby producing a pleasure that is different from the one expressed in the image of bliss.

Narratively, Barthes's bliss concerns the hold of the story, the desires it kindles, the delays that it stretches out, the solutions and values that it ultimately delivers. However, this suspense is ever entangled with the possibility of suspension, when the story progressing through and over the text finds an obstacle in its course, arresting its steady development. Sexually, bliss articulates the climax of narrative, orgasm as narrative, as expressed in the phallic image of bliss. However, bliss also allows for the possibility of pleasure emerging at moments and in shapes other than the image of bliss demands. The din caused by the shuddering and shimmering of the textual layers of "leaves"/"pages" bespeaks an alternative vision of ejaculation.

As to gender, bliss shows how narrative partakes of the differentiation between people, women and men, fathers and sons, and how such differences are invested with desire and pleasure. In part, bliss articulates the appropriation, the predominantly oral consumption and consummation of the text, conceived as the maternal body, or, when narrativized, as the voyeuristic pleasure of watching the well-timed procedure of the striptease. However, bliss also implicates the possibility that the dormant and hidden body of the father, which forms the ground of the narrative, suddenly moves into focus, flashes in the text, thereby rendering moot the status of paternity and, hence, the differences between people calibrated with that norm as their joint reference point. While pleasure, in its narrow sense, is angled toward feminine bodies as conventionally seen (the mother, the stripper), Barthes's articulation of bliss is largely projected toward male bodies, possibly even the father's, bringing up what he describes as a "dialectic of tenderness and hatred." Thus, bliss also allows for other masculine pleasures in relation to feminine bodies.

Semiotically, pleasure may cathect to the phraseology of fixed notions and calcified assumptions in the text, the *semina* of culture. Or, it can happily trace the wandering seeds that escape them. That these alternative options, in different dimensions, are continuously and simultaneously present, available, or, alternately, so entangled with each other that they can hardly be distinguished is, in the final analysis, precisely the perspective on pleasure, gender, and meaning that bliss makes possible and insistent. For, bliss, as Barthes repeatedly claims, is never sure nor safe.

NINE

DISSIMULATING THE SUPREME SPASM

Derrida

JACQUES DERRIDA'S *Dissemination* is a book about male orgasm, ejaculation, and semen. Of course, it is also about the tenuous place of the foreword in relation to the literary or philosophical exposition it precipitates ("Outwork"); about a treacherous, liquid element contaminating from within what is philosophically, as philosophy, defined by its exclusion ("Plato's Pharmacy"); about the impossibility of a thematically cohering interpretation of the works of Mallarmé ("The Double Session"); and about a numerically charged rhythm or cadence working to structure, as well as to fracture, signification ("Dissemination"). But it should be noted that the various essays and arguments that make up the book are repeatedly and consistently informed by, worked through, a reconsideration of ejaculation and semen in relation to philosophical and literary meaning.

For example, "Outwork," the first text in the volume, dispels the notion that the preface should be thought of as the seat of the single cell or germ spawning the totality of the book it announces. In "Plato's Pharmacy," sperm takes its place in the series of "pharmakological" fluids at stake, such as medicine, poison, ink, paint, and perfume. "The Double Session" proposes a gestural, spasmodic—that is, orgasmic—writing performance, which bypasses mimeticism and referentiality, as well as an understanding of the seminal white that, in Mallarmé, both grounds, blots out, and multiplies textual markers. Hinging between singularity and plurality, finally, semen forms the occasion for a rethinking of the logic of numbers in "Dissemination." In this chapter, I trace the implications and consequences of this insistent presence of semen and ejaculation in the different essays that make up Derrida's book.

TRANCE

The fact that precisely semen should form the viscous trace that makes the four essays of the book stick together is perhaps not a big surprise. A short fifth text, titled "Trance Partition," offers a series of citations that are all, in some way or other, closely related to ejaculation and orgasm in the book's further argument. Performing the "refolding" [*reploiement*] that is one of the key terms in the book, this text is folded, like a separate, loose, and supplementary leaflet, into the book, as if casually inserted between its pages. The first sheet appears on page 172, right in between "Plato's Pharmacy" and "The Double Session"; the second and last page appears on page 286, where it sits between the latter and "Dissemination."[1] Hence, "Trance Partition" serves as a belatedly added user's guide for the book as a whole, one that is only intelligible as such after reading the book, and, moreover, one that only functions indirectly, by supplying a series of quotes ranging from Hegel to Artaud.

As it happens, *Dissemination* lacks a preface or introduction where one would expect authorized directions for how to read and use the book. "Outwork," the book's opening essay, offers no professions of personal motivations, no programmatic remarks, and no introductions of the three texts that follow. Offhandedly, almost contemptuously, Derrida throws in a couple of general statements on the titular notion of "dissemination" between parentheses, before dispensing with such a summarizing and regulating presentation altogether (see, for instance, 7, 11). Instead, "Outwork" largely reflects upon the incongruity of the preface through a reading of ambiguous introductory gestures in writings by Hegel, Marx, Lautréamont, Novalis, and Mallarmé.

However, that absence is partially made good by the "Trance Partition" that partitions the book into separate pieces. *Trance*, I take it, here connotes both a cut or slice (as a pun on the French *tranche*) and a reconnection, transport, or crossover between diverse elements (as "trans-").[2] The separating as well as crossing feature that this text consistently highlights turns out to be ejaculation. For together the quotes form a rudimentary narrative of male orgasm.

The first quote is by Hegel, and refers to "the philosopher's stone" supposedly hidden "within Nature herself" (172). Erect and solid, that stone is the phallus. As Derrida asks (and answers), "But *what is* the stone, the stoniness of the stone? Stone is the phallus" (40, n. 39). The second quote, by Sade, begins as follows: "The Moravian brothers put people to death by tickling" (172). Elsewhere, this "tickling" condenses the frenzy of murder, suicide, and orgasm—"supreme spasm!"—in the mimicry of Pierrot, which Derrida reads in one of Mallarmé's texts, titled "Mimique" (199–201). Apparently, the phallic stone is "tickled," that is, pleasured and irritated, until it falls.

Consequently, the next and third quote, from Mallarmé, no longer alludes to the philosopher's stone, but to a *fluid* "philosopher's elixir," liquid being the element of sperm and the *pharmakon*, Derrida argues (152). In the last quote, by Artaud, Harlequin the mime introduces himself with the words "I HAVE COME / TO HAVE THEM EXTRACT FROM ME / THE LAPIS PHILOSO / PHALLUS" (286). The accompanying director's note specifies that the line be delivered with increasing silences after each segment (where I have inserted slashes). Thus, narratively, "Trance Partition" moves from the solid stone of the phallus to the liquid substance of semen, and from a hidden presence pledging the fullness of power and truth to an extraction and extension due to breaching and rupturing silences. In these terms, then, orgasm and ejaculation are theorized and thematized.

Such rupturing, silencing instances also inform the makeup of the book. *Dissemination* reads like a menu without a main course, or like a *coitus interruptus*, offering much by way of fore- and after-play, yet no proper intercourse. Indeed, the book lacks a main part to organize and hierarchize the other ones. The "Outwork" or *Hors Livre* presents itself as an appetizer or starter, as an *hors d'oeuvre*. It ceases, or rather, *seizes*, on a section densely and excessively playing on two French words. These are *la coupe*, for "cup" or "glass," as well as for "cut," "slice," or "incision"; and *le coup*, for "thrust," "kick," or "blow."

While the cup, like a grail of sorts, akin to the philosopher's stone, promises the culmination or plenitude that the preface should anticipate, the cut indicates a renewed severance; and the thrust or rhythm of the two transgresses or crosses the threshold between preface and main exposition. Thus, Derrida suggests, points of departure and points of arrival become intricately entangled: start and finish, the kick-off and the final reward of the gold cup (from *coup d'envoi* to *coupe d'or*, 58–59), foreplay and "the climax of pleasurable fulfillment" (57–58), the spermatozoon's generative cell or head and its dispensable tail.

From there, the book moves on to "Plato's Pharmacy," which is entirely dedicated to the section on writing in Plato's *Phaedrus* that its narrator offers as an appendix; as "an amusement, an *hors d'oeuvre* or rather a dessert," Derrida observes (73). The text opens with a dictionary entry listing the meanings of the Greek *kolaphos*, for "blow," "knock," or "slap." It seizes on another opaque scene, which has Plato deliberating whether or not to answer insistent knocks on his door (169–71).

Subsequently, "The Double Session" is presented as an interval or pause. It moves "into/inter/antre/in-two of" Mallarmé, lavishly punning on the French *antre*, *entre*, and *entre-deux* (181, n. 9; 182). Once more, its ending takes up the thread of the blow or thrust, now rephrased as a "throw of dice" (285). Finally, the epigraph of "Dissemination" considers the motion of a "successive bumping" (289) and then moves on to a discussion of the "triggering" that prompts discourse before it properly begins (290), and ceases at the suggestion of an urgent restart, of beginning all over again (366).

Hence, the linear, logical, and temporal progression of the book is repeatedly arrested and interrupted by cuts, tickles, strokes, thrusts, kicks, blows, knocks, slaps, bumps, and throws. All these imply, first, an indexical, gestural, and motioning hand (or foot). Additionally, this indexical extremity exerts only a severely qualified control over what it pushes or presses into motion: its movement triggers events and consequences that it cannot entirely predict or oversee. Finally, the hands-on gestures imply the chance and unpredictability of intimacy and violence, of tickling, stroking, slapping, and cutting. Hence, no doubt, the many references to qualified bodily gestures or motions in the book: fingers getting caught (63), hands being dealt (67), silent pointings being made (177), strokes being roughly marked (183), amputations being carried out (184), feet being tickled and stroked (201), leaps being made with both feet (201), strings being pulled (350).

It appears that the writing in and of *Dissemination* is, like Proust's, masturbatory. For, in "Dissemination," the shot, throw, or blow of *le coup* is given explicit ejaculatory bearings, projecting and parting "the seed" (340).[3] Hence, a frantic hand strokes, rubs, halts, slaps, motions, and seizes, without being able to control or securely time the effects it brings about, be they pleasurable or meaningful, literary or philosophical, let alone the dispersion of sperm that is projected, ejected, into the book. There, however, a sticky trace of semen persists, crossing and coursing through the pages, from essay to essay, from cover to cover. Thus, this particular kind of writing performs "dissemination" as much as it discusses it, treats it, handles it. Not merely the topic being repeatedly addressed, but also the operation through which the book proceeds, ejaculation is a highly intricate and intimate concern or burden informing the book's argument as well as its performance.

LUCKY WORD

Indeed, the title and main concept at issue in the book, dissemination, entangles semen and meaning (*sēma* is Greek for "sign"). "This word," Derrida states, has "good luck":

> It has the power economically to condense, while unwinding their web, the question of semantic differance (the new concept of writing) and seminal drift, and the impossible (monocentric, paternal, familial) reappropriation of the concept and the sperm.[4]

Hence, the felicity of the word does not depend on the simple analogy between sperm and meaning, the rather banal comparison between the scattering of semen and the proliferation of meaning. Nor does it offer a direct, oppositional critique of the ideological tendency to connect the ejaculate with significance to begin with, patriarchy's tender cherishing of the precious substance as a privileged and exemplary instance with respect to all possible relevance and signification.

Rather, dissemination attempts both to condense and to unwind the two from within their seat inside patriarchy, disturbing the monocentric, paternal, and familial appropriation of the semen and the sign. In this respect, the term threads a fine line between continuing, extending, and undoing the linkage between the two. If a heightened or exemplary significance and semen are already closely associated with each other in the patriarchal tradition, then that tradition may be strategically best attacked precisely by following up on and by following through the supposedly seminal aspects to meaning. Simultaneously, the critical strategy of dissemination remains caught up in the terms of the traditional equation, so that its luck may indeed soon run out.

A third reference of the term, next to semen and *sēma*, gives the "seminal drift" concrete spatial and temporal bearings. In *The Ear of the Other: Otobiography, Transference, Translation*, Derrida discusses the biblical story of the tower of Babel. Since the people erecting the edifice are the descendents of Shem, one of Noah's sons, he terms their "scatter[ing] . . . abroad upon the face of all the earth" (Genesis 11:9)—the very thing they wanted to prevent by building the tower ("And they said, Go to, let us build us a city and a tower, whose top may reach unto heaven; and let us make us a name, lest we be scattered abroad upon the face of the whole earth"; Genesis 11:4)—a "disschemination."[5]

A translator's note explains that the word condenses no fewer than four notions: dissemination, deschematization, de-"Shemitizing," and a derouting or diverting from a path (*chemin*, for "path" or "road") (103). It would seem that dissemination challenges autochthony, the claim to a proper and rightful place, be it of semen, of meaning, or of people. The term envisions a spatial and quasi-historic "diaspora" taking place inside and through both meaning and semen, akin to the scattering of the Shem people across the earth. If dissemination implies an unmooring of the three from their original and proper anchorage in the terms of a monocentric patriarchy, it also suggests a spermatic hyperproductivity or hyperpotency, which may well work to augment the proliferating power of the seed.[6]

However, this sense of seminal abundance or potency is countered in two ways. The particle *dis-*, from the Latin *bis* and the Greek *dis*, originally meant "two" or "in twain," as the *Oxford English Dictionary Online* specifies. Its first meaning is "apart," "asunder," "abroad," or "away" (as, for example, in "dissent"). The second meaning of the particle, however, is privative, denoting removal, aversion, negation, or reversal (as in "disown"). In a third meaning, *dis-* can also serve as an intensifier for this privative aspect, signifying "utterly" or "exceedingly"; an example is "disannul." Therefore, dissemination adds a double, intense negation to the proliferation of the sperm. Hovering between excess and privation, the outpouring of too much and of nothing at all, the term suggests a de-seeding, seminal nonproductivity or impotence, as much as the hyperbolic dispersion of seed.

In sum, then, dissemination imagines an ejaculation that extends, ruptures, crosses, augments, scatters, and negates meaning. To what precise extent, if at all, does this view of male orgasm and semen inform Derrida's understanding of masculinity, the gender so intimately at stake here, however exponentially, implicitly, extensively, or contingently? What are the consequences of this specifically disseminative view on ejaculation for the proposed or implied formation of manhood?

MASCULINITY: DESIRE AND HYSTERIA

But for the many and obvious references to ejaculation and semen, it is not immediately clear how Derrida's dissemination can criticize and reimagine traditional masculinity. *Dissemination*, the book, does not meet the matter head-on; masculinity is hardly explicitly addressed in its pages. However, the book seems burdened with the question of masculinity at several dense and convoluted instances.

The first instance where masculinity is at stake concerns the suggested visual mode of the appearance of the male body and the interests that it may compel in Derrida's reading of the Platonic dialogues in "Plato's Pharmacy." At one point in the essay, Derrida argues that Platonic ideology conjures up a vision of masculinity in the shape of the looming, ever-present, yet invisible Father. Of this father, the origin and calibration-stone for all possible meaning and value, it is impossible to speak "simply or directly," because "it is no more possible to look [him] in the face than to stare at the sun" (82). Trying to do so will only cause a blinding "bedazzlement" (82). This paternal appearance partakes of the same kind of alluring imperceptibility as Hegel's philosopher's stone hidden within nature, and as Lacan's veiled phallus. However, elsewhere in the text, seemingly unconnected to the bedazzling Father-Sun, Derrida discusses two scenes from the Platonic dialogues in which the paternal spokesman and initiator of young charges into Platonic ideology, Socrates, is himself thoroughly bedazzled by the appearance of his pupils. Hence, Socrates' own affective, sensual, and sexual body becomes visible, palpable, through and owing to the desirous looks that he casts at his students. That is why I read the scenes as an implicit critique of, or alternative to, the invisible and glittering stature of the Father-Sun that Derrida reads in Plato.

The two scenes feature in the same vein as Lacan's play with the veil and Barthes's consideration of flashes of skin, momentarily appearing and disappearing between two edges of clothing. They replace invisibility with the play of vision, with the irritability and seducement of the look. In *Charmides*, Derrida observes, the titular youth, suffering from headaches, is brought before doctor Socrates, who may be able to prescribe a cure. Yet initially, Socrates' interest lies elsewhere:

> When Critias told [Charmides] that I was the person who had the cure [*pharmakon*], he looked at me in an indescribable manner, and made as though to ask me a question. And all the people in the palaestra crowded about us, and at that moment, my good friend, I glanced through the opening of his garment, and was inflamed by his beauty. Then I could no longer contain myself. . . . But still when he asked me if I knew the cure [*pharmakon*] for the headache . . . I replied that it was a kind of leaf, which required to be accompanied by a charm [*pharmakon*] . . . (quoted in Derrida, *Dissemination*, 124–25)

Derrida notes that this scene involves "a certain *pharmakon*": the cure, the leaf and the charm, peddled to Charmides (124). His reading largely follows up on that aspect, with the text showing the original Greek *pharmakon* for "cure" or "charm" at several points, without fully taking into account the rest of the scene. For here the *pharmakon* seems uncertain: Charmides charms Socrates at least as much as the other way around.

A single glance or peep destroys Socrates' self-containment, perhaps even his "continence." "Inflamed," Socrates may be blushing, stuttering, panting, or otherwise perceptibly aroused. Yet he prescribes his cure, though "*still* . . . I replied" cannot but indicate some acute awareness of an already lost medico-paternal authority or dignity. Moreover, Charmides may well have seen it coming, as his "indescribable" look and the unasked question suggest. If so, then Charmides has not been charmed at all. The effective pharmakon at play is not the empty, preemptively discredited cure, but instead the fabric of Charmides' garment, irregularly folding and opening, compelling a glance and surprising the eye. Like the tickling, this pharmakon inflames, penetrates, contaminates, and draws out the paternal self-containment of Socrates. Additionally, it brings out the male body into a possibly vulnerable visibility. The pushy crowd may well have noticed Socrates' embarrassment in public.

Derrida links this fragment to another cloak scene from *Phaedrus*. Again, Socrates glances at the garment of one of his impressionable charges; yet what now appears is not a piece of skin, but something else. When Phaedrus attempts to deliver a speech by heart, Socrates is quick to call his bluff: "Very well, my dear fellow, but you must first show me what it is that you have in your left hand under your cloak, for I surmise that it is the actual discourse" (quoted in Derrida, *Dissemination*, 72). Hidden under Phaedrus' cloak is the written text of the speech he tries to present, but does not know entirely by heart; Socrates prompts him to produce it, to bring it out into a material visibility.

A little later, Phaedrus makes a comment on Socrates' present diversion from his usual city ways, his stubborn refusal to leave the polis (the party has retired in the countryside). Then Socrates quips, ironically,

> Yet you seem to have discovered a drug for getting me out. A hungry animal can be driven by dangling a carrot or a bit of greenstuff in front of it; similarly if you proffer me speeches bound in books I don't doubt you can cart me all around Attica, and anywhere else you please. (quoted in Derrida, *Dissemination*, 71)

Here, Socrates can only be half-ironic. The ultimate irony must be on him. For Socrates has in fact already left behind his usual city haunts, driven, like a "hungry animal," by suggestive, seductive presences, partially hidden under clothing, dangled or proffered to him. If not, he would not have noticed the book under Phaedrus' cloak to begin with. The fact that he has indicates that Socrates was already ogling Phaedrus's clothes before, perhaps hoping for another flash of skin to inflame him. As Derrida interprets, a completely "unveiled, naked" speech would not have had the same result (71). Only words that are "deferred, reserved, enveloped, rolled up" are able to seduce him, drawing "Socrates . . . out of his way" (71).

Put more strongly, I would argue, only words carried close to the male body, worn against the warm skin, are able to form an irresistible lure, an effective draw, for Socrates. Derrida hardly comments on this homoerotic aspect of the scene. But the close theatrical analogy between this scene from *Phaedrus* and the previous one from *Charmides* that Derrida does notice and point out cannot but imply an understanding of textuality, of writing, that revolves around promising and deferred, dazzling, appearances of the male body. The scene from *Charmides* prompts the whole discourse on the true remedy that is temperance; the one from *Phaedrus* triggers the consideration and ultimate condemnation of writing. In both cases, an instantaneous glance at what is partially hidden under a cloak, be it skin or text, skin as text, or text as skin, ushers in lengthy discursive excursions.

Thus the two scenes, present and intimately connected in Derrida's exposition, propose the entanglement of the male body and philosophical meaning in a dazzling texture of folding and visuality. The fabric of writing enfolds, folds around, the possibility of the appearance of the male body, alternately drawing toward it and withdrawing from it. With respect to its withdrawing aspect, Socrates quickly regains his confidence and promotes dialectical wisdom as a panacea in *Charmides*; in *Phaedrus*, Socrates eventually condemns the same written text that he could not but notice under Phaedrus' garment.

The fact that Derrida, too, is drawn to these cloak scenes, yet does not follow up on their consequences with respect to masculinity and sexuality, implies that his own reading, to this precise extent, follows in Socrates' footsteps. The opening out of the male body into textuality—its theatrical production, in Thomas's vein, bringing out on the scene, or staging—allows for his own insistent and consistent scrutiny of orgasm, ejaculation, and semen throughout *Dissemination*. Perhaps, then, the Father-Author cannot be directly seen as he hides behind the bedazzling and blinding sun. But that does not preclude the fact that he himself, from behind the glittering light, looks or glances at men's bodies with a mixture of curiosity, irritation, and desire, so that he is nevertheless drawn out into a cautious, yet vulnerable, visibility, bedazzled rather than bedazzling.

The second juncture in the text of *Dissemination* where masculinity seems to be at stake is far less clear. This lack of clarity may be symptomatic. At the third restart of "The Double Session," Derrida specifies that its beginning, a listing stating the essay's programmatic move *into*, *inter*, *antre*, and *in-two* (of) Mallarmé, should be "pronounce[d] without writing" in order to make the most of the French pun (*l'entre*, *l'antre*, *l'entre-deux*) (182). A long note shows that Derrida sees it coming: his detractors will gleefully point out his dependence on the spoken voice after all (181–82, n. 8). Tersely, he cites from his own work, arguing that it was never his point to privilege writing over speech to begin with.

This largely imagined reaction is "symptomatic," Derrida goes on, "and belongs to a certain type":

> Freud recounts that when he was having trouble gaining acceptance for the possibility of masculine hysteria, he encountered, among those primary sorts of resistance which do not reveal mere foolishness or lack of culture, the resistance of a surgeon who *expressly* told him: "But, my dear fellow, how can you pronounce such

> absurdities? *Hysteron* (*sic*) signifies 'uterus.' How then can a man be hysterical?" . . . This note, this reference, the choice of this example are placed here merely to herald a certain *out-of-placeness* of language: we are thus introduced into what is *supposed* to be found *behind* the hymen: the hystera . . . , which exposes itself only by transference and simulacrum—by mimicry. (182, n. 8)

The precise reference to Freud is not given. Hence, the parenthetic "*sic*" may have been inserted either by Freud or by Derrida. It is added, presumably, because *hysteron* does not mean "uterus"; *hystera* does. *Hysteron* signifies that which is "lower," "behind," "later," or "weaker." Thus, I take it, the surgeon betrays his own symptomatic and hysterical attachment to the view that women are lower, inferior, and hysterical in his disavowal of the possibility of masculine hysteria. Here, hysteria entails the frantic and stubborn clinging to the received oppositions between men and women, and between speech and writing, as based on the hierarchization of what is supposedly upper and lower, before and behind, earlier and later, stronger and weaker.

In contrast, the recognition of the "*out-of-placeness of language*" resituates both language and gender at the "hymen" itself, the boundary, thin sheet, or screen, separating outside from inside. The hidden interiority this hymen presupposes only "exposes itself" in the transferences, simulations, and mimicries that are issued at its reflexive, bouncing surface, including that of the surgeon's. The surgeon's mistaken recourse to the Greek nevertheless partakes of Derrida's own favorite game of etymological speculation. "[T]he presumed origin of a concept or the imagined etymology of a word," Derrida argues, is often held up to ward off its reconsideration "without any regard for the fact that what was being utilized was precisely the most vulgar sign most heavily overladen with history and unconscious motivations" (182, n. 8). How then can this same judgment not apply to Derrida's own coinage of "dissemination," playing on semen, *sēma*, and Shem, and escape from the vulgar, historic, and unconscious word game that repeats rather than undoes patriarchal ideology?[7]

It cannot. Hence, the thrust of the argument can only be that men do not need a womb to be hysterical; it suffices that they ejaculate. Elsewhere, again in a note, Derrida writes that "dissemination [the operation? the concept? the book?] reads, if one looks closely, as a sort of womb," now extending the surgeon's projection (49, n. 47).[8] That is to say, *Dissemination* figures in a thematic of masculine hysteria. To the extent that it pits swarming semen against bouncing hymen, to the extent that it etymologically—read: historically, vulgarly, unconsciously, ideologically—connects semen with signification, with its excess and its loss, the book itself is a hysterical text. To push the point, here is another rendition of the surgeon's expressed sentiment, now as returned to Derrida: "But, my dear fellow, how can you pronounce such absurdities? *Dissemination* (*sic*) signifies 'semen.' How then can a woman be implicated in dissemination?" Masculinity cannot but show itself, entering into textuality as a mode or form of hysteria.

The pun on *hysteron/hystera* participates in the first of three rhetorical strategies I want to present together as the third and last way in which masculinity is implicitly but insistently at stake in *Dissemination*. This first strategy entails the flipping of temporal, spatial, and apparential bearings, such as between beginning/ending, before/after, back/front, head/tail, origin/aftereffect, and so on. If this strategy works to unhinge the anatomy of the book, its corpus, it must also do so with regard to male anatomy. For example, unlike the properly differentiated body of the *logos* or living speech, as calibrated in the Platonic dialogues, the male body has "neither head nor tail," Derrida writes (79). It may be moved in parts, irrespective of the whole, and from the outside, when the responsive penis becomes rebellious, disobedient, and maddened (154). Additionally, Mallarmé's generative or germinative titles do not so much stage the seminal "head," Derrida notes, but rather display the fleeting wink or flick of the spermatic "tailpiece" (178).

The second strategy involves a metonymic lateralization: the "histological" move from "anything upright" to the horizontal threads connected to it or supporting it; or, from the vertical phallus to the lateral text. The meaning of the Greek word *histos*, given as the epigraph to "Plato's Pharmacy," metonymically moves from a ship's "mast" to the "sail" or "canvas" attached to it (63). In Mallarmé's poetic "wet dream," for instance, the "masthead ... blots itself into abysses of lost veils, sails, and children" (267). An uncredited quote in "Dissemination" specifies the operation as follows:

> In place of phalli, says Herodotus, they came up with other objects about a cubit long, which had a thread attached; these were carried by women who, by pulling on the threads, were able to make the objects stand upright, a reproduction of the male genital organ, almost as big as the rest of the body. (341)

Note the augmentation of scale: from the approximate length of a forearm ("cubit") to nearly the size of a body—until, of course, the women let go of the ropes. In these cases, the vertical masts and phalli are reframed in a textuality that both erects them and pulls them down again. Thus the stature of masculinity is thoroughly textualized, made out to be dependent on the erecting, extending, and paying out threads that manipulate and move it around like a puppet.

The third strategy consists of the breaching and broaching [*entamer*] of anything supposed to be solid: phallus, column, or stone.[9] These are being cut up and passed around like so many pieces of cake. For example, "Plato's Pharmacy" refers to the Egyptian myth of the dismemberment of Osiris. Osiris' fourteen body parts are scattered to the wind and, eventually, reassembled by his spouse Isis, save for the penis that is swallowed by a fish (90). Throughout the book, furthermore, stones, pillars, and columns are continuously reduced to "gravel," to scattered "pebbles" (e.g., 358).

In these three related ways—the male body appearing and disappearing into textuality, the hysterical projection of masculinity's burden onto femininity, and the various rhetorical strategies that suggest a reconfiguration of male anatomy—masculinity is intimately, yet implicitly, at stake in *Dissemination*. Nevertheless, the notable underthematization of gender in the book in relation to the marked overthematization of ejaculation and semen can well be said to accommodate a renewed mystification of the seed, in which semen still features as something highly significant, thus continuing its exemplary status with regard to meaning.

At the same time, the enactment of the masturbatory dissemination in the book by Derrida's narrator (as I have argued with reference to the rupturing instances that revolve on ejaculatory blows, strokes, and shots, as well as to the book's recurring and insistent trace of viscous semen) may suggest that the book and the concept speak most eloquently to gender when they obliquely, abstractly, mutely, articulate it by gesturing or motioning toward it, by simulating, miming, or acting it out. In the following sections of this chapter, I inquire into the co-implications of masculinity and dissemination as intimated, propositionally, performatively, or gesturally, in the four essays of *Dissemination*.

Dissemination does not offer a single perspective on meaning, masculinity, and ejaculation. Instead, it treats this tangled knot of values from several different angles. The book reflects on the liquid element of sperm, and hence, on its infiltrating, contaminating, and penetrative propensity: its "pharmakology" ("Plato's Pharmacy"). Furthermore, it considers the numerical aspect of semen, swerving between singularity and innumerability ("Dissemination"), as well as its color, an opalescent white that Derrida views as layered and folded ("The Double Session").[10] In addition, it offers a critique of the generative power inhering in the single cell of sperm, its head ("Outwork"). These considerations will surface in the remainder of this chapter. I will begin with Derrida's understanding of the mimed motion of an androgynous, but not sexless, writing performance that is orgasmic and spasmodic, as read by him in the poetry of Mallarmé ("The Double Session").

SUPREME SPASM

"The Double Session," the book's third text, suggests the relevance of a specific constellation of the phallus, the hymen, and semen for the poetry of Mallarmé. Through Derrida's interpretation, however, these all-too-familiar elements, which readily suggest a thematic or dynamic of marriage, intercourse, and consummation, are unrecognizably reconceived.

When Derrida detects a "*phallic* allusion" in the many pens, pennae, birds, beaks, wings, feathers, quills, and needles that feature in the poet's oeuvre, he quickly notes that these innumerably multiplied avatars of the phallus are never able to penetrate a hidden interiority (274, 242, 240). Instead, they string, tack, scratch, and bounce on and against a malleable, yet stubbornly impenetrative, surface (240). The phallic penna merely "plies" this surface, "applies it, stitches it, pleats it, and duplicates it" (272). In "a sort of lateral movement," moreover, this particularly Mallarmean phallus-as-penna cannot mark or demarcate its presence—it can only drift and spin. Like a ballerina's pointed toe, it endlessly turns on its point, its motion suspended between where it presently "is," whence it came, and to where it moves (241).

The surface that both grounds and blocks the phallus's repetitive motions is the hymen. This hymen, however, is never broken, crossed, or pierced (215). Hence, the Mallarmean hymen does not offer access to the hidden interiority it usually presumes. Like a mirror, the hymen blocks and bounces back the gestures issued at it, returning them to sender as so many simulacra or mimicries (206). As a textile membrane, tissue, or pellicle, it is folded by and enfolds the needlework applications of the phallic penna, translating them into the many curtains, screens, and veils that accompany the phallus in Mallarmé's texts (213, 180). Denoting both "virginity" and "marriage," and thus entangling the opposition between the two, the hymen stands as a pure and irrevocable medium between fusion and confusion, between a prospective desire and its eventual fulfillment (209). Consequently, the semen never reaches its goal or telos behind the hymen. Rather, it gets lost, caught up, in the intricate pleats and folds that make up the hymen's surface (267). At most, the semen remains as a pearly and glittering "lustre," multiplying and fracturing the singular masculine presence it should embody, "skimming" and "frothing" against the hymen (244, 267).[11]

Hence, the consummation of marriage and intercourse that should, temporally and spatially, move from a before, then through, and ultimately behind or after the hymen is entirely suspended. In Mallarmé, Derrida argues, the trajectory of consummation is resituated, leveled, flattened, or lateralized, on and against the mediating surface of the hymen. If there is any consummation left, then that consummation is, indeed, "all-consuming," affecting the phallus and the semen as much as it does the hymen and the womb (213). In this suspended spatiality and temporality, Derrida avers, orgasm takes place.

In "The Double Session," orgasm crops up when Derrida addresses a short prose text by Mallarmé, entitled *Mimique*. The piece is reproduced in full at the opening of the essay. Though the text does not specifically mention orgasm, it refers in a quote to the contiguous hymen, "tainted with vice yet sacred, between desire and fulfillment, perpetration and remembrance" (175). Additionally, Mallarmé's narrator explicitly refers to another text, Paul Margueritte's *Pierrot Murderer of His Wife*, in which the "supreme spasm" of orgasm is intricately at stake. Thus, Derrida takes this second text as a relevant intertext or quasi-internal "graft" (202).

A written account of a mimed, hence mute, performance, Margueritte's text recounts the murder of Columbine by her husband Pierrot. Suspecting her of adultery, Pierrot kills Columbine by tickling her feet. As Pierrot acts out both parts in his performance, the crime is mimed "doubly," androgynously, Derrida comments (201). After her spasmodic death, Columbine rises from the dead and, taking her revenge, in turn tickles Pierrot to death. At the conclusion of the mimed drama, her portrait erupts in raucous laughter. Margueritte's rendition of the moment of simultaneous pleasure and death runs as follows:

> She (he) bursts out in a true, strident, mortal laugh; sits bolt upright; tries to jump out of bed; and still her (his) feet are dancing, tickled, tortured, epileptic. It is the death throes. She (he) rises up once or twice—supreme spasm!—opens her (his) mouth for one last curse, and throws back, out of the bed, her (his) drooping head and arms. Pierrot becomes Pierrot again. At the foot of the bed, he is still scratching, worn out, gasping, but victorious. . . . (quoted in Derrida, *Dissemination*, 201)

Note the subtle difference between the unique, singular, and instantaneous spasm, and its temporization through iterability: the mime "rises up *once or twice*."

Working this scene into Mallarmé's *Mimique* and back again, Derrida undoes an extensive series of oppositions, such as masculinity and femininity, speech and writing, intercourse and masturbation, action and language, present and past, and reality and representation. However, these oppositions do not simply disappear or amalgamate into something else. Rather, the dynamic of the hymen and the spasm forces the terms together, makes them connect or interact, and then returns them as intertwined and entangled, yet still different:

> It is the difference between the two terms that is no longer functional. The confusion or consummation of this hymen eliminates the spatial heterogeneity of the two poles in the "supreme spasm," the moment of dying laughing.... Thanks to the confusion and the continuity of the hymen, and not in spite of it... difference inscribes itself without any decidable poles, without any independent, irreversible poles. (209–10)

Oppositional differences, thought of as wide apart, as spatially distinct and separate, are reinscribed as interdependent and reversible, repositioned at the hymen or in the spasm.

Playing the roles of Pierrot and Columbine, murderer and victim, the mimic is poised and wavers between gendered opposites (201). And, since there is only the one actor, the one mime, who switches between two parts, the performance simulates both masturbation and intercourse, both suicide and murder (201). Because the mimicry proceeds in utter silence, but can only be reproduced and accessed by Margueritte, Mallarmé, and Derrida in the shape of a written text, the mime's act hovers between silence and language (175). Mallarmé remarks on the scene as a "stilled ode" or "mute soliloquy," framed between two silences: from its opening phrase ("Silence, sole luxury after rhymes") to the conclusion of "there reigns a silence still, the condition and delight of reading." This silence the poet attempts, dares, to write, to "translate!" (quoted in Derrida, *Dissemination*, 175).

Since Pierrot only acts insofar as he simulates actions, and because that simulation wavers between self and other, and between a silly pleasure and a serious death, he does not actually *do* anything. Derrida writes, "nothing happens that could be grasped as a present event, a reality, an activity, etc. The Mime doesn't *do* anything; there is no act (neither murderous nor sexual), no acting agent and hence no patient. Nothing *is*" (216). Neither does the mime play his parts on the basis of a preexisting text or script that predetermines them. Margueritte's and Mallarmé's writings are put down only *after* the performance has been completed. As Mallarmé specifies, the scene is "composed and set down" by Pierrot himself *as* he enacts it (quoted in Derrida, *Dissemination*, 175). Thus, Derrida quips, "In the beginning of this mime was neither the deed nor the word," but the embodied *gesture* in between the two (198).

Consequently, the mime's medium is a purely gestural writing. As "white as the yet unwritten page," notes Mallarmé, the mime, "by simulacrum, writes in the paste of his make-up, upon the page he is," Derrida explains (175, 195). Derrida concludes: "The Mime ought only to write himself on the white page he is; he must *himself* inscribe *himself* through gestures and plays of facial expressions. At once page and quill, Pierrot is both passive and active, matter and form, the author, the means, and the raw material of his melodrama" (198).

Additionally, the mime renders moot the ontological and temporal opposition between a thing and its representation. According to Derrida, this hierarchical opposition underlies Plato's understanding of mimesis. That is why he links up Mallarmé's *Mimique* with the section from Plato's *Philebus* that views pictures and images as secondary (175). Secondary, because, to Plato's mind, the thing itself comes before its representation, both ontologically and temporarily (192). Hence, Platonic mimesis, Derrida claims, preserves the primacy, anteriority, and precedence of the thing (192).

However, the mime's mimicry disturbs this mimetic hierarchy. For the act has already taken place when Pierrot mimes it, which, in fact, implies that he should be dead, killed in return by Columbine (200). Yet he enacts the crime in the present, as it is happening, and not through a retrospective narration. At the same time, the miming anticipates and carries out Pierrot's own spasm, his death by orgasm. Like Mallarmé's hymen, then, the performance stands between "desire and fulfillment, perpetration and remembrance: here anticipating, there recalling, in the future, in the past, *under the false appearance of a present*" (quoted in Derrida, *Dissemination*, 175).

If the present and presence of the mimicry merely constitute a "false appearance," then the mime's simulations cannot be relegated to an anterior reality. Derrida concludes: "What is marked in this hymen . . . is only a series of temporal differences without any central present, without a present of which the past and the future would be but modifications" (210). Thus, the hymen and the spasm are temporal, do occur in time, but do not allow this temporality to be securely distinguished and differentiated. Without the temporal hierarchy between (primary, preceding) thing and (secondary, belated) representation, the distinction between these opposites falls, too. Perpetually, the mime's expressions and gestures allude to something, to narrative characters and events; that is his business. However, this allusive something does not come before, and does not remain after, the immanent play of the expressions and the gestures. Additionally, the crucial spasm suggests both the tender and the violent, the playful and the serious, the pleasurable and the murderous (210). Hence, the mime alludes without breaking the "mirror" that separates representation from reality, "without reaching beyond the looking glass" (206). The act of Pierrot, Mallarmé writes, "is confined to a perpetual allusion without breaking the ice or the mirror" (quoted in Derrida, *Dissemination*, 175). This "speculum," Derrida adds, "reflects no reality; it produces mere 'reality-effects'" (206). Ultimately, what Pierrot mimes is nothing but imitation itself (219).

When these oppositions make contact with each other, are flattened onto each other, and rubbed together (male/female, self/other, speech/silence, event/nonevent, active/passive, past/present/future, thing/representation) through and due to the hymeneal spasm, what results is a curious condition or state, which Mallarmé describes as a flowing "Dream," a "fiction," and "a pure medium" (quoted in Derrida, *Dissemination*, 175). Derrida understands this dreamlike "medium," which he characterizes as a kind of "waking wet dream," as a "middle," a state not reducible to the either/or of binary oppositions, as well as an "element" in its own right: "ether, matrix, means" (211, 283). Presumably, the grammatical meaning of medium, as a self-reflexivity in between the active and the passive voice, is also implied. This state can only be understood, oxymoronically, as an immanent medium, as specified in the three senses above; immanent, in the sense that this medium does not enable communication or transfer between the oppositional poles, but relocates them, flattens them, at its surface. Hence, this superficial medium does not translate or convert the one to the other in a three-dimensional spatiality, but entangles them two-dimensionally.

This immanent medium allows for the articulation of an "ecstatic hilarity," ushering in what Derrida describes as a "purely gestural, silent sequence, the inauguration of a writing of the body" (201, 199). Once more, here is Pierrot the mime, as appearing in Margueritte's *Pierrot Murderer of His Wife*:

> Ow! that hurts! (He strokes his foot) Oof! That hurts! It's not serious, it's better already. (He keeps on stroking and tickling his foot.) Ha! ha! No, it makes me laugh. Ah! (quoted in Derrida, *Dissemination*, 201)

As I have argued, Derrida repeats—that is, mimes, simulates, or motions—this same gestural, indexical hilarity in the writing of *Dissemination*, the book that, at so many instances, ceases and seizes in passages that, densely and obscurely, play on strokes, tickles, blows, and pushes. Hence, it is the body, a body, that is doing the talking, or the writing, there.

Derrida draws on the mime's simulation of an orgasmic spasm in order to understand writing and literature anew. In doing so, he cannot but offer a specific understanding of male orgasm. First, Derrida undoes the "colonial" imagination that rules ejaculation: the phallus pierces the hymenal veil, and, in depositing the seed in the womb, takes up occupancy there. This view of things establishes a consummation in which man consumes woman, forging a marriage based upon the stabilized hierarchization of opposites. But now this constellation is recast as the frantic needlework applications and ballerina pirouettes of the phallic avatars on a surface that will not give; that instead enfolds these movements and their ejaculations in a multifaceted, bouncing, and lustrous textuality; and that only works to divert, fracture, and return the presence they would establish.

Second, the flaunted instant of the orgasmic spasm can only be "supreme," because it is internally riven by iterative, uncontrollable motions. The moment is rendered as highly significant and calibrated as a privileged mode of culmination; however, it is simultaneously voided by rupturing silences and non-sense. Orgasm is an act that does not quite happen, a simulation that remains immanent. It is neither something that one does, nor something that befalls one, but something in between that offers no secure bearings on the ideological active/passive scale. Throwing oneself back on the self, orgasm is masturbatory; yet it cannot proceed without some other, real or imagined, or something in between. And this other cannot be orgasmically possessed, as little, in fact, as can the orgasmic self. Happening in the now, seemingly pledging a pure present, orgasm is nevertheless sandwiched between anticipation and retrospection, about to happen and already over, and caught between its instantaneity and its iterative displacement.

Finally, Derrida and Mallarmé's spasmodic medium can be brought to bear on other representations of orgasm and ejaculation, exposing the ways in which these ambivalently acknowledge the immanent medium of orgasm, and/or attempt to disavow it by restoring and recuperating the entangled oppositions. Narrative film pornography's cum shot comes to mind here, the genre that shows "the real thing" that can only be simulated, mimed, and written; that narrates the supreme moment that is immediately repeated and looped. Both the reality and the narrativity of orgasm are then resituated in an excessively gendered constellation that separates the active from the receptive, the abjecting from the abjected. If this piece is largely about the immanence of orgasm, the next work I consider is about its material counterpart, other, and effect: liquid sperm.

SEMEN AS PHARMAKON

In "Plato's Pharmacy," Derrida argues that Plato's Socrates is consistently stern on liquid substances. Fluids such as perfume and paint add a false, sensory appearance to something that, because of them, can no longer be known in its verifiable essence; perfume and paint hinder the true knowledge of a thing by offering up diverting and seductive smells or colors (129, 136, 142).

This condemnation also counts for ink. In Plato's mind, according to Derrida, writing departs from the quest for truth that ideally takes place in the live and exclusive conversation between men, between philosophers and their pupils. Teaching should not proceed through the reading of written texts, because these can be made out to mean just about anything to anyone, and be put to indiscriminate uses. Without the living voice of the author or teacher to guide and correct him whenever necessary, the inexperienced reader of a text may be led astray (77, 81). True, a written text may serve as a handy support for one's memory. But that memory aid might also overrule the preexisting knowledge that can only be "remembered," brought up and out, in and through the conversation between wise men (Plato's *anamnesis*) (112). Hence, wisdom should be taken to, and learned by, heart.

In contrast, writing, the circulation of books and pamphlets, is democratic (144). Thus writing undermines the philosophers' aristocracy that Plato imagines. Rather than the exclusive conversation between wise men that the dialogues themselves mimic, Derrida argues, writing is continuously relegated to the "orgy, debauchery, flea-market, fair" or "bazaar," where indiscriminate sexual, commercial, and social contacts take place (145). And these, he adds, cannot proceed without "some sort of urgency or outpouring of sperm" (150).

Sperm, then, becomes specifically and especially urgent in Derrida's text in the opposition and rivalry between two homosocial arrangements: on the one hand, the steady and aristocratic friendship between dialectical philosophers and their pupils, and, on the other hand, the promiscuous and democratic exchanges between men at the orgy or marketplace. At stake in the Platonic judgment on writing and ink, then, are masculinity and authority, or rather, a senior masculinity based on epistemological authority, on a supposedly privileged access to truth. Rather than reading on their own and hanging around at the marketplace, the young men of the polis should attend philosophical lectures and take the orally delivered lessons to heart. In what Derrida terms the "politico-familial violence and perversion" of Platonic ideology, the control of teachers over their pupils, fathers over their sons, older men over younger men, must be rigorously maintained (150).

At the same time, Derrida claims, Plato depends on what he condemns. The judgment on writing is delivered *in* writing, *as* writing. In addition, Plato's argument, at critical junctures, takes recourse precisely in metaphors of writing: for instance, when he claims that the dialectical lessons should be "written in the soul" of the philosopher's pupils (148). The same remedy or medicine for forgetfulness that writing initially seemed to be, but that was quickly revealed to be a mere poison with respect to the joint search for truth, hence turns out to be an integral and essential element of dialectical philosophy and pedagogy. When Plato characterizes writing as a *pharmakon* (Greek for both "medicine" and "poison"), he cannot but bring into play the ambivalences inherent in his own teaching, condemning and promoting writing as a proper medium for the transfer of knowledge. What is excluded is already inevitably, essentially and necessarily, included in the philosophical and pedagogical stance that Plato himself advocates.

Listing the various liquids discussed so far, Derrida characterizes the infiltrating propensity of the pharmakon as follows:

> Sperm, water, ink, paint, perfumed dye: the *pharmakon* always penetrates like a liquid; it is absorbed, drunk, introduced into the inside . . . soon to invade it and inundate it with its medicine, its brew, its drink, its poison. In liquid, opposites are more easily mixed. Liquid is the element of the *pharmakon*. (152)

Here, Derrida notes a structural equivalence between the fluids: all are termed pharmaka throughout the Platonic dialogues. However, this pharmakological equivalency has several consequences that Derrida does not explicitly address. First, the comparison between sperm and paint or perfume implies that sperm, too, must be sensorially attractive, appealing, seductive. Second, the analogy between ink and sperm suggests that the latter must have a rhetorical status and function as well, similar to the ambiguously condemned writing. Apparently, semen argues, plays, leads on, persuades. Finally, the series of pharmakological equivalences implies that sperm, again like writing, forms an integral and essential element or medium within dialectical teaching. Somehow, semen is as urgent in the philosophical teaching of pupils by their teachers as it is in the frowned-upon marketplace or orgy.

That this is so becomes clear when Derrida juxtaposes Plato's condemnation of homosexuality in *Laws* with the idealization of dialectical teaching in patently homoerotic terms in *Phaedrus*. In the former, Plato argues that one should abstain from "congress with our own sex," because of its "deliberate murder of the race and its wasting of the seed of life on a stony and rocky soil" (quoted in Derrida, *Dissemination*, 152–53). Immediately, he cautions that this particular law may not quite impress the young. "Yet should some young and lusty bystander of exuberant virility overhear us as we propose it," Plato concedes, "he might probably denounce our enactments as impracticable folly and make the air ring with his clamor" (quoted in Derrida, *Dissemination*, 153). As *Phaedrus* makes clear, however, the laughter of this lusty bystander may soon die down, once he realizes that the point of the matter is the extension and maintenance of paternal control over him by way of the penetrative sperm or seed:

> The dialectician selects a soul of the right type, and in it he plants and sows his words founded on knowledge . . . words which in-

> stead of remaining barren contain a seed whence new words grow up in new characters, whereby the seed is vouchsafed immortality, and its possessor the fullest measure of blessedness that man can attain unto. (quoted in Derrida, *Dissemination*, 155)

Hence, rather than reading by themselves and cruising around at the market, young men should wholeheartedly swallow the philosopher's sperm and allow themselves to be impregnated, presumably guaranteeing their teachers' blessedness and immortality rather than their own.

Yet the ringing laughter of the bystander may also continue, even increase, as soon as he realizes that the philosopher's stern professions boil down to a competitive attempt at his seduction, a transparent bid for his favors. Implicated in the attempt to control the bodies of the young is a measure of awareness of the qualified controllability of the bodies of the teachers. In contrast to the written text, Derrida argues, speech or *logos* is characterized as a living organism in the Platonic dialogues: it is or has "a differentiated body proper, with a center and extremities, joints, a head, and feet" (79).

The male body, however, is precisely not such a properly differentiated body. Philosophically and ideologically, it would be preferable if the male body were only to be put into motion in its entirety and from within itself, if it were to act and react in a formation both totalized and automotive. But the male body allows for a partial and externally exerted motion. From Plato's *Timaeus*: "worst of all is that which moves the body, when at rest, in parts only and by some agency alien to it" (quoted in Derrida, *Dissemination*, 100). In parts, the male body may respond to alien agencies, and this makes it both internally other and fragmentable.

Consequently, the penis and semen, the hallmarks of masculinity, do not fit the proper, organicist, logocentric body, either. Again, from *Timaeus*:

> The marrow . . . we have named semen. And the semen, having life and becoming endowed with respiration, produces in that part in which it respires a lively desire of emission, and thus creates in us the love of procreation. Wherefore also in men the organ of generation becoming rebellious and masterful, like an animal disobedient to reason, and maddened with the sting of lust, seeks to gain absolute sway. (quoted in Derrida, *Dissemination*, 154)

This suggests, finally, that the ultimate pharmakon disturbing the (phallo)-logocentric authority and stature of masculinity is, precisely, the male body itself.

SINGULAR PLURAL

The differentiation and fragmentation of the male body continues in the last essay of *Dissemination*. "Dissemination" considers sperm numerically: Does semen embody singularity or multiplicity? What is sperm's elusive number? Philippe Sollers's *Numbers*, Derrida's object-text in the chapter, offers a heterogeneous narrative that proceeds by numbers rather than by events. Its sections, Derrida observes, follow each other up on the basis of two numerical series: the one periodical, moving from 1 to 4, the other linear, running from 1 to 100 (307).[12]

Derrida's interest in this aspect of the novel is clear. Relating to each other rather than to anything external to them, the graphic numbers have no obvious or absolute signified or referent. "This is why," Derrida claims, "they don't show anything, don't tell anything, don't represent anything, aren't trying to say anything" (350). Additionally, the nonphonetic numerals also work to disturb phonocentrism. Graphic numericity, Derrida argues, "suspends the voice, dislocates self-proximity, a living presence that would hear itself represented by speech" (331). However, the living voice is not simply done away with.

For the sequenced numbers compel their melodic chanting out loud in a sort of song, "beat[ing] out the measures of all the marks in *Numbers*" (331). Hence, the numbers not only expropriate the voice by graphically suspending it, but also operate "*within* voice" itself, extending and spacing out the voice into a resonant bodily cadence, melody, or pounding (333). This thrusting rhythm "gives voice," Derrida states, "to an authorless voice, a phonic tracing that no ideal signified or 'thought' can entirely cover" (332).

Thus, Derrida continues, Sollers's numbered and chanted sequences reinscribe the presence of the atomistic "|" as both "I" and "1" (305). Now both singularity and individuality must take leave from "the 'primitive mythical unity' " that they assume (305, 304). Moreover, the extension and sequentiality by and through the numbers also fractures the supposed singularity of the phallus and the semen. In the following quote, Derrida concretely imagines the presence of the atomistic "|" in the shape of an erection, which appears as proximate to the hand that would rule it and to the eye that beholds it:

> What is called "present"—that which erects itself freely before me, upright, close at hand, that which is appearing—can be given as such, as a pure upsurge owing to nothing, only in a mythical discourse in which difference would be erased. If account be taken of what divides it, cuts it up, and folds it back in its very triggering, then the present is no longer simply present. (303)

This erectile differentiation, division, intercutting, or refolding returns in the many ballistic references in "Dissemination": unpredictable triggerings, recoilings, ricochets, repercussions, reverberations (303, 305, 307, 325). It also looms large in the allusions to castration, circumcision, and decapitation; for example, in Sollers's severed heads brandished and toted around on poles, his rows of "pointed teeth" (302). Finally, it affects the rigidity and verticality of the various architectural, textual, and physical columns. Each monolithic pillar is reduced to so many scattered pebbles, to "gravel" (358). The columns that make up a text are endlessly refolded, grafted, and interspersed. In another uncredited reference to Freud, spinal and phallic columns are lateralized and moved in intimate relation to others: "The column of faeces, the penis, and the baby are all three solid bodies; they all three, by forcible entry or expulsion, stimulate a membraneous passage . . ." (340).

Hence, "Dissemination" proposes a view of ejaculation that allows for no atomism or singularity. Ejaculation comes to operate as the "shot/throw/blow [*le coup*]" that parts the sperm in the very moment that "*projects* it" (304). Breaking the path for "the" seed, Derrida claims, ejaculation "produces (itself) and advances only in the plural." Thus, semen embodies "a singular plural, which no single origin will ever have preceded," either discursively, textually, or "in the case of some 'real' seed-sowing" (304). Indeed, the essay's central invocation is to try "to think the unique in the plural" (365).

Again, Derrida's argument implies the entering, the opening out, of the male body into textuality. This mode of appearance, Derrida suggests, also involves and affects the reader (290). It does not entail a kind of full disclosure, a straightforward revelation (291). Bodily, affectively, and resonantly partaking of the numerical cadence that structures and fractures Sollers's novel, the reader can no longer situate himself apart from and before a text that is already written, completed. "Because [the reader's] job is to put things on stage," Derrida writes, "he is on stage himself, he puts himself on stage. The tale is thereby addressed to the reader's body, which is put by things on stage, itself" (290). In mounting the text, the reader is simultaneously mounted *by* the text. There, he finds himself "not displayed, but given play, not staged but engaged, not demonstrated but mounted" (291).

Ultimately, then, the reader cannot reappear as the text's *deus ex machina*. For he himself enters into the textual machinery, "[p]lugging it in and triggering it off" (292). Each textual and anatomical term, "germ," or "member," each graphic and physical part, any and each of these plugs, cogs, and shunts, Derrida writes, "depends at every moment on its place and is entrained, like all the parts of a machine, into an ordered series of displacements, slips, transformations, and recurrences that cut out or add a member in every proposition that has gone before" (300). Such a textual triggering, then, envisions a male body that is plastic, fragmentable, and responsive, entrained in a mechanical motion that is ordered, yet never hierarchized.

THE SPERM'S TAIL AS SUPPLEMENT

Throughout *Dissemination*, Derrida questions the originating power supposed to inhere in a single cell or germ of textual seed, whether this generative nugget is presented in or as a title, a preface, or an epigraph: "The staging of a title, a first sentence, an epigraph, a pretext, a preface, a single germ will never make a beginning. It *was* indefinitely dispersed" (43). "The Double Session," for example, reflects on the double suspension of the title, both put above or over the text as its putative head, chief, center, or *archon*, and put in suspension, cordoned off from the text by a white interval (178, 179). The function of the title as a productive resource for Mallarmé may be widely acknowledged, Derrida claims, but the poet himself already remarks on the title as "the invitation proffered by the wide white space expressly left at the top of the page as if to mark a separation from everything, the already read elsewhere . . . " (quoted in Derrida, *Dissemination*, 180). From the text, Derrida continues, the title is to expect and receive "all—or nothing" (179). Hence, he reconceives the titular, seminal head of a text as the fleeting wink, flick, or motion of a textual tailpiece (178). Front and back, center and margin, high and low flip places.

What Derrida describes as the "question of the preface as *seed*" comes up in "Outwork," *Dissemination*'s opening essay (44). Two of Derrida's cases are specifically relevant here. The first concerns the Comte de Lautréamont's *Songs of Maldoror*. In this text, Derrida finds a "hybrid" or "renegade" preface, which cannot be subsumed into the greater project of the book (44). Instead, the preface overrules the book (36). In the sixth song, Lautréamont's narrator discounts the previous five, by far the greater part of the book, as mere "frontispiece," a "preliminary explanation" (quoted in Derrida, *Dissemination*, 36).

The sixth song itself, however, fails to make good on the expectations thus raised. According to Derrida, it merely offers a sudden cessation of the narrative, as well as the figure of an encroaching textuality in the image of a spider. Hence, the *Songs* enact a "totally different partition" (43). They replace the anatomical boundary between preface and main text with elusively placed "effects of opening and closing" (36). This alternative placement or topology follows on the many gratings, columns, squares, and stones that punctuate Lautréamont's book (39). These work to extend and displace the monolithic presence suggested by the stone and the phallus, Derrida claims.

In a lengthy note, Derrida reflects on the solidity and verticality of the phallic stone as the twin effects of a mitigated male anxiety in a discussion with Freud's reading of the Medusa myth (39–41, n. 39). Her head crowned with coiling snakes, Freud's Medusa reveals the absence of the phallus on her body and, in doing so, turns her petrified victim to stone (41). In that way, the absence of the phallus is acknowledged as well as mitigated, since the stiffening at least reassures the viewer of the enduring presence of his own penis, even though in death (41). In Freud's reading, then, the solidity and uprightness of the phallus are seen as the effects of fear and consolation. Yet, Derrida obtusely adds, "[d]issemination would always arrive on the scene to threaten signification" (41). How?

What Derrida seems to imply is that the solidification and rigidification of the male body function to ward off its dissemination, its fracturing and scattering, rather than the phallic absence. Hence, apotropaically, the lapidary phallus precisely serves to disavow ejaculation. The phallus does not function as the solace or compensation for castration, as Freud argues, but for ejaculation. That the disseminative ejaculation has, in fact, already taken place is attested to by the many, *too* many, stones, bricks, and pebbles that litter and punctuate the text of the *Songs*. Because of their very excess, they can no longer serve as secure signposts for presence. Instead, Derrida observes, they "glut . . . the gorgonized reader's examination. So many stones!" (40).

The conventional preface, then, is not so much the seat of the originating sperm cell, or the vehicle for its generative power. Rather, the preface attempts to reclaim and reinternalize the seed that has already been disseminated into textuality. Otherwise, there would not have been a text to begin with. Welled up and lost in "seminal differance," Derrida concludes, the already dispersed sperm must be "reappropriated into the sublimity of the father," the author (44). Thus, the preface stages the author's pathetic and breathless attempt to reclaim the spawned text as his:

> As the preface to a book, it is the word of the father assisting and admiring his work, answering for his son, losing his breath in sustaining, retaining, idealizing, reinternalizing and mastering his seed. The scene would be acted out, if such were possible, between father and son alone: autoinsemination, homoinsemination, reinsemination. (45)

The second case study in which the "question of the preface as *seed*" is intricately at stake pertains to Novalis's *Encyclopedia*. Unfinished, this book exists only as an aborted program, a preface without the main text it should introduce. The "genetic pro-gram" of the encyclopedia, Derrida notes, is to cover and regenerate totality. "Everything must be encyclopedized," Novalis states (quoted in Derrida, *Dissemination*, 50). Additionally, the book "should become a scientific Bible . . . and the germ of all books" (quoted in Derrida, *Dissemination*, 52). In this way, Derrida claims, Novalis reinstalls "the seed in the *logos spermatikos* of philosophy" (50).

Subsequently, Derrida argues that philosophy has so far treated semen under the heading of nostalgia:

> the *philosophy of the seed*, conceived as an enrichment in the return-to-self, is always substantialist, and also derives from a romantic metaphorism and a myth of semantic depth, from that ideology . . . in reference to sperm and to gold. The treatment which they undergo in dissemination should break away from all mythological panspermism and all alchemical metallurgy. (50, n. 50)

A parenthetic remark specifies how:

> As the heterogeneity and absolute exteriority of the seed, seminal differance does constitute itself into a program, but it is a program that cannot be formalized. For reasons that *can* be formalized. The infinity of its code, its rift, then, does not take a form saturated with self-presence in the encyclopedic circle. It is attached, so to speak, to the incessant falling of a *supplement to the code*. Formalism no longer falls before an empirical richness but before a queue or *tail*. Whose *self*-bite is neither specular nor symbolic. (52)

Hence, the genetic "pro-gram" or lonely preface to the unwritten *Encyclopedia*, Derrida suggests, has failed to generate anything not so much because of the complexity and variety of the world, its richness, but because the generative force dormant in the headpiece, the preface, the sperm's head—seeking to cover everything and to regenerate all—is forced back on itself by the supplementary and dispensable tail. Apparently, the minute motions of this spermatic tail suffice to throw out of whack the totalizing circularity that would saturate the book with presence and reason. Before this tail, the head will always fall.

CLOSING OPENING

Derrida's reticence with regard to gender and sexuality has exasperated critics. Arguably, his noncommittal stance has furthered the idea that sex and sexuality are below, or somehow not good or important enough for, philosophy, even for the deconstructive philosophy that claims to attack the metaphysical and ideological hierarchies that relegated them to their low standing. In *Male Matters*, for example, Calvin Thomas reproaches Derrida for consistently viewing writing as something less, something more, in any case something different, than a material, sensory, tangible trace or marking (139).

In holding onto and withholding Heidegger, Thomas argues, Derrida has ended up acting out an anal retention, which renders him unable to articulate a body that is productive, male, and Jewish (131). Hence, Derrida cannot but reinstate the opposition between speech and writing in the specific division that, according to Thomas, haunts all "hegemonically masculinized writing" (145). This split, Thomas continues, inheres "between the intentional and expressive auto-affection of orgasm and the always excrementalizable di(visibility) indicated by ejaculation" (145). Never fully embracing the latter—Derrida's traces and marks never seem to cling to a body—he inevitably ends up in the former category, Thomas concludes.

I am sympathetic to this criticism, and must admit to more than casual annoyance and impatience in the face of Derrida's refusal to explicitly address masculinity in the book titled, of all things, *Dissemination*. To me, this seems intolerably demure and coquette at the same time. For, as I have argued, this asymmetry might well renew the mystification of the seed as something extraordinarily significant.

However, that was before I thought through the mime that sits in the middle of the book, and whose obscene gestures, motions, and expressions flit across its pages. Now it seems to me that the book overwhelmingly matters to gender and sexuality, though in a mode that is (dis)simulative rather than propositional. A viscous trace of semen makes the pages of *Dissemination* stick together; without it, the book would fall apart. Further, the book writes by, through, ejaculatory instances, by strokes, blows, and shots. The book abounds with male appearances, dazzling, hysterical, and rhetorical. The immanent medium of the orgasmic spasm enables the articulation, the nonphonocentric voicing, of a senseless yet sensual hilarity or ecstasy, chanted aloud in a pounding rhythm. The mimed act requires an audience: Derrida, Mallarmé, and Margueritte watching Pierrot come. Semen is considered in its materiality, in its element, its color, and its number. Hence, the mime signifies even more, perhaps best, when he is mute on the matter. Perhaps his greatest con or simulation was to make people believe that his act was serious, that it was all about philosophy.

Even Thomas's favored anality, what he views as the "dead end" of philosophy, is fleetingly at stake. Just the one time; yet, from there, it inevitably grinds itself into the whole of the book, itself so much about opening and closing, insertion and expulsion, membranous passages, motions, and pleasures:

> From where you stand, please note, in an angle of the graph paper (*The Park*), in the checkerboard squares (*Drama*), in the squares or

> cubes (*Numbers*), *this opening paradoxically wrought like a thing that closes*, the one playing itself off against the other. The necessary exit lays siege; it surrounds the text indefinitely, and also imperfectly, by referring—by exiting—toward another text. A false exit extends out of sight. The mirror is shown the door. Or squared. The enclosure—the grille—in *The Park*, *Drama*, and *Numbers*, is shaped like an *opening*, a *little opening* where the key can be inserted, an innumerable opening since it is but a grid (a relation between the lines and angles in the network). It is therefore both necessary and impossible. Urgent and impracticable, literally obsessive, as this will already have been situated and reserved in the *Park*: "Flat on my belly, my face buried in the pillow, I must attempt the experiment again. All the elements, if I wish, have been known for some time; I know, I can know; I could get out, find *the imperceptible crack*, the way out that nobody before me has been able to attempt." (336, emphasis added)

Ultimately, then, this angle, exit, enclosure, little opening, or crack refolds the predominantly genital and seminal business of the book in the anus, in anality. Hence, one must try the experiment again, as this passage cautions, and reread the book, starting from, and with, the back.

TEN

ANXIETY AND INTIMACY OF EXPENDITURE

Bataille

I BEGIN THIS THIRD AND LAST CHAPTER on available concepts of ejaculation, following Barthes's bliss and Derrida's dissemination, with a reading of André Masson's *Acéphale [Headless]* (Figure 12). This drawing adorns the cover of *The Bataille Reader;* hence, it can be taken to function as the visual shorthand or logo for Georges Bataille's philosophical project in general, much as *The Ambassadors* does for Lacan's. The concept at stake is Bataille's *dépense,* for seminal "expenditure" or "waste." Masson's drawing bears the same name as the obscure secret society that Bataille founded in 1936, and it adorned the cover of the first issue of the magazine by the same title associated with the group.

The figure's outstretched and frontal position recalls Leonardo's *Vitruvian Man* (see Figure 9), discussed in chapter 4. In Leonardo's image, masculinity strikes a pose, achieves form. Indeed, the image offers a stable vision of wholeness, hierarchy, symmetry, proportionality, and secure contours. The framing circle and square fix the body in place. In Masson's drawing, however, such stability seems forfeited. Gone are the figure's head and face. At the figure's center, the skin is opened up to reveal an intricate tangle of intestines, which works to repudiate the mathematical or geometric architecture Leonardo ascribes to the masculine anatomy.

Additionally, the skull, haunting the male subjects from a centrifugal angle in Holbein's *The Ambassadors* (see Figure 6 in chapter 3), has moved inside the body and is resituated at the figure's crotch. "Headlessness," it appears, entails a triple displacement: the figure's head has disappeared from the top of the body; it has become a dead skull; and it is moved to the lower body, replacing the penis. Thus what Holbein depicts as the externally anamorphic materializes inside the morphology of the male body in Masson's image. Vanitas is no longer an obsession that burdens the scene from an oblique margin, but inhabits a constitutive center.

In my reading of *The Ambassadors,* I have stressed the relationship be-

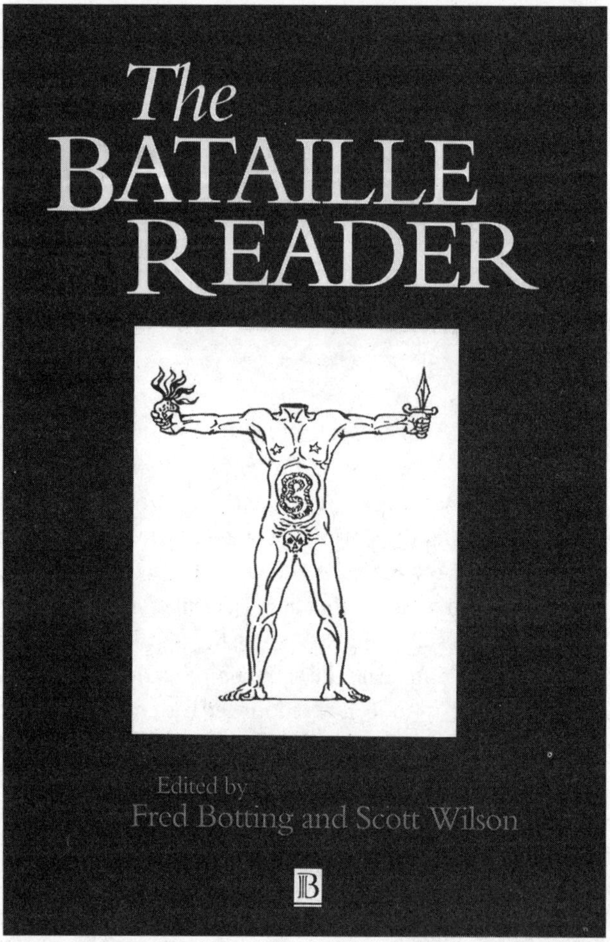

FIGURE 12. *The Bataille Reader*, showing André Masson's *Acéphale*, 1936.

tween the skull and the crucifix in the painting. Centrifugal to a similar extent, they suggest opposing attitudes on the mortality of the flesh. If the skull is there to remind the viewer of the reality of death, then the crucifix pledges the mercy of the afterlife of the soul. At the same time, this antithesis is susceptible to the reversal of its values. Where the crucifix shows the viscerality of the body in Christ's protracted suffering, the bald skull has lost its flesh, its substantiality. Hence, the frame that these two features establish implies the consideration of the appearance of masculinity as sandwiched between the materialization and the transcendence of the body. As it turns out, Hegel, the philosopher always at the background in Bataille's writings, puts forward exactly the skull as a suitable representation of what is ultimately unrepresentable: Spirit.

In *Male Matters*, Calvin Thomas comments on the figure of the skull in Hegel's *Phenomenology of Spirit*. Asserting that "the being of Spirit is a bone," Hegel quickly cautions that its inflexible materiality should be disregarded: "Of course, the intention here is not to state that Spirit, which is represented by a skull, is a Thing; there is not meant to be any materialism . . . in this idea" (quoted in Thomas, *Male Matters*, 55). The analogy between Spirit and skull only holds if the latter is understood as pure concept or notion (*Begriff*), as wholly defleshed and dematerialized. "The material boniness of Spirit's being is thus recognized and sublated," Thomas concludes (55). Precisely because the flesh of the face has rotted away, to push the point, the bleached and smooth skull can become the apt vehicle to represent Spirit.

The simile becomes more complicated when Hegel moves on to denounce the dependency of the human mind on representation, the brain's capacity for "picture-thinking," in favor of purely conceptual reasoning. The fact that the same mind can think in concrete images and in abstract concepts, and that these two cognitive faculties are obstinately entangled with each other, Hegel characterizes as "the same conjunction of the high and the low which, in the living being, Nature naïvely expresses when it combines the organ of its highest fulfillment, the organ of generation, with the organ of urination" (quoted in Thomas, *Male Matters*, 56). Thus, the distinction between the high mind and the low organ is reiterated on both sides: between high conceptual reason and low representational thought in the mind, and between high generation and low urination in the male organ.

The development from picture-thinking to conceptual reasoning entails an abstracted *Aufhebung*: the latter mental capacity succeeds, elevates, and subsumes the former in dialectical history. Simultaneously, this *Aufhebung* is, implicitly though no less concretely, imagined as erection, because that is what enables the movement from low to high in the subsidiary and analogous case of the male organ. Urine secretes downward with the penis in its flaccid state; semen surges upward with the penis in its tumescent state. Thus, erection is the hidden and motivating representation for conceptual *Aufhebung*. Paradoxically, the development from representation toward reason and conceptuality is informed by the image of erection. Irreducibly, conceptualization remains linked to representation. Lacan, it appears, was not far off the mark in his pun on the notion (see chapter 2).

Betting that nature might not be as naïve as Hegel has it, Thomas rereads the distinction between the penis as organ of generation and of waste as an attempt to elide the relevance of sperm. If generation must be analogous to conceptual reason, then it follows that the unnamed substance must disappear from the equation lest the mere mention of it conjures up an image or picture, which would spoil the clarity of the distinction between reason and representation. I quote Thomas at some length for his clarity:

> I submit that the difference Hegel is alluding to is one he could neither speak nor name: not that between semen and urine but that between *invisible and visible semen*. It is a sort of purely speculative money shot, unspeakable as such, that Hegel negotiates here, for in evoking the ambiguity of the male organ, Hegel clearly alludes to the two different substances that pass through the same urethral defile. Quite significantly, however, he *names* only the one that he has already aligned with visibility and hence degraded. He never names that substance whose emission leads (or can lead) to life's "highest fulfillment." In Hegel's passage, the word *semen* never appears, as if even to commit the thought to writing would call forth an image and thus align that precious substance with the very picture-thinking that Hegel relegates to the *pissoir*. (59)

The series of distinctions in Hegel's conceptual edifice rests on the elision of the name and image of sperm, which it must nevertheless invoke, because it puts generation at the top of the hierarchy. In the same way that *Aufhebung* denotes a conceptual reason situated beyond visuality and representation, while it simultaneously remains wedded to the image of erection, this spiritual generation or productivity remains linked to the material substance and image of semen.

Nevertheless, semen ostensibly survives as something that is purely conceptual and spiritual, the immaterial *spiritus* of the Aristotelian tradition (chapter 1), which allows for life's fulfillment through generation. "The being of Spirit thus is not a bone," Thomas puns, "it is the imageless *Begriff* of a boner. In Hegel's conceptual/copulative scenario, this 'boner' brings its vital inward essence up from the depths and allows it to spill out into the material world" (60).

Thomas's reading of Hegel associates masculine iconophobia, the historical invisibility of the male body and its processes in our culture, with transcendentalist, idealist thought. It also enables one to reconsider the audacity of Masson's drawing. If Holbein's anamorphic skull serves as a *memento mori*, Masson's skull, in contrast, raises the specter of a Hegelian *Aufhebung* in the picture. The dead head may have moved to the site of the penis, but since Hegel himself recognized a naïve duplicity between the high and the low in that organ, that in itself is not saying much. Then again, the image, with the penis noted for its absence, seems to claim a triumphant virility within or beyond castration.

What seems truly subversive, however, is that the disappeared penis and the displaced head are not so much combined, for instance, in some new and phantasmic organ, say, a talking penis, or compared metaphorically, but embrangled or entangled at the same place. Hegel's analogy between modes of thinking and distinguishable capabilities of the penis is subjected to a metonymic slide or contagion that, like wild flesh, has made both aspects grow together. Thus, Masson forges the exposure of the conjunction of, or the slippage between, the high and the low that irks Hegel, and which he attempts to erase.

Additionally, because the tangle of viscera is presumably wired straight into the skull's oral cavity, *Acéphale* proposes the structural simultaneity, or isotropy, of mouth, penis, and anus. Not only semen and urine, but also speech and excrement are discharged through the same orifice, and therefore cannot but contaminate each other. The production of these forms of human output—logocentric speech, generative semen, and digestive waste products like urine and feces—all originate from the same dark and meandering knot of intestines. Consequently, the (Hegelian) "spirit" of distinction is countered in the image. Indeed, in Bataille's writings, semen may occasionally be ejaculated. But, it may just as well be vomited, spitted, pissed, or shitted.

Masson makes intelligible what can be described as a cloacal configuration of the body that is specifically masculine. According to Freud, the *cloaca* (Latin for "sewer") is a fixture of the sexual theories of young children, in which the distinction between the vagina and the anus is not yet recognized. Thus, the theory pertains particularly to the female body: "The clear-cut distinction between anal and genital processes which is later insisted upon," Freud writes in *Three Essays on the Theory of Sexuality*, "is contradicted by the close anatomical and functional analogies and relations which hold between them. The genital apparatus remains the neighbor of the cloaca, and actually 'in the case of women is only taken from it on lease' " (quoted in Laplanche and Pontalis, *The Language of Psychoanalysis*, 70).

The importance of the distinction between genitality and anality (to which psychoanalysis, incidentally, has greatly added), which is "clear-cut," yet uncomfortably close or adjacent ("neighbor"), and even grafted onto each other ("on lease"), may thus be threatened in the cloacal imagination as focalized by children, and as (wrongly) assigned to women. Now, children may not be capable of telling the difference just yet, but they are understood to do so in due time, if they are to become proper individuals. In the meantime, the female body ideologically serves as perennially insufficiently differentiated stuff, as a morphological mess. Both parties, children and women, then, play a contrasting role for the valuation of the mature man, a man like Hegel (or, for that matter, Freud), who sees things as they are, who is able to tell the difference, and whose body, accordingly, must be properly differentiated in its functions and processes.

But, as Hegel's exasperation shows, the cloaca may be not only a figure through which children imagine the female body, but also a philosophical burden imposed on man by a naïve nature, since it combines the functions of high generation and low urination in one male organ. *Acéphale* raises the stakes: genital and anal, as well as mental and discursive processes, are not so much shown as adjacent or connected, but rather as indistinguishable. They are all circuited through the same tangle of viscera, and they all exit through the same orifice, the skull's oral cavity. Hence, these various processes are all, to borrow Freud's phrase, "on lease" from the cloaca to a similar extent. Moreover, the figure's crotch opening, simultaneously anal, genital, and oral, survives as the only possible place of input.

Masson's cloacal drawing of a male figure is thus triumphantly regressive (it relegates the masculine body to a putatively infantile past) and gender-transgressive (it transposes a supposedly feminine trait onto the male body). Canceling the oppositions between up and down, life and death, front and back, inside and outside, Masson's vision of masculine headlessness suggests an (anti)logic that is bent upon "undifferentiation," indistinction, or de-hierarchization. As we will see, this dynamic is highly germane for Bataille's writing; I will return to Masson's drawing in due course.

Through Bataille, this chapter discusses the "matter" of semen, its substantiality as well as its relevance (how much it matters). It will move between the vertical hierarchy of the high and the low, and the surprising effects that come to matter when that distinction is countered, upstaged, or wrongfooted. From one angle, semen makes all the difference for meaning and for masculinity; from another, this established difference is met with a steady, sometimes aggressive, indifference. The ejaculatory surge may reach an imaginary zenith or pinnacle, or go flat.

The two other object-texts in this chapter, the porn movies *The Uranus Experiment* and *Flyin' Solo*, as their titles indicate, show a marked design to make sperm escape from gravity, to levitate into space. However, these two movies simultaneously encapsulate different imaginations of what semen might be, do, or mean. A related perspective is offered by the contrast between the vertical relations between fathers and sons, and horizontal or lateral relations between men, comrades, or brothers. The chapter will conclude with a close reading of the "cum-shots" in Bataille's own novella *Story of the Eye*. In the next section, I inquire into the Bataillean notion that is most obviously related to a nonfulfilling, nongenerative perspective on sperm: *dépense* ("expenditure" or "waste").

HOSTILE EXPENDITURES BETWEEN MEN

In the spirit of Hegel, the phrase "concept of ejaculation" is, on the one hand, an oxymoron. For, conceptuality itself is grounded on the elision of semen, of substance and representation. On the other hand, the phrase is pleonastic or redundant, because conceptual reason is as fulfilling and generative as ejaculatory impregnation is, provided that the sperm remain immaterial and invisible. Bataille can be understood to seize on exactly that paradox, coining *dépense* as a notion highly susceptible to ejaculatory elaboration. In Masson's *Acéphale*, the mark, or rather, the blur, of expenditure is the conjunction, to the point of indistinction, of the usually opposite processes of production and waste, or, in Hegel's terms, generation and urination. The prospect of achieving life's "highest fulfillment" seems moot, if sperm may be wasteful, urine generative; if the two are not properly differentiated to begin with.

It would seem, then, that Masson and Bataille are dedicated to the debunking of masculinity and the economy of hierarchies that conventionally sustains it. That is not the case, however. For notwithstanding the castration and reconfiguration of the male body in Masson's drawing, the figure nevertheless pledges a raw sense of power and hypermasculinity, with the mythical knife and the flame in the figure's stretched-out hands as its prominent emblems. In his writings, correspondingly, Bataille insists on the virtues of virility at a nearly hysterical pitch. The Bataillean paradox, then, entails the double movement of both rejecting and championing masculinity. In Bataille's essays on expenditure, this paradox is readable in his celebration of pure and absolute loss even as he remains equally obsessed with the acquisition of "glory." Glory, it turns out, is the elusive commodity to be harvested from intense intermale rivalries: between father and son, between one man and his rival, and within a fraternity of comrades. Glory functions as the replacement of the highest fulfillment, the symbolic zenith or crown, that Hegel locates in generation and reason. Expenditure may lead to a pseudo-aristocratic glory, waste to culmination.[1]

Bataille's "The Notion of Expenditure" starts with a critique of the principle of "classical utility."[2] This idea, according to Bataille, has led to a series of quantitative, flat, and ultimately untenable values, understood to propel and motivate life: acquisition, conservation, and reproduction. Only a reduced or moderate pleasure is allowed to serve as "a subsidiary diversion" (168). In this picture of the world, Bataille continues, it has become nearly impossible to entertain the idea "that a human society can have . . . an interest in considerable losses, in catastrophes that, *while conforming to well defined needs*, provoke tumultuous depressions, crises of dread and, in the final analysis, a certain orgiastic state" (168).

Hence, Bataille proposes a principle of loss to supplement and criticize the dominant one of utility. In a move that no doubt inspired Barthes's critical pairing of pleasure and bliss (chapter 9), Bataille distinguishes between two modalities in consumption. The first one, consumption proper, is intent on investing a relative minimum of energy, time, and objects to secure the maintenance of life. The second one, or "unproductive expenditure," however, capitalizes on the maximization of loss, which "must be as great as possible in order for that activity to take on its true meaning" (169). Examples are jewelry, sacrificial cults, competitive games, art, and "perverse sexual activity (i.e., deflected from genital finality)" (169).

The two principles of consumption oversee respective economic orders: a "restricted" economy based on scarcity and measured consumption, and a "general" economy predicated on excess and waste. The hierarchy between the two orders is complex but clear: the latter frames, precedes, and impinges on the former. The general economy frames the restricted economy, because it encompasses it. The first also antedates the second in "primitive" societies in which squandering rituals like potlatch and ritual sacrifice are paramount, so that profitable production can be said to be "secondary" or "derivative" (172). Bataille identifies the Protestant individualization of property as the latter-day establishment of the narrow economy (175). Finally, the general economy punctures through the restricted one, because unproductive expenditures have stubbornly persisted in the new order.[3]

The intricate entanglement of the two economies suggests that any activity or sign should be evaluated in both. The sign may produce meaning within the bounds of the narrow economy in that it succeeds to get its message across with a minimum amount of trouble. The sign may also prompt excess meanings that are not deemed profitable. Similarly, sperm may lead to a secondary or derivative fulfillment through the generation of offspring, or, alternatively, "take on its true meaning" by being squandered, diverging from "genital finality" (169).[4]

If the general economy that Bataille puts forth abolishes the hierarchy between acquisition and loss by giving the latter a greater and more archaic force, it also introduces a new value, or reinstates an old one, liable to immediate rehierarchization. That value is alternatively characterized, with suitable masculinist pathos, as "glory," "power," or "honor." "[T]he most absurd of [unproductive values], and the one that makes people the most rapacious," Bataille writes, "is glory" (180). Glory, it turns out, can only be reaped from fierce, antagonistic rivalries between men. The first of these plays out between father and son.

"[P]ersonal experience," Bataille writes in the essay, gives the lie to the dominant conception of the narrow economy, at least "if it is a question of a youthful man, capable of wasting and destroying without reason" (168). This young man mirrors the lusty bystander of the Platonic dialogue, who makes the air ring with his laughter when he learns of the interdiction against homosexuality that the philosopher proposes (chapter 9). Subsequently, the conflict between economic orders is explicitly compared to the struggle between the older and younger man, father and son, adult and minor, in a terminology that recalls Hegel's characterization of nature as "naïve" and Freud's coinage of "infantile" sexual theories:

> In the most crushing way, the contradiction between current social conceptions and the real needs of society recalls the narrowness of judgment that puts the father in opposition to the satisfaction of his son's needs. This narrowness is such that it is impossible for the son to express his will. . . . In this respect, it is sad to say *that conscious humanity has remained a minor;* humanity recognizes the right to acquire, to conserve and to consume rationally, but it excludes in *principle non-productive expenditure.* It is true that this exclusion is superficial and that it no more modifies practical activities than prohibitions limit the son, who indulges in his unavowed pleasures as soon as he is no longer in his father's presence. (168)

Like the son, it seems, humanity should simply grow up by spending the father's capital, thus expressing its will. The distinction implicitly called upon is the one between the masturbating son, spilling his seed, and the reproductive father. That such an arrangement entails something more than a typically bourgeois domestic quarrel becomes clearer when Bataille explains the success of Christianity through its central image: "the theme of the son of God's ignominious crucifixion, which carries human dread to a representation of loss and limitless degradation" (170). The implication must be that the son or humanity can only self-destruct when the paternal legacy is done away with.

The promised, and indeed necessary, "development of a conception that is not guided by the servile mode of father-son relations" remains undelivered when Bataille moves on to his second example of intermale rivalry (169). Potlatch, a practice of northwestern American Indians, may take the shape of either gift giving or the destruction of wealth (172). One chief presents his rival with a spectacular gift, or destroys his own property while the rival is watching, killing slaves, burning villages, and smashing canoes with abandon (173). The object is to humiliate, defy, and obligate the rival to retaliate in kind; the ideal is to make the scale of the gift or the destruction so great that the possibility of return action is preempted. For Bataille, here loss is constituted as a "positive property—from which spring nobility, honour and rank in a hierarchy" (173). Power is defined as the "power to lose. It is only through loss that glory and honour are linked to wealth" (174).[5]

While the winner basks in his glory, the loser of the game is relegated to the status of abject objecthood. For him is created "a category of degradation and abjection that leads to slavery" (177). Contemporaneously, this categorical condition is reserved for the proletariat, whose revolutionary antagonism has been co-opted by those who strive for equality and emancipation. In the United States, Bataille continues, such a co-optation has been greatly facilitated by the presence of a class of people who cannot enter the game of inimical rivalry, "the preliminary existence of a class held to be abject by common accord, as in the case of the blacks" (177). This mode of abjection Bataille subsequently explicitly connects to anal sadism: "In unconscious forms, such as those described by psychoanalysis, [expenditure] symbolizes excretion, which itself is linked to death, in conformity with the fundamental connection between anal eroticism and sadism" (173).

Thus, expenditure functions as the social dynamic through which the other becomes, indeed, expendable, turned into shit. So far, then, the notion is uncomfortably sandwiched between a stereotypically youthful indulgence that is easily allowed (adding to rather than undermining the system) and a sadistic abjection through which the other-as-rival becomes the other-as-shit, expelled from the economic system altogether. That expenditure might suddenly switch from being not all that serious into something all too serious seems to be the rule of the game. Therefore, if Masson's *Acéphale* must be seen as a triumphant portrait of the knife-wielding victor, one should perhaps imagine the shadow-figure of a humiliated slave prostrated at his feet.

The third and last example of rivalrous expenditure is performed rather than described by Bataille. "The Use-Value of D. A. F. de Sade (An Open Letter to My Current Comrades)" stages Bataille's defection from the ranks of the surrealists. The letter is addressed to the necessary witnesses of the defection; the erstwhile comrades are trashed rather than engaged.[6] Bataille's former "so-called intimate friendships" are recanted as he blames a number of writers for imparting a "vulgar impotence" to the memory of Sade: "The behavior of Sade's admirers resembles that of primitive subjects in relation to their king, whom they adore and loathe, and whom they cover with honours and narrowly confine" (148).

Bataille, however, restores the figure of Sade to its radical dignity. Refusing to deal "with individuals like those I already know," he concerns himself "only with men (and above all with masses) who are comparatively decomposed, amorphous and even violently expelled from every form" (146). At the end of the essay, these masculine masses turn out to be "the blacks," as Bataille forecasts "the probable intervention of blacks in the general culture" (158). For only from such an intervention can "institutions . . . develop which will serve as the final outlets (with no other limitations than those of human strength) for the urges that today require worldwide society's fiery and bloody Revolution" (158). The abjected blacks will return with a vengeance. Again, expenditure functions within a context of fierce antagonism, rivalrous violence, and the promise of bloodshed.[7]

Thus, Bataille's dehierarchization, *contre* Hegel, of what is deemed high and what is condemned as low initially turns the existing hierarchy upside-down, but then supplements it by the immediate rehierarchization of men under the heading of a rapacious glory. Hegel's distinction between sperm and urine pinpoints a differential *within* man, within one organ, which Bataille negates, but then redistributes *between* men, between the glorious and the abject. The men who lose precisely because they cannot afford to, or are not prepared to, lose more are made expendable. Crowned with glory, however, even the victors are subjected to the overhaul of the morphology of the masculine body. In the name of masculine glory, then, masculinity is decisively reconfigured.

Masson's drawing, in combination with Bataille's professed identification or solidarity with "decomposed" or "amorphous" men, points to a different understanding of male "matter" in its double sense: first, the place of the substantiality of the male body in the conception of masculinity, and, second, the ways in which that body is made to matter, to make a difference, once its various processes are forged within a hierarchy, and ascribed respective relevance and meaning through the calibration of proper form. To anticipate a specifically Bataillean understanding of masculine materiality and the forms it can take, the next section proposes a reading of a peculiar porn movie in which the materiality of sperm is exactly what is at stake, what matters, in the story.

GLOBULAR DROPLETS

The Uranus Experiment, a science-fiction porn movie in three parts, is among the industry's big-budget extravaganzas. The movie sports a professional soundtrack composed by members of the mainstream dance bands Massive Attack and Prodigy. With some controversy, the film's script was nominated for a Nebula Award, sponsored by the Science Fiction and Fantasy Writers of America. The novelty or gimmick with which the movie was successfully marketed consists of images of ejaculation in conditions of weightlessness. To achieve that end, the movie crew reportedly used the same techniques that were employed during the filming of the mainstream space movie *Apollo 13*. A sharp dive of an airplane from 11,000 meters up creates twenty to twenty-five seconds in which the force of gravity is briefly suspended. It was up to performer Nick Lang to manage to ejaculate in that narrow margin. The resulting cum shot was trumpeted on the movie's box covers and its advertisements: "Private [Media] proudly presents the first cum shot in real zero gravity."

Apparently, Private Media and Millerman were bent on the representation of ejaculation and semen beyond the constraints of gravity, thus upping the ante for its elevation or *Aufhebung*. However, this endeavor cannot but betray the implicit admission that conventional cum shots, never mind the surges of semen they do portray, do not offer "real zero gravity" to begin with. And, even if the scene accomplished the desired effect, it must also be said that its manufacture was tenuous at best, and moreover provoked an odd but telling reverse materialization of the substance charged to reach the stars. This move can already be gauged from the publicity that accompanied the trilogy's initial release.

"Insiders described the filming process," the Web site www.space.com reported, "as particularly messy from a technical and logistical standpoint." Another article added: "Purportedly, one of the biggest difficulties in filming under such situations is dodging globular droplets of semen that scattered in all directions during filming" (see www.talkingblue.com).[8] At the occasion of the movie's DVD release, *Adult Video News Online* reviewer Ken Michaels finally called Private Media's bluff: "More disappointing is Private's continued trumpeting of the supposed 'first-ever cum shot in zero gravity.' Sorry folks. The 'zero-g' footage is all earthbound—as is obvious from even casual observation of Private's own 'Making Of' featurette."[9]

Such, then, are the stances taken in the reception of *The Uranus Experiment*: on the one hand, the fantasy of a weightless ejaculation, a trajectory of sperm that is not earthbound, a flight of fancy capturing the imagination; on the other hand, the gleeful debunking of the trick or hoax, exposing the images as the result of mere technical and montaged construction. Punching through both alternatives, however, is the possible emergence of a third take on what semen might be or do if the forces of gravity are temporarily circumvented: the messy scattering of the globular droplets of semen in all directions.

"In all directions": the airborne packets of seed are imagined as neither attempting to reach the stars, nor forced by gravity to soil the floor. Instead of moving either up or down, they disperse freely, sending the cast and the crew in an uproar to dodge their unpredictable paths. Hence, the attempt to make the sperm fly higher, to elevate itself more freely, and to escape gravity, has effectively vacated or annulled the vertical axis of high and low on which the meaning of semen, following Hegel, should be situated. What is *aufge-*

hoben (elevated, sublated), then, is not so much the materiality of sperm, to be subsumed into a principle of a higher order, but rather the vertical logic that underpins the notion of *Aufhebung*. Due to the semen's arbitrary dispersion through space, as invoked by the publicity responding to the movie, sperm may manage to escape both the high and the low, the transcendental and the abject, glory and slavery, the immaculate stars and the dirty floor.

I must emphasize that this alternative vision of ejaculation and sperm is merely a conjecture brought up by the wording of one response to the film. The fact of the matter is that *The Uranus Experiment* emphatically does not offer footage of scattering sperm, neither in the three movies themselves, nor in the "Making of" feature that accompanies the second installment of the series. Astonishingly, the movie seems much more about the capture of sperm than about its escape or flight.

Part one of the trilogy starts with images of a bird flying over the opening credits. A launchpad moves into the shot; a space shuttle is shown to be ready for departure; and then the countdown begins. A series of scenes set at NASA, the Oval Office, Russian and American ground control rooms, and media stages all heighten the excitement. We are awaiting the joint launch of Russian and American spacecrafts, named the *Resolution* and the *Reunion*, respectively. Their mission is to make contact in space. Incidentally, the American crew is all-male, while the Russian crew consists exclusively of female members.

As the countdown continues, the movie pauses to insert several retroversions, all revolving on a KGB plot to study "the effects of weightlessness on the production of sperm." Exactly why this should entail a crucial piece of intelligence for the Russian spy organization is left unexplained.[10] We see Russian intelligence officials considering potential crew members for the *Resolution*'s upcoming mission. Sexologist Olga Wiberova comes highly recommended, it transpires, because she experiences "no sexual feelings whatsoever" due to a strict religious upbringing. Next, we witness Wiberova at her place of work, a clinical research facility with stern white walls and flickering computer screens. She is preoccupied with timing and observing a copulating couple. As the camera zooms in on the action, the unfazed Wiberova looks away, concentrating instead on the data her instruments deliver. Her attitude of scientific detachment is complemented by the KGB operatives, who observe Wiberova through a one-way mirror.

Wiberova dismisses the woman guinea pig, and instructs her male counterpart that she will now need a sperm sample, please. He complies and masturbates into a test tube held up for him by Wiberova, his sperm mottling the glass. Unceremoniously, she cleans her hand with a tissue and takes the man's pulse. Her understated reaction contrasts with the usual behavior of the female performers in porn, who exhort and welcome the visual advent of sperm with vocal and facial ecstasy. Next is a scene in which Wiberova's detached and objective attitude is contrasted with the disposition of a frisky assistant, who jeopardizes the research results with her unprofessional interest in the male guinea pig.

The motive of capturing sperm for investigative purposes continues in the second set of retroversions. Since the goal of the Russian female space travelers is to investigate whether or not sperm production is affected in space, they need comparison data from samples taken in earthbound conditions. Female spies have been sent to America to obtain these, and subsequently we witness these women's seductions of two of the male members of the American crew. They are repeatedly shown sealing the obtained sperm samples in transparent plastic bags. Hence, the first, prelaunch part of the movie centers on the capture or appropriation of semen for reasons of research and intelligence.

The mission of the female operatives thus adds another layer of probabilization for the cum shots. The semen must not only be grasped visually on celluloid or video to secure the convention of the cum shot in the genre, but it must also be captured materially in accordance with the plot, adding an unusual twist to this trope's economy. The question is whether the genre can sustain the double burden thus imposed on semen. What initially emerges is the uncanny affirmation of sperm in its capacity of substance. Indeed, semen has become an appropriable and quantifiable object, a prop, rather than the privileged sign that signals and performs the culmination of the hard-core scenes or numbers.

In the second part of the movie, footage of the launches of the spacecrafts, blasting into orbit in an apparently effortless defiance of gravity, begins to counteract the double confinement of sperm, visually and narratively, that the first part establishes. The *Reunion* and the *Resolution* dock in space, and the two crews make each other's acquaintance to the general excitement of television audiences, control room personnel, and presidential and KGB offices. A mock newscast offers slapstick footage of the attempts of the crews to enjoy a joint dinner: cutlery, foodstuffs, and amorphous globes of liquid float over the table, continuously escaping the hands and mouths of the dinner guests. The implicit promise seems clear: similar imagery of sperm to come.

Then, it is the first night in space, and a member of the Russian crew readies herself to hunt for sperm samples of the American crew to complete the research. As she seduces pilot Frank Stone, she is unaware of the fact that live video feeds beam their contortions to control rooms and news channels down below. The bodies of the two performers intermittently bob and float through the air.

Yet the cum shot that follows fulfills none of the expectations raised by the movie's figure of anticipation (the levitating drops of water at the dinner table) and its prepublicity ("the first cum-shot in real zero gravity"). Quite transparently, the shot is simply edited upside-down, and thus shows no genuine weightlessness or the multidirectional scattering of sperm. For a moment, it seems that the trajectory of semen will escape the force of gravity, only to then cathect securely on the female performer's skin and stay there. Peculiarly, the woman scientist fails to take a sample. Over and over again, the produced cum shot is rerun to the amazement and concern of the varied audiences in the movie.

The third and last part of the movie centers on the ramifications of the public relations disaster following the inadvertently broadcasted space encounter. Typifying pornographic narrative, the story line starts to meander and digress in order to include as many hard-core numbers as possible. An American intelligence officer assures the president that all necessary security measures have been taken. A flashback qualifies this particular claim as he is seen to be seduced effortlessly by a Russian spy. At the KGB research facility, an aphrodisiac drug is now being tested. The movie arbitrarily concludes with an orgy of three American officers and three Russian spies at the Houston ground control offices.

The dissipation of the story line, readily discarded after its scrupulous setup, may reinforce the judgment that porn's narrativity is obligatory and inconsequential. One might also speculate that the inconclusive ending serves to facilitate a sequel, which in fact did materialize. However, I would argue to the contrary, for if one is prepared to leave aside the anecdotal narrative, narrative in its narrow sense, another and double narrative dynamic can move into focus.

MALE GUINEA PIGS

As I have argued, following Linda Williams, the narratives of porn are often explicitly or implicitly antagonistic: two parties express and resolve conflict in the framing narrative and the series of hard-core numbers that puncture it; for example, the workers versus the bosses in *Lunch Hour*. Here, the relevant conflict plays out between the Russians and the Americans, and between the women scientists and the male guinea pigs, involuntarily subjected to sperm testing.

Frequently, the sense of an ending in porn is achieved indirectly through a resolution number, which relieves or allays the animosity that moves the plot. *Lunch Hour*'s hero Spinelli, for instance, escapes the brutal sexual politics of the workplace in a reciprocal scene with his lover. In a similar vein, the renewed Cold War in *The Uranus Experiment* loses its ferocity in the final orgy scene. For, the quantity and variation of positions and combinations offer an abundant spectacle that deflates binary enmity. Promiscuity, the ending appears to suggest, can satisfactorily deal with antagonism.

A second narrative that I want to propose concerns the changing status of sperm in the course of the film. Though the team of female characters, intelligence operatives, scientists, and cosmonauts, is enlisted to participate in conventional hard-core scenes and cum shots, and though their agency is qualified by the power of the burly KGB officers whose orders they obey, they are nevertheless involved in a conspiracy with its own agenda: to steal, appropriate, and exploit sperm. Because of the women's actions, semen becomes a material object or prop, captured in test tubes and sealed in plastic bags. The men the women cheat out of their seed are only the first and most obvious victims of that move.

For the fundamental casualty must be porn's mode of storytelling, of narrative, as calibrated in and through the cum shot. The cum shot usually functions as a narrative trigger. Invariably, it completes the hard-core numbers and shunts the movie back to the framing story line in which they take place. Thus, sperm acquires a signaling functionality in the larger agency of the narrative. In this way, the power of narrative itself is invested in the sperm. The agency of the external narrator or focalizer collapses with the embedded character-bound narrators or focalizers, who are always male. Thus, each time a male character comes, the movie "comes" as well: the hard-core sequence culminates and finalizes. This structure of collapse works to outwit and disenfranchise the female characters: their bodies do not hold the capacity to wield control over the narrative; they lack the access to the narrative switch.

Unless, that is, the female characters, like those in *The Uranus Experiment*, manage to seize the privileged substance for their own purposes, appropriate it from the male characters, so that the masculine agency in the narrative becomes qualified. The decisive figure of the story, the signal that controls the story, is brought down in the story, becomes entangled with it, and is controlled and acted upon by the female characters. Therefore, the relevant antagonism here involves a gendered conflict over the significance and functionality of sperm in the genre. The women work together to disown, capture, and appropriate the power of narrative itself. This confiscation of the seminal fluid is shown in the scenes in which the cum of the male performers mottles a test tube from within, or clings to the see-through plastic of the sample bags. These scenes impart a tangible viscosity to the sperm. The detached and scientific view of ejaculation that the women show illustrates this alternative perspective on sperm, in which it is robbed of its power and privilege.

If it is true that the conflict of the movie entails the narrative power invested in ejaculation, then how is that antagonism ultimately resolved? Before the movie makes an attempt at such a resolution, it fleetingly raises the possibility of another perspective on sperm. At the dinner table of the first encounter between the crews in outer space, we briefly see weightless pockets of fluid moving through the air, continuously changing their shape and their course as they go along. The guests, control room officers, and international television audiences look on with amazement. This vision of matter, finally, corresponds to the imagination that one of the articles responding to the movie's release phrases so suggestively: "globular droplets scattering in all directions." These droplets of moving matter can neither be appropriated as a sticky and tangible prop, nor be elevated or subsumed to control the narrative engine. Resisting capture, this matter will effortlessly continue morphing, floating, dispersing, and escaping, until the moment that gravity returns.

But it is not sperm. As if only temporarily entranced by this alternative vision of materiality, the movie quickly restores the matter by returning to a proper and conventional cum shot. The anticipation that this brief scene brings up is not followed through in the movie. Instead of a genuinely weightless ejaculation scene, we see an utterly conventional cum shot, edited upside-down, in which the traces of matter safely land on the female performer's skin. And, although the capture of sperm was understood to be this operative's objective, she omits to do just that. This time around there is no plastic bag or test tube to enclose the fluid.

One could choose to dismiss these elements of the film as mere accidents. The desired and planned weightless cum shot has, one might speculate, in fact failed during the complex filming process, so that an emergency surrogate became necessary. The odd failure of the Russian spy to take the sperm sample can well be written off as a continuity error. But as the movie is, edited and released for public consumption, these details cannot but have their effect on the viewer.

The point seems to be that sperm manages to elude *both* female capture as elaborated in the story line *and* the visual possibilities of true weightlessness. Consequently, the usual switch of values in the cum shot can take place without further contestation: the male performer ejects, projects, or abjects bodily matter on the surface or ground of female skin. Hence, the female body becomes the dumping ground for what is deemed low in masculine self-expression. While the male performer accedes to glory, the female performers are made expendable, much like excrement or urine. What is secreted, displaced, is male matter itself, or rather, any remaining materiality in the idea of masculinity. Consequently, male matter only matters insofar as it is subsumed into agency, identity, or form; masculinity does not appear in the decomposed and amorphous shape that Bataille advocates. Thus, *The Uranus Experiment* raises two possibly alternative perspectives on sperm: semen as an appropriable prop in the story, and semen as escaping capture because of its morphing and dispersing propensity, both of which are ultimately arrested by the timely return to the conventional cum shot.

On the one hand, hard-core porn delivers an image of what Hegel views as the natural but naïve conjunction of the high and the low, their obstinate entanglement. The genre presents a representational, therefore low, image of what Hegel exempted from the chain of analogies: high semen, which should remain notional or spiritual. To that extent, cum shots are, indeed, cloacal figurations, combining the high (semen) and the low (visual representation) in one figure. On the other hand, the cum shot also repeats the Hegelian imperative, because it redistributes the high and the low between the genders. What Hegel acknowledges as an exasperating ambivalence in the mind and in the male body is displaced as a narrativized distinction between men and women. Nevertheless, *The Uranus Experiment* also entertains the fleeting vision of semen, the scattering, globular droplets of liquid, that cannot be reduced to this powerful hierarchy. Through the movie, then, it becomes possible to conceive of bodily matter as not ending up on either side of the scale, up or down, but as extending horizontally, multidirectionally, centrifugally; as amorphous, scattering, and active on its own accord. Such a vision of matter, and of what matters to masculinity, lies at the heart of Bataille's materialist philosophy. In the next section I outline Bataille's understanding of materiality, to then consider another porn movie as a critical counterpart to *The Uranus Experiment*.

INTIMACY OF EXPENDITURE

In "The Notion of Expenditure," Bataille defines matter as "nonlogical difference" (180). In "Base Materialism and Gnosticism," Bataille expands on that idea. Matter is nonlogical because it escapes the philosophical and binary opposition between form or identity and substance, a structure he decries as "metaphysical scaffolding."[11] Binarism actually rests on a "monistic Hellenistic spirit," Bataille argues, in that all second terms are only accredited as "degradations of superior principles," or, one might add, as obstacles to be overcome and sublated dialectically (160). To clarify the issue, Bataille turns to Gnostic and Zoroastrian dualism, in which matter is conceived as active, creative, autonomous, and external (162). In that sense, substance is irreducibly other, something that "The Use-Value of D. A. F. de Sade" describes as "the (heterogeneous) *foreign body*" or "*das ganz Anderes*"

(150–51). In this view of materiality, then, matter is "base," that is, both basic and low.

Bataille cautions that his brand of materialism should not be taken to imply an ontology, the implication that matter is "the thing itself" ("Base Materialism and Gnosticism," 163). I cite his explanation in full for its anti-Hegelian eloquence and for its emphasis on the dynamic or operational value of base matter:

> For it is a question above all of not submitting oneself, and with oneself one's reason, to whatever is more elevated, to whatever can give a borrowed authority to the being that I am, and to the reason that arms this being. This being and its reason can in fact only submit to what is lower, to what can never serve in any case to ape a given authority. Also I submit entirely to what must be called matter, since *that* exists outside myself and the idea, and I do not admit that my reason becomes the limit of what I have said, for if I proceeded in that way matter limited by my reason would soon take on the value of a superior principle (which this *servile* reason would be only too happy to establish above itself, in order to speak like an authorized functionary). Base matter is external and foreign to ideal human aspirations, and it refuses to allow itself to be reduced to the great ontological machines resulting from these aspirations. (163)

Hence, baseness does not so much imply reveling in what is dirty and low, but rather the refusal of elevation, a move that can only be described, oxymoronically, as "submit[ting] to what is lower." Bataille's intervention thus entails a double movement: first, to privilege the second term, to lower to scale; second, to cancel the vertical and hierarchical order that enables even that counteracting privileging. And, since one cannot get below what is already base, the movement ends up with the leveling of the hierarchy that makes the distinction between high and low possible. The point is not only to flip the scale, but also to abolish it. In that latter, ultimate sense, "base" means *flat*.

The idea of base materialism is taken up in *Formless: A User's Guide*, by art historians Yve-Alain Bois and Rosalind E. Krauss. The entry on the concept explains it as a desublimating gesture or operation of "de-class(ify)ing," the simultaneous "lowering and liberating from all ontological prisons, from any '*devoir être*' (role model)" (*Formless*, 53). As Bois's "Introduction" clarifies, "It is not so much a stable motif to which we can refer, a symbolizable theme, a given quality, as it is a term allowing one to operate a declassification [*déclasser*], in the double sense of lowering and of taxonomic disorder" (18).

Additionally, Bois considers one substance liable to such a movement: spittle. He recalls Michel Leiris, one of the contributors with Bataille to the *Dictionary* that appeared in the pages of the magazine *Documents*. Leiris observed that saliva "lowers the mouth—the visible sign of intelligence—to the level of the most shameful organs" (quoted in Bois and Krauss, *Formless*, 18). Term for term, Leiris's description of spit is appropriate to sperm, if not for sperm's long history of idealization. Indeed, both substances enjoy a measure of inconsistency, humidity, indefinite contours, and imprecision of color, which together work to challenge proper form (18). Can sperm lower the penis in the same way that saliva lowers the mouth?

The lemma in *Formless: A User's Guide* on "horizontality" elaborates on the flat aspect of base materialism. Especially in the works of David Siqueiros and Jackson Pollock of the mid 1930s, Krauss argues, the "floor had become a production site that was set in direct opposition to the vertical axis of the easel of the artist's studio, or the wall of the bourgeois apartment, or the high-cultural ideals of the museum" (93). With the artist's canvas lowered to the ground, it can now receive the dribblings and dumpings of paints, oils, and enamels, which work to challenge the elevation of matter into vertical form. High art is lowered horizontally. At ground level, the artistic image is materially "urinated" into being rather than idealistically or quasi-spiritually generated vertically, a gesture Warhol would take literally in his *Oxidation* paintings of the 1970s.

Reportedly, the artist's friends relieved themselves on metallic surfaces, so that the uric acid would produce intriguing whorls and shapes by oxidation in due time. In that way, moreover, the hyped machismo of the circle of action painters became inevitably recoded. As Krauss argues: "For Warhol's 'urinary' reading of Pollock's mark was insisting that the verticality of the phallic dimension was itself being riven from within to rotate into the axis of a homoerotic challenge" (102). Artistic creation is drawn into the orbit of, say, the intermale pissing contest or circle jerk. In turn, that move is taken literally in the second porn movie that I introduce here.

If *The Uranus Experiment* shows how the attempt to elevate sperm further into outer space prompts its inevitable reverse materialization, then Paul Barresi's *Flyin' Solo* pinpoints the same effect by lowering the scale. Two effects are pertinent here. Paradoxically, both go against the movie's title. "Solo" is a generic term, indicating that the hard-core scenes of the movie show masturbation. The performers masturbate together, though, so that Bataille's stress on rivalrous practices can be supplemented by the emphasis on homosocial intimacies. Additionally, the movie is obsessed not so much with flying as it is with shooting and bombing, so that, certainly in the latter case, ejaculation is accorded gravitational weight.

Flyin' Solo is set at a navy base, where a class of would-be fighter pilots receives instructions from captain Dick Leaky. "This practical applications course deals with the proper use of fire, maximizing your fire power, and ultimately increasing your kill ratio," Leaky informs his charges at the beginning of the film. As the captain's discourse indicates, the movie hijacks military vocabulary and conventions for a pornographic parody. Leaky's speech capitalizes on every occasion for sexual innuendo: he points out the available "fire power at hand," talks about "dropping your payload," compliments one participant's excellent "four finger ball tuck" and another's "high-caliber piece," distributes "government-issue ball huggers," offers incisive instructions as to "tool utilization" and "manual technique," and so on. The object for the masturbating team members is to hit the enemy, a poster image of a black silhouette of a human shape with target circles.

Taking turns, the men ejaculate on the target. At their own discretion, they have the choice between shooting, when the target image is pinned or held up vertically, and bombing, with the target image held or laid down horizontally. Accompanied by extradiegetic sounds of airplane motors, each ejaculation is inspected for its precision and quantity. Each shot is lavishly complimented by Leaky. The emphasis is on the need for cooperation "out there," on mutual dependence, trust, and protection, on "saving each other's asses." As the captain explains, "Each cock should be in unison, working together as one well-oiled machine, capable of destroying the enemy, still returning home with a full payload." The movie ends with a double, joint ejaculation at the target. As an air siren wails in the distance, Leaky dismisses his class, saying, "A good day for a war!" All the cum shots of the movie are repeated during the end credits, while a disembodied voice performs another countdown: "T minus 19, T minus 18, . . . ," and so on.

Like the first part of *The Uranus Experiment*, then, *Flyin' Solo* pulls ejaculation down to the narrative plane. On the one hand, the availability of a simple pun, "shooting," imparts macho militarism, violence, and control to ejaculation. On the other hand, it allows for the scrutiny of sperm in its substantiality, its visibility and tangibility. In that sense, the images of the sticky, messy target posters of *Flyin' Solo* are directly comparable to *The Uranus Experiment*'s mottled plastic evidence bags and test tubes. Like Pollock's congealed drippings and Warhol's urinary whorls, these images show traces of a materiality that resists proper form.

Hence, the semen becomes visible in exactly the terms that Leiris reserves for saliva: inconsistent, humid, indefinite of contours, imprecise of coloring, a potential that the grid of the target circles cannot completely erase. The phallus is rotated horizontally, lowered. Semen becomes base in its double sense. Low, because it drops on a target beneath. Even the semen shot at the vertically held target posters slowly but inevitably trickles downward. Flat, because sperm clings to, and becomes part of, a two-dimensional image.

Moreover, *Flyin' Solo* adds the social axis that *The Uranus Experiment* cannot consider, and that Bataille can only entertain in terms of a death-crazed rivalry: a homosocial and homoerotic intimacy. The "other" of the group of military apprentices is the target poster: a flat and black silhouette of a man. In relation to that figure, the men bond; the mute silhouette organizes all their efforts. In that way, the poster becomes the ground, both literal receptacle and figurative foundation, for the men's joint achievements, replacing the skin and face of the female performers in straight porn. Together, the men extend and inscribe themselves on the silhouette poster, thus negating the solidification of the hierarchical perspective that the military situation easily could have supplied. The black and flat posters, smeared with semen, become the image of the base materialism that the men confront and engage.

This intimate leveling also draws in the (male) viewer. Both movies discussed here offer a figure that compels and interpellates the viewer: the countdown, the measured timing of the crucial event. *The Uranus Experiment* shows its countdown at the beginning of the movie: the audience revels in the launches of the spacecrafts, as well as in the ideological theme it illustrates. *Flyin' Solo* supplies the countdown at that movie's conclusion, repeating all the cum shots shown before, so that the viewer is invited to participate in the ejaculatory dynamic of the movie as a whole. In that way, the viewer may become "one of the guys," one of captain Dick Leaky's eager apprentices.

Hegel's hierarchies, between representation and conceptual thinking, waste and generation, urine and semen, appear rigid and immobile, although it is exactly their conjunction that exasperates the philosopher. The porn movies I have discussed, in a Bataillean vein, seize on the narrow margin left open by these hierarchies. Indeed, *The Uranus Experiment* and *Flyin' Solo* both push the point, with similar effects. The former forces sperm to go higher than high, and ends up with a scattering motion of matter it can barely acknowledge. The latter goes for lower than low, traces of sperm sticking to the flat poster image, and culminates in the leveling of matter and men, or rather, of men in relation to each other and to matter. Both suggest the rotation of the vertical axis, opening up a dimension that entails the lateralization and flattening of meaning and manhood.

Let us take one last look at Masson's *Acéphale*. Despite all the subversive implications it offers to the idea of hierarchy (the displacement of the head, the replacement of the penis, and the opening up of the abdominal cavity) the image nevertheless celebrates the triumph of verticality through the figure's erect posture, his glory. The artist Jean Fautrier, who, like Masson, cooperated with Bataille and illustrated some of his publications, offers a counterimage that, while similar to Masson's drawing in some respects, goes much further. Of his *L'homme ouvert* (1928–29), Sarah Wilson writes:

> Fautrier was working an encaustic, waxy material, mixed into his paint, that became analogous to flesh. For *L'homme ouvert*, like a real anatomist himself, Fautrier worked on the flat—as though above a veritable corpse, physically engaging, as it were, with the entrails of his life-size victim.[12]

Thus, *L'homme ouvert* conveys the horizontal pull of matter more strongly than *Acéphale*. The work replaces the distanced, frontal vision of the glorious victor with the intimate and engaged concern for the slain victim. Hence, whereas Masson mediates between Leonardo's *Vitruvian Man* and Fautrier's *L'homme*, the latter offers the most uncompromising vision of male matter as conceived "on the flat."

THE EYE OF THE STORY

In two ways, the following description of a frenzied orgy scene in Bataille's *Story of the Eye* is programmatic for the ejaculations in the novella:

> But the explosion of totally drunken guffaws that ensued rapidly degenerated into a debauche of tumbling bodies, lofty legs and arses, wet skirts and come. Guffaws emerged like foolish and involuntary hiccups but scarcely managed to interrupt a brutal onslaught on cunts and cocks. (17)

First, male orgasm does not occupy an exempted or exalted place in a hierarchy of values. Though the bodies "tumble," the legs and arses are equally "lofty," and "wet skirts and come" are unproblematically heaped together. "[D]ebauche," then, pinpoints an impersonal and nonvertical indifference. To further scandalize the Hegelian sentiment, throughout the story, ejaculation and urination take place sequentially, sometimes, impossibly, simultaneously, and at other times are virtually indistinguishable from each other (e.g., 21, 41–42).

Second, male orgasm here does not have the power of climax or culmination. For the involuntary, pulsating, and iterative "guffaws" and "hiccups" do not succeed in interrupting the flow of the proceedings. If that is the case, then how does this pornographic novella manage to end? Can Bataille's *Story* supply narrative's requisite sense of an ending?

At a literal, anecdotal level, *Story* does not end or finalize. Abruptly and arbitrarily, the last line of the tale reads, "and we [the narrator, Simone, and Sir Edmund] set sail towards new adventures with a crew of Negroes" (67). At another level, Bataille supplemented the story with a biographical essay, titled "Coincidences," in which he discusses some of the events from his life that inspired it. Finally, the Penguin Classics edition of the tale offers Bataille's "Outline of a Sequel to *Story of the Eye*," which accompanied the 1967 edition. Hence, *Story* ends with a protracted series of convulsive hiccups, forfeiting a definite ending. However, after reading the tale, one is nevertheless struck by the impression that something has halted, a sensation that there is little need for further happenings. How can this be?

In her defense of French avant-gardist pornography such as Bataille's *Story* and Pauline Réage's *The Story of O*, titled "The Pornographic Imagination," Susan Sontag comes up with an answer. She ascribes to Adorno the idea that pornographic fiction cannot be literary, because it lacks the required, Aristotelian, and organic structure of "beginning-middle-and-end." Paraphrasing that view, she writes, "A piece of pornographic fiction concocts no better than a crude excuse for a beginning; and once having begun, it goes on and on and ends nowhere."[13] Subsequently, Sontag argues that *Story*, in contrast to the works of Sade, does have an ending, if not a realistic one. The principle that informs Sade's fiction is static: his narrative is like a "catalogue or encyclopedia" (99). Instead of moving toward an ending, "Sade stalled. He multiplied and thickened his narrative; tediously reduplicated orgiastic permutations and combinations," Sontag writes (108).

Bataille, however, does offer the sense of an ending, albeit one of exhaustion rather than of culmination or fulfillment. Noting that *Story*'s narrative is "thing-based" rather than character-driven, Sontag concludes:

> [Bataille's] principle of organization is thus a spatial one: a series of things, arranged in a definite sequence, are tracked down and exploited, in some convulsive act. The obscene playing with or defiling of these objects, and of people in their vicinity, constitutes the action of this novella. When the last object (the eye) is used up in a transgression more daring than any preceding, the narrative ends. (110)

That final transgression, incidentally, is the insertion of a priest's eye in Simone's vagina. Gazing at the narrator, it sheds tears of semen and urine, offering a "dreamy vision of disastrous sadness" (Bataille, *Story of the Eye*, 67). As shocking as that image may be, it does not really surprise after all the creative abuses happening to eyes in the preceding pages. Indeed, the story follows a steady course of incrementation that is utterly predictable. Yet Sontag aptly characterizes the mood of exhaustion that characterizes the ending of this short novella (only sixty-seven pages): "tracked down," "exploited," "used up."

In "The Metaphor of the Eye," Roland Barthes offers a similar analysis. Whereas, again, Sade's narrative is "encyclopedic," pervaded by a bookkeeper's spirit of accounting and tallying, Bataille manages to void meaning: "Using metonymical interchange, Bataille drains a metaphor, which although double is by no means saturated in either chain."[14] According to Barthes, *Story* consists of two chains of metaphors, each of which is "*varied*" or "*declined*" (120). The first chain includes globular objects such as "eyes," "eggs," "saucers of milk," and "testicles" (121). Through a metonymic switch (container-content), the second series is made up of "tears," "yolk," "milk," and "semen." In turn, that chain dissolves into the various modalities of the appearance of moisture: "from 'damp' to 'streaming,' all the varieties of 'making wet' complement the original metaphor of the globe" (121). The workings of these two chains are so encompassing that they even implicate the sun, Plato's symbol for the patriarchal *logos*. Here, it shines with "liquid" and "urinary" rays (122).

The point of drainage occurs when the two chains are not so much combined ("break an egg," "put out an eye"), but rather crossed through metonymic association ("put out an egg," "break an eye"), thus establishing "a kind of general contagion of qualities and actions" (124–25). Hence, Barthes concludes,

> [T]he metaphor that varies [the associations] exhibits a controlled difference that the metonymy that interchanges them immediately sets about abolishing. The world becomes *blurred*; properties are no longer separate; spilling, sobbing, urinating form a *wavy* meaning, and the whole of *Story of the Eye* signifies in the manner of a vibration that always gives the same sound (but what sound?). (125)

However, if *Story* emits such a vibration or wave of blurry meaning, then it would not be a story proper, because a story needs events, and hence, change. Instead, it would be a poem, as Barthes suggests, rather than a *histoire* or a *récit* (120). The novella conjures up a shimmering and alternating set of images of contagion rather than a plot or story line. Nothing really happens; consequently, the story cannot deliver the sense of an ending, just more waves.

But *Story* has an ironic surprise in store for the reading that Barthes formulates. Strikingly, the tale performs a preemptive strike, an *a priori* voidance, of the structuralistic reading that Barthes presents. Barthes has little to teach the bedridden Simone, who gives the trick away:

> Upon my [the narrator] asking what the word *urinate* reminded her of, [Simone] replied: *terminate*, the eyes, with a razor, something red, the sun. And *egg*? A calf's eye, because of the colour of the head (the calf's head) and also because the white of the egg was the white of the eye, and the yolk the eyeball. The eye, she said, was egg-shaped. . . . She played gaily with words, speaking about *broken eggs*, and then *broken eyes*, and her arguments became more and more unreasonable. (34)

Bataille, too, revealed the engine of his story. In "Coincidences," he writes, "The entire *Story of the Eye* was woven in my mind out of two ancient and closely associated obsessions, *eggs* and *eyes*," only professing a belated surprise when it dawns on him that the proficient testicles take part in this association as well (71). Finally, the narrator of *Story* sums up the repetitive and predictable associations, all variations on the same theme, that make up most of the novella's action, with a devastating "etc.":

> Nothing would be easier, at least for the time being, than to have Marcelle living in Simone's room secretly like myself. We would simply be forced to share the bed (and we would inevitably have to use the same bathtub, *etc.*). (38, emphasis added)

If the story were to end with a similar "etc.," then the analyst's discourse, like Simone's, would become "more and more unreasonable," excessively reveling in what is obvious. What *Story* seems to drain or vacate, then, is the structuralist's approach to narrative meaning, ridiculed *avant la lettre*. Does narrative cease when the structuralist has only one thing left to say: "etc."?

To his credit, Barthes also suggests a different thematic, one that I want to take up:

> The imaginary world unfolded here does not have as its "secret" a sexual fantasy. If it did, the first thing requiring explanation would be why the erotic theme is never directly phallic (what we have here is a "round phallicism"). . . . *Story of the Eye* is not a deep work. Everything is on the surface; there is no hierarchy. The metaphor is laid out in its entirety; it is circular and explicit, with no secret reference behind it. . . . The narrative is simply a kind of flow of matter enshrining the precious metaphorical substance. (122–23)

Hence, Barthes suggests that *Story* is not so much about ejaculation, but rather itself, in a way, ejaculatory ("flow of matter"). But is the sperm then still "precious"? Additionally, the superficiality and lack of hierarchy of the narrative that Barthes notes point to the flatness and lateralization discussed above. Can there be found in Bataille a subjectivity and an erotic apart from, or beyond, the "directly phallic," alternatively figured as "round," or as secreting and flowing "superficially"?

DRAINING MASCULINITY

In this section, I want to suggest a different way of reading the novella. I contend that *Story* is, indeed, a story; that something happens and changes in it; and that it ends. The chain of eyes, eggs, and testicles may occupy the center of the narrative, but only so in the sense that it forms the "eye of the storm." For the same thing happens to them over and over again—they are pierced, liquid oozes out—which is tantamount to saying that nothing much happens to them. They are not characters who cause or experience events.

The end of the story, taken in its double meaning of "aim" and "finale," is, in Sontag's resonant verbs, to track down, exploit, use up, and exhaust the dominant convention of masculinity and the hierarchy that sustains it; *that* is the story's ultimate protagonist as well as its most pathetic casualty. When, to all intents and purposes, that objective has been achieved, the narrative concludes. The story engages and drains, empties out, several figurations of masculine subjectivity and desire. Meanwhile, it promotes an alternative masculinity that is testicular and ejaculatory rather than erect and phallic; participatory rather than distanciated and voyeuristic; liquid rather than solid; and formless rather than formed.

The first figuration of masculine sexuality that *Story* debunks and reinscribes is stereotypical enough: the gun. However, that weapon delivers none of the values typically associated with it: a violent will, an instrumental control, a secure aim. In a bid to liberate the institutionalized Marcelle, the narrator and his consort Simone arrive at the hospital during a stormy night. Soon the narrator finds himself alone and out of his wits. Inexplicably, he removes his clothes, first down to his shirt, which partial state of undress he earlier, at the sight of another male participant to the orgy, decried as a "ridiculous" look, and then down to his shoes, probably making an even more farcical appearance (Bataille, *Story of the Eye*, 16).

The mood is one of frenzy ("aimlessly," "haphazardly," "erratic," "anxious," "hurriedly") (25). At the sudden sight of a fleeing woman, the narrator charges after her, brandishing the gun, though its exact use initially eludes him:

> I did not know what to do with the gun which I still held, for I had no pockets left; by charging after the woman who had run past me

> unrecognized, I would obviously be hunting her down to kill her. The roar of the wrathful elements, the raging of the trees and the sheet, also helped to prevent me from discerning anything distinct in my will or in my gestures. (25)

The weapon suggests, teaches, its usage to the narrator, who acts at its disposal. "Excited by [his] revolver"; hence, "I would obviously be hunting her down to kill her," he concludes. The instrument controls the agent rather than the other way around. So, how will it fire?

Grabbed from behind by Simone, the narrator simultaneously ejaculates and fires his gun:

> I scarcely had time to spin around when my come burst in the face of my wonderful Simone: clutching my revolver, I was swept up by a thrill as violent as the storm, my teeth chattered and my lips foamed, with twisted arms I gripped my gun convulsively, and, willy-nilly, three blind horrifying shots were fired in the direction of the château. (26)

Because the two events happen at the same instant, their descriptive terms cannot but bear on each other. Chattering, foaming, and twisting, the narrator's body executes no instrumental control or agency over either the gun or the penis ("willy-nilly"). Though manual pressure on the weapon is increased (it is first "clutched," then "gripped"), the ambivalent shots are executed without subject: "three . . . shots were fired." Blind, the shots lack a calculated aim; they only manage to go off in the general direction of the institute.

Most important, however, is the temporal instantaneity of the ejaculation. There is hardly time to turn around, and yet the narrator's semen ends up in Simone's face. This orgasm is modulated by the three targetless, convulsive, and iterative shots. Indeed, they produce a protracted series of hiccups or guffaws rather than a singular climax. Term for term, aspect for aspect, then, this description of ejaculation empties out, negates, the status of ejaculatory climax.

In a later chapter, the gun returns in an imagined, daydreamed threesome with Marcelle. Now it is notable for its utter harmlessness. Even the moment of shooting is omitted. What is more, the potentially hard and penetrative qualities of the lead bullets are substituted for by the play with oozing, seminal *crème fraîche* and urine:

> I would arouse [Simone's] breasts from a distance by lifting the tips on the heated barrel of a long service revolver that had been loaded

> and just fired (first of all, this would shake us up, and secondly, it would give the barrel a pungent smell of powder). At the same time, she would pour a jar of dazzling white *crème fraîche* on Marcelle's grey anus, and she would also urinate freely in her robe or, if the robe were ajar, on Marcelle's back or head, while I could piss on Marcelle from the other side (I would certainly piss on her breasts). Furthermore, Marcelle herself could fully inundate me if she liked, for while I held her up, her thighs would be gripping my neck. And she could also stick my cock in her mouth, and what not. (33)

In this staccato series of proceedings and positions, simultaneity and sequentiality are hard to distinguish ("at the same time," "and," "or," "while," "furthermore," "while," "and"). What seems clear is that the penis only enters the scene as a negligible afterthought, and is even then immediately dissolved by another "etc." ("and what not"). At the beginning of the fantasy, the revolver has already been shot; at its conclusion, the male organ appears, but emphatically not in the way to anticipate climax; in the meantime, urine and dazzling white cream are equally eroticized.

If the first image through which masculinity and ejaculation are reconceived, the revolver, stands out for its utter predictability, the second one seems highly improbable. It is a bicycle, of all things. Yet that mundane mode of transport can be taken to follow up on the problematization of the mechanical, technical, and instrumental view of sexuality that was indicated by the revolver. Forced to flee the scene after their aborted attempt to free Marcelle, Simone and the narrator hurriedly mount their bikes, offering "one another the irritating and theoretically unclean sight of a naked though shod body on a machine" (29).

This galling spectacle is presented to the eyes of both parties here ("one another"), but subsequently the scene first isolates the narrator's concerted look at Simone, who drives ahead:

> A leather seat clung to Simone's bare cunt, which was inevitably jerked by the legs pumping up and down on the spinning pedals. Furthermore, the rear wheel vanished indefinitely to my eyes, not only in the bicycle's fork but virtually in the crevice of the cyclist's naked bottom: the rapid whirling of the dusty tire was also directly comparable to both the thirst in my throat and the erection of my penis, destined to plunge into the depths of the cunt sticking to the bicycle seat. (30)

The motion of jerking, pumping, spinning, and whirling, at the collapse of the body and the machine, strikes the narrator as the "goal of my sexual licentiousness: a geometric incandescence (among other things, the coinciding point of life and death, being and nothingness), perfectly fulgurating" (30).

The sight of the wheel, churning indefinitely into the crevice of Simone's crotch, offers an image of the *perpetuum mobile* of desire. It is "directly comparable" to the narrator's erect penis, which must plunge into the incandescent vanishing point to fulfill its destiny ("destined"). This apparent destination of the penis could well bring into play a linear and climactic dynamic, rivaling and offsetting the circular, repetitive, and mechanical whirling of the bike's rear wheel. Then again, how is one to come, to arrive at a destiny, which fulgurates, and where opposites coincide? It appears that the penis can only be grafted on, caught into, this indefinite motility. Thus, its only proper destiny is to vanish.

The next step would be to implicate the narrator and his body in the imagery of mechanical desire. The scene does precisely that by entertaining a return look by Simone at her male consort, even if this look is wholly focalized by the narrator, who specifies that Simone cannot really see him:

> Now it was difficult for Simone to see [the absurd rigidity of my penis], partly because of the darkness, and partly because of the swift rising of my left leg, which kept hiding my stiffness by turning the pedal. Yet I felt I could see her eyes, aglow in the darkness, peer back constantly, no matter how fatigued, at this breaking point of my body. (30)

Through a vision imagined by the narrator, the male organ becomes part of the fulgurating machinery, indefinitely rising and turning, appearing and disappearing. Hence, its destiny cannot but be lost. Small wonder, then, that the scene fails to proceed toward penetration and ejaculation, but stops short with an accident.

As if to punish Simone for witnessing the breaking point of the narrator's body, she comes to suffer: "her nude body was hurled upon an embankment with an awful scraping of steel on the pebbles and a piercing shriek" (30). In this anticlimax to the scene, the narrator's next action is to "cover" and "[lie] down next" to Simone's unconscious body. Whereas Simone is relatively unharmed ("no injury, no bruise marked the body"), the narrator will become the bike's—desire's—most crushing casualty:

> I threw myself upon the lifeless body, trembling with fear, and as I clutched it in an embrace, I was overcome with bloody spasms, my lower lip drooling and my teeth bared like a leering moron. . . . I lay down next to Simone's body just I was, soaked and full of coagulated dust, and soon I drifted off into vague nightmares. (30–31)

Together the gun and the bike, when taken as figurations of masculine sexuality, empty out most of the gender's stereotypical aspects. Instead of penetration, we have the indefinite movement of fulguration, of vanishing and drifting. In contrast to ejaculatory climax, we find iterative and involuntary hiccups. These movements concern the narrator, the I who tells the *Story*.

But the exhaustion of tropes of masculinity that drives the narrative also pertains to the other male characters. Two of them, the young priest Don Aminado and the bullfighter Granero, meet with accidents, too, though these unhappy occurrences seem less accidental when they are read as the necessary and inevitable disqualifications of specific tropes. Both involve the high: hierarchy, verticality, elevation. In the priest's case, that trope turns out to be the upturned eye, the look at the heavens, the desire for transcendence.

In a baroque church in Seville, Simone and the narrator, accompanied by Sir Edmund, make the acquaintance of Don Aminado as he appears from a confession booth:

> a blond priest, very young, very handsome, with a long thin face and the pale eyes of a saint. His arms were crossed on his chest, and he remained on the threshold of the booth, gazing at a fixed point on the ceiling as though a celestial apparition were about to help him levitate. (57)

Whether it is because of his blondness, youth, or beauty, or alternatively, because of the spiritual tendencies that transfix his look up on high ("ceiling," "celestial," "levitate"), the appearance of the priest inspires the threesome with a frenzied desire to humiliate and debase him. The narrator revels in selected terms of abuse, all designed to cut the priest down to size: "sordid creature," "larva," "cadaver," "pig," "swine," "monster," "naked cadaver" (57–64). Cleverly co-opting the priest's masochistic desire for martyrdom, Simone, Edmund, and the narrator draw him into a series of perversions that culminates when he is strangulated to the point of simultaneous death and orgasm (65). An annoying fly buzzing in a sunbeam over the body is waved away by Simone. Then,

> Something bizarre and quite baffling had happened: this time, the insect had perched on the corpse's eye and was agitating its long nightmarish legs on the strange orb. (65)

The final insult to heavenward vision arrives when Simone plucks out one of Don Aminado's eyes and inserts it into her vagina. Streaked with tears of urine and come, it gazes back at the narrator, offering him a "dreamy vision of disastrous sadness" (65). Arguably, this is Bataille's own look at Hegel.

Fellow *libertine* Sir Edmund is not dispensed with in the same manner as Don Aminado and, as we shall see, Granero, the bullfighter. However, the narrator delivers one disapproving description of his behavior, strongly contrasting with his own attitude. The narrator and Simone fully participate in the promiscuous promenade of sexual encounters in Seville. Yet, the same let-go disposition does not animate the Englishman:

> Usually, Sir Edmund would follow at a distance in order to surprise us: he would turn people, but he never came close. And if he masturbated, he would do it discreetly, not for caution's sake, of course, but because he never did anything unless standing isolated and almost utterly steady, with a dreadful muscular contraction. (55)

Distanced, isolated, steady, and masturbating with "a dreadful muscular contraction," Sir Edmund's stance stands in contrast to the sense of abandonment and self-loss celebrated by the narrator.

The last male character I want to discuss is Granero. The matador is exclusively and excessively drawn in vertical lines. Only twenty years of age, he is "extremely popular, being handsome, *tall* and of a still childlike simplicity"; he comes across "like a very manly Prince Charming with a perfectly elegant *figure*" (49, emphasis added). The narrator remarks that the spectacle of bullfighting offers a coital image to its audience: the bull "makes its quick, brutal, thrusts over and over again into the matador's cape, barely grazing the *erect line* of the body" (47, emphasis added). In this respect, he continues, "the matador's costume is quite expressive, for it safeguards the *straight line* shooting up *so rigid and erect* every time the lunging bull grazes the body and because the pants so tightly sheathe the behind" (50, emphasis added). Granero's straight, rigid, and erect appearance is complemented by a long, thin sword.

When Simone, Edmund, and the narrator witness Granero's first fight, he performs in close accordance with the vertical logic that animates his stature and his outfit: "The young man sent the furious beast racing around him in his pink cape; each time, his body was *lifted* by a sort of spiraling *jet*, and he just barely escaped a frightful impact" (50, emphasis added). When the bull is killed, the narrator and Simone briefly withdraw to an outer courtyard for a frenzied copulation. As they return, the narrator's penis remains "stubbornly rigid," as if inspired by the vertical and phallic dynamic of the bullfight (51). A present awaits Simone on her seat: a plate with the peeled testicles of the bull finished off just before. She wants to sit on the plate, she says, but Edmund and the narrator, worrying about the attention they are drawing from other audience members, forbid her to go ahead. Even so, the narrator admits to feeling unsettled by the "renewed desire" that the plate of balls inspires in him.

As the afternoon goes on, Simone and the narrator reach a curious state, morose, stupefied, and dissociated, due to the combined effects of the raging sun, the violent spectacle before their eyes, and the boredom that comes from being prevented from acting on their impulses. Then, suddenly but expectedly, the scene and the chapter end in a series of cross-cut images: Simone bites into one of the balls; Granero advances toward the bull; Simone inserts the other ball into her vagina; Granero is wedged against the balustrade; a horn pierces his right eye and penetrates his head; Simone comes violently and suffers a nosebleed (53).

These events, the narrator warns, while "actually" related, seem to him to occur "without transition or connection," because of his absentminded and dissociated state, and because of the fact that they happened "in just a few seconds" (53). Yet, the improbably fast and accurate cutting between the two scenes, the one playing in close up, just at his side, the other at some distance in the arena, cannot but betray his judgment: a fitting and appropriate ending for the man who was too vertical, too phallic, to begin with.

His right eye dangling from its socket, Granero is carried out of the arena. Exit the masculinity he embodies. Again, a vertical or hierarchical masculinity, elegant though it was, has come to ruin. At the story's final page, after all that has happened to, as well as through, the gun and the bicycle, and what has befallen Don Aminado and Granero, there is little left for the narrator to deconstruct. Thus, *Story* offers the sense of an ending through the exhaustion, voidance, or drainage of the masculinity that only matters to the extent that it be erect, rigid, and phallic.

CONCEPTS OF EJACULATION

Reassociating the phallus with ejaculation, or replacing the former with the latter, resituates male subjectivity in narrative. Whereas the phallus, indirectly, implicitly, and invisibly, looms over the narrative rather than participating in it, ejaculation forges a temporal and visual dimension that can only be accounted for in and through a story, the focalized rendition of what happens and what remains. Indeed, through ejaculation, masculine subjectivity is forced to come to terms with an event, something that happens, and with the consequences of that event, something that materially remains.

Both the event and the effect challenge the formation of a masculinity that, in the case of the phallus, can remain outside the story while forming its imagined shadow, anchor, calibration stone, ground, origin, or telos. In sharp contrast, stories of ejaculation forge the account, the making sense, of the event of orgasm, as well as the consideration of an image of the male body and its products. Narrative forces the issue: it makes masculinity relate to the bodily event and to its substantial effects. The invisibility and solidity of the phallus is contingently narrativized, replotted, so that masculinity becomes visible and fragmentable in its various aspects.

According to Barthes, the event of orgasm may be reified as the pleasurable culmination of the narrative, serving as its destiny or fate. At the same time, Barthes also makes way for the possibility that the event, ill-timed, sudden, and intermittent, might derail the narrative that prepares for its timely climax, so that other images of the event become visible and intelligible. Derrida locks orgasm into an immanent mediality that contracts the story, and relevels it at the screen or mirror, which the mime's orgiastic simulations ceaselessly address, but never break. Bataille replaces the climactic event with iterative hiccups and guffaws that extend over the narrative, thus voiding climax in a throbbing entropy.

Additionally, Barthes, Derrida, and Bataille seize on different aspects of the event of ejaculation, which in itself already speaks for its heterogeneity. Barthes's focus is largely on temporality and timing, hence on narrativity and its discontent: the oscillation between the affects of pleasure and bliss, between the well-timed and properly narrative orgasm, and a bliss that always arrives too late or too soon. Derrida concentrates on semen's impossible number, both singular and plural, an approach that returns in the various perspectives he discusses under the single heading of dissemination. Hence, dissemination is not one thing or operation, but splits apart in the different aspects he distinguishes. Bataille puts most stress on the materiality of semen, which he describes as "base," thus canceling and flattening the philosophical and gendered hierarchies that give matter its place.

With respect to masculinity, Barthes makes that gender come across as insecure and embarrassed, unable to wield the reins of the horses of pleasure and bliss without getting them mixed up. Derrida's masculinity is plastic, responsive, and fragmented. Its limbs and organs are entrained, plugged in and let go, in a textual machinery that runs its course without care for the formation of a properly differentiated masculinity. While angling for glory, Bataille's masculinity submits to what is low, leveling and lateralizing its shape against a two-dimensionality that allows for no elevation or erection of value or form. Thus, masculinity must find its image in formless, flattened shapes.

Conceptually, Barthes alienates ejaculation by splitting it in two, pleasure and bliss, while that distinction remains ever insecure. In turn, Derrida alienates ejaculation through its multiplication, layering aspect on aspect, so that it becomes dense and overdetermined. Finally, Bataille alienates ejaculation through indifference, its indiscriminate association with processes and functions usually thought of in contradistinction.

In that sense, "concept of ejaculation" is not only a Hegelian contradiction, but also a Bataillean one. For in Bataille's world ejaculation and semen no longer command a distinct force or value. Bataille works and exhausts semen and ejaculation to their complete unraveling. Mixed up with urine, saliva, and a host of other moist and formless substances, sperm loses its power of distinction, its capacity to matter, to make a significant difference. Serialized and reiterated as hiccups without consequence, ejaculation forfeits its power of conclusion, climax, culmination. Hence, both dissolve. Precisely because of the persistent and obsessive attention paid to ejaculation and semen, then, they disappear as tropes of masculine distinction. Indeed, ejaculation and semen are smeared out, smudged away, horizontally, narratively, and conceptually. Thus, the ultimate and paradoxical consequence of the sustained conceptualization of ejaculation is that it can no longer support a concept.

PART FIVE

LITERATURE

ELEVEN

MISPLACED THIGH

Proust

IN THE NEXT THREE CHAPTERS, I turn to literature, to three intricately worded scenes of ejaculation that are part of the first books of Marcel Proust's *In Search of Lost Time.*[1] Intriguingly, these scenes encapsulate temporal modulations of male orgasm other than the discrete point of climax. Additionally, they offer ejaculations that are all nonpenetrative, ranging from a wet dream to masturbation to an involuntary climax during a wrestling game. Finally, the scenes consider and perform what can be seen as initializing acts of pro-ductivity, in the sense of Thomas: the origination of writing, tapping into the libidinal, energetic thrust that will generate the series of books; first-time masturbation and ejaculation, where traces of semen figure as writing; and the dense initiation of the male subject in various homosocial groupings of men, paternal, connoisseurial, and amical and/or erotic.

In all, the becoming-writer of the speaking subject is at stake. Indeed, ejaculation not only is the obvious theme of these passages, but also serves as the instance through which the subject considers writing and begins to write, with writing conceived of as both a material process and a product. I will begin with the curious wet dream that appears at—possibly *as*—the beginning of *Combray*, the first installment of the series of novels.

BEGINNINGS

Where does *Combray* begin? As often noted, the book starts twice over, which suggests that its origin is suspended between two places, two chapters, or that the book cannot be said to originate properly at all. Initially, the childhood memories of Combray that form the subject matter of the book emerge in the oscillation between sleeping and waking that opens the book.

By the end of the first chapter, however, these recollections are discredited as merely superficial and partial. For the narrator is able to observe "no more of [Combray] than this sort of luminous panel, sharply defined against a vague and shadowy background, like the panels which the glow of a Bengal light or a searchlight beam will cut out and illuminate in a building the other parts of which remain plunged in darkness" (1:49). Yet when the narrator consumes a tea-soaked piece of pastry, the madeleine, Combray's past rises up in its entirety and reveals itself to him, now "taking shape and solidity" (1:55). Hence, the double beginning of *Combray* sets up a frame for the novel that moves from two-dimensional and partial imagery to three-dimensional and complete shapes.

Chapter 2 opens on a distanced, panoramic, and perspectivized view of Combray ("Combray, at a distance, from a twenty-mile radius") (1:56). The play of the horizon and shadows quickly gives way to a richly descriptive approach. This second beginning switches from a "flat" superficiality to a "deep" perspective, and from partiality to totality. Nevertheless, the "luminous panel" of the first opening returns in the many allusions to the colors of painting and the fickle projections of the magic lantern (1:56). Thus, the second and "now-for-real" start of *Combray* cannot completely overrule the first and failed one. *Combray*'s actual beginning, it would seem, remains elusive.

According to Malcolm Bowie in *Proust Among the Stars*, the book energetically starts with a nocturnal emission that does not quite happen, precariously poised between sleeping and being awake. This third and alternative origin is enfolded in and overrules the other two. As Bowie comments, "From the threshold of an orgasm that did not occur, there extends an interminable desiring itinerary." The withheld ejaculation announces "[t]he huge exploratory programme of the novel." [2] Proust writes:

> Sometimes, too, as Eve was created from a rib of Adam, a woman would be born during my sleep from some misplacing of my thigh. Conceived from the pleasure I was on the point of enjoying, she it was, I imagined, who offered me that pleasure. My body, conscious that its own warmth was permeating hers, would strive to become one with her, and I would awake. (*Lost Time*, 1:3)[3]

Bowie's reading signals the "touristic" significance of ejaculation ("itinerary," "exploratory") in accordance with the images of travel and journey that balance the lack of movement in the opening pages of *Combray*. This bedside tourism partakes of the typical Proustian attitude of mobile immobility, a bodily sedentariness supporting frantic movement of the mind and the imagination.

However, Bowie's reading opens up the question of scale. The orgasm that does not happen engenders an energy capable of sustaining a program or journey that is huge, even interminable. Generally, Bowie explains, sexuality in Proust is "subject to displacement and endlessly transferable" (*Proust Among the Stars*, 211–12). In order for orgasm to be able to access nothing short of infinity, to span the whole of the novel and the itineraries it traces, it apparently cannot have happened. To engender the book, the ejaculation must remain suspended at its threshold. Only by staying latent can it form the inexhaustible source of energy for *Lost Time*.

Bowie takes up the point later, offering what he calls the "quizzical cost-benefit analysis" of the wet dream from *Sodom and Gomorrah*. "[W]hich of us, on waking," Proust writes, "has not felt a certain irritation at having experienced in his sleep a pleasure which, if he is anxious not to tire himself, he is not, once he is awake, at liberty to repeat indefinitely during that day" (quoted in Bowie, *Proust Among the Stars*, 239–40). Such, then, is the economy of ejaculation at stake: withheld, it can access totality and infinity; completed, it brings about only irritation and fatigue. Hence, Bowie locates male orgasm in the economy that Bataille terms "restricted," that is, belated, derivative, and liable to the cost-benefit analysis that seminal expenditure would trump. This view of ejaculation is stereotypical enough, conforming to the conventional idea that orgasm drains vigor and strength.

But the passage does not so much narrate the suspension of ejaculation as it suspends the question of whether or not orgasm has occurred by cutting out the moment of its happening. "Conceived from the pleasure I was on the point of enjoying, she it was, I imagined, who offered me that pleasure." The pleasure jumps from nearly happening ("on the point of enjoying") to already happened ("offered me that pleasure"). The sentence skips from something about to occur ("the pleasure") to something over and done with ("that pleasure"). In the meantime, *this* pleasure, pleasure as it happens, disappears in an ellipsis.

This suspension of the moment is underscored by the passage's overall temporality. "Sometimes," the paragraph starts. Hence, the narrator is talking neither about a topical and singular occurrence nor about infinity. Far from being a one-off happening or an endless flow of energy, these emissions are both momentary and sequential. Thus, if this ejaculation forms the point of origin of *Lost Time*, preceding and puncturing through Combray I and Combray II, nocturnal reverie and madeleine, one must take into account that it is simultaneously elided and dispersed over repetitive instances. Thus, it cannot be fixated. Indeed, its timing is lost. The origin of *Lost Time* is lost.

Nevertheless, a genesis or creation is taking place, phrased in a biblical and mythological register: "Sometimes, too, as Eve was created from a rib of

Adam, a woman would be born during my sleep from some misplacing of my thigh." The instant of ejaculation may be lost, but that does not prevent it from being productive. The woman is imaginary, but her administrations carry results that persist after waking: "my cheek was still warm from her kiss, my body ached beneath the weight of hers" (1:3). Hence, this creation is real, and the woman enjoys existence and agency, temporary as they may be. Her birth is triggered by "some misplacing of my thigh." Admittedly, this scene can easily be pictured in a fairly realistic and crude way: a man is asleep, his thigh moves, an organ gets stuck or rubbed; *voilà*, there she is. However, the rhetoric of the sentence warrants more attention, particularly the simile in which "a rib" is compared to, as well as displaced by, "a thigh." As it turns out, this thigh is misplaced, displaced, in more ways than one.

ADAM'S RIB

The reference to Adam's rib is to Genesis 2:21–22. There, God puts the first-created human being in a deep sleep, "and while he slept [God] took one of his ribs and closed up its place with flesh; and the rib which the LORD God had taken from the man he made into a woman and brought her to the man" (Revised Standard Version). Where the King James Bible already names the first human being as "Adam" at this point, the Revised Standard Version uses the more ambivalent "man" for "mankind." This ambiguity may relate back to the earlier story of human creation in 1:27, where man and woman are created simultaneously and equally in God's likeness.

In the follow-up or retelling in Genesis 2, however, "man" is created first out of dust or clay and brought to life by receiving God's breath (2:7). The second being is created out of the first one's rib, is not given divine breath, and is only then named "woman" by the first being. The proper name "Eve" is not mentioned until Genesis 3:20. Further sexual ambiguity is arrested in readings that ascribe secondary, derivative, and inferior status to "woman" under the name of "Eve."[4]

The problem is deceptively simple: since man and woman form a binary pair, they define each other. Hence, there can be no properly male being before the existence of a female being. In *Lethal Love: Feminist Literary Readings of Biblical Love Stories*, Mieke Bal argues that "man" or "Adam" should be taken as a yet sexually undifferentiated being. It is neither androgynous nor bisexual, for sex as such does not exist at this early stage. Its Hebrew name, *ha'adam*, Bal explains, is not a proper name that indicates sexed individuality. A common noun derived from *ha'adama*, for "clay" or "dust," it only denotes a species.[5] Only *after* the second being is specified as "woman" can a third being be differentiated as male out of the original one. Proper names arrive later, finally turning the belatedly sexed beings into characters.[6]

Not that the passage refrains from using explicitly gendered language, such as personal pronouns. But this after-the-fact language may nevertheless be burdened with the attempt to come to terms with a different antestate. For example, Genesis 2:24 mentions parents, while these seem anachronistic at this early stage: these humans neither are nor have parents. Then again, the reference works to bring imagery of maternal and paternal reproduction into play, even if the creation of Adam and woman, strictly speaking, does not occur along those lines.

In Genesis 2:21–22, *ha'adam*, the human being created from the earth, designates an ambivalent entity without sex or character. How is woman produced from it? God puts the entity to sleep. Its rib is removed and molded into a second being. If one insists on the creature's masculinity, "rib" may be read as a displacement of the penis (like the usual "feet" for "testicles" in the Bible), a more likely reproductive organ. Yet some biblical scholars, Bal adds, read "side" for "rib," so that it euphemistically stands for "belly" or "womb" (115). There is little need to decide: the rib condenses both possibilities, metonymically and metaphorically. God acts as a midwife, or as a sculptor busy with human bone and flesh, as earlier in the text God acted as a potter with dust or clay. With "rib" serving as a double displacement, the act of creation becomes thoroughly sexually ambivalent in accordance with the first being's still-undifferentiated state.

Several modes of production are conflated here. Before bringing them to bear on the Proustian creation in the quoted passage, I will differentiate them according to agent, material, and manner. First, in Genesis 2:7, God creates the human being out of the earth's dust, breathing into its nostrils to give it life. Second, in 2:21–22, God creates woman out of the first being's rib, a piece of flesh and bone, by way of a surgical intervention and a sculptural construction. More breathing is apparently no longer necessary. Third and alternatively, now understanding "rib" as "womb," God acts as a midwife, helping the first being give birth to woman from its body.

The Semitic god who creates the world by speech acts here appears to act more like a hands-on producer, fabricating human beings ceramically, sculpturally, and surgically. But the pinnacle of creation is performed by way of the breath that also carries God's voice. God's body does not seem to be part of the proceedings, except in the form of manual agency. However, once the dust is turned to flesh courtesy of divine inspiration, it acquires self-generative potential. With life of its own, the rib generates offspring without further need for God's life-giving breath. In the third case, God becomes more of a mediator, a midwife, rather than an autonomous creator. In this way, the reproductive power of the body moves to the fore: creation becomes a thing of the flesh.

In the passage from Proust, both the narrator and Adam are asleep. A woman is born from the former's body, while the speaker also takes the place of the creating God. Hence, creative agency and creative material collapse in one body. The woman is not produced thanks to an outside agency, God's breath, but conceived from the body's own pleasure. As the thigh replaces the rib, it takes its duplicitous potential with it: the woman is both ejaculated into being *and* given birth to. If this wet dream forms the place of origin of *Lost Time*, then its conception is indeed double, male and female, or rather, ambivalently poised between the two modalities of reproduction, between ejaculation and gestation.

When the narrator talks about the book he is writing, here still as an apprentice at the task, metaphors of pregnancy and gestation abound, while ejaculating, as we will see, figures as writing, too. Perhaps giving birth concerns the book as a product, whereas ejaculation involves the process of writing. In the description of the wet dream, they are conflated into one, perhaps because the book is already written, and yet about the process of its writing. Proust's graft on Genesis highlights the generative, productive body: literary creation is about matter as well as about agency and inspiration. In Thomas's vein, writing is *pro-ductive:* "to cause to appear and be made to appear" (*Male Matters*, 34). What is rendered visible is the writing body and its output: traces of sperm, text; a birth, the book.

JUPITER'S THIGH

Again, the switch from rib to thigh can easily be dismissed realistically. A rib cannot implicate the dormant penis in the same way that a thigh can. However, the thigh cannot but help to bring another mythical intertext into play, one that further underscores the complicated process of creation that is being described here. The reference to the thigh brings in the myth of another god: Jupiter giving birth to his son from his own body.

The story: Semele, impregnated by Jupiter, is manipulated by a disguised Juno into requesting to see her lover in his actual shape. Jupiter, bound by a promise to grant Semele everything she asks for, must comply. What happens next is told by Ovid in *Metamorphoses:*

> But Semele's mortal frame could not endure the exaltation caused by the heavenly visitant, and she was burned to ashes by her wedding gift. Her child, still not fully formed, was snatched from his mother's womb and, if the tale may be believed, the feeble baby was sewn into his father's thigh till the months for which his mother should have carried him were fulfilled. (*Metamorphoses* 3:82)

The story seems curiously out of place in a book dedicated to telling "of bodies which have been transformed into shapes of a different kind" (*Metamor-*

phoses 1:29). Jupiter's shape-shifting during his philandering is a common theme (Leda and the swan, Danae and the golden rain). *Metamorphoses* recounts Jupiter's rape of Europa in the form of a bull shortly before the Semele story. But the Semele myth is ostensibly not about another transformation. Instead, the god will for once show his true form to a human.

As a result, another transformation must be at stake here. Replacing the scorched Semele, the omnipotent high-god changes into a mother. The masculine god shows his actual shape and immediately turns into a mortal mother: such is the irony of the story. Perhaps to underscore his double birth, Bacchus will be invested with androgyny for life; his characteristic epithet is "twice-born." Just as in Proust's reworking of Genesis, Jupiter both impregnates and gives birth to his offspring. This move may boil down to an appropriation of feminine reproduction. Alternatively, it can be taken to betray an ambivalence at the heart of masculine reproduction, an ambiguity that triggers endless replotting, a narrative spanning the series of books.

FROM WET DREAM TO BAD DREAM

Like Bacchus, *Lost Time* is twice-born. So, what about the ending of *Combray*? The book concludes with another awakening and with the setup for *Swann in Love*, the second book in the series. Through the chain of recollections and associations, the taste of the tea and the madeleine brings to mind Swann's love affair with Odette, which took place before Marcel's birth (1:223). *Combray*, meanwhile, ends with another nocturnal event, a nightmare of sorts, offering a blistering antidote to the exalted and creative imaginings of the wet dream at its beginning. At the book's opening, a woman is generated through circularity: she is born from a pleasure that she herself administers. But the pleasure is all the narrator's, and she exists only in his imagination.

Swann's nightmare that closes *Combray* clearly has orgasmic overtones, partially because of its imagery: waves are "surging," his heart is "anxiously beating." Just before Swann wakes, "the speed of these palpitations" redoubles (1:458). The greater significance of the nightmare, however, lies in its hard-nosed debunking of the creative potential of ejaculation that was celebrated before, establishing a negative mirror image of the wet dream. The divine creation of *Genesis* is now substituted for by the evolutionary divisions of lower organisms. If the rib/thigh earlier served as productive flesh and creative agency, this time "the warmth [of Swann's] own palm" models its imaginary offspring into being. Proust writes:

> For, from an incomplete and changing set of images, Swann in his sleep drew false deductions, enjoying at the same time, momen-

> tarily, such a creative power that he was able to reproduce himself by a simple act of division, like certain lower organisms; with the warmth that he felt in his own palm he modelled the hollow of a strange hand which he thought he was clasping, and out of feelings and impressions of which he was not yet conscious he brought about sudden vicissitudes which, by a chain of logical sequences, would produce, at specific points in his dream, the person required to receive his love or to startle him awake. (1:457)[7]

This person turns out to be his valet: "Sir, it's eight o'clock, and the barber is here. I've told him to call again in an hour" (1:458). In this blistering rewriting of the nocturnal emission, Eve is replaced by a manservant, myth by prosaic detail. And, while the narrator's cheek was still wet from the woman's kisses after waking, no such validation is granted Swann: "He touched his cheek. It was dry" (1:458).

From a glorious wet dream to an anticlimactic nightmare, *Lost Time* narrates its own origin through the figure of ejaculation. Its dispersive force is such that it cannot be placed. Instead, it opens up a series of possibilities that play out a creative productivity as suspended—misplaced like the thigh—between spirituality and materiality, body and agency, masculinity and femininity, ejaculation and gestation, creation and evolution, gods and lower organisms, reality and imagination, truth and falsity, power and simplicity. This wavering is narratively signaled by the temporal ellipsis and dispersion that mark ejaculation. It is not told, yet puts the narrative in motion. It cannot be placed temporarily, yet it modulates the novel as a whole. It hints at an exalted lost origin, yet it ends with banal delusions.

Indeed, the wet dream that forms the starting place of *Lost Time* concatenates masculine reproduction, punctual and virtual, with feminine reproduction, durative and material, into an iterative series of nocturnal emissions that entangle ejaculation and gestation, high creation and low evolution. The ellipsis of the moment at which ejaculation happens allows it to garner more weight, temporally and materially, as to its productive potential. The switches from penis to rib to thigh to womb impart a paradoxical motherliness onto ejaculation. Ultimately, this is why its timing cannot but be lost.

Hence, the beginning and the ending of *Combray* fold together hierarchized oppositions into a writerly, embodied productivity that opens and generates the series of books. The figuration of the wet dream and the nightmare partake of the same entanglement of values that Aristotle, if not for the unfortunate necessity of the "business" of reproduction, prefers to remain separate; that Lacan apprehends as the "concatenation" of the phallus and the signifiable, and as the hybridization or bastardization of the resulting effect of meaning; and that Hegel views as the "naïve" duplicity that nature imposes on the male organ and the mind. Ejaculation, misplaced or displaced, can form the starting place of writing. But it does so only on the condition that it stretches out to enfold notions and values that stand in contradistinction to it. Thus, ejaculation escapes the narrow economy that sanctions its place, garnering excessive associations and connotations. Precisely this duplicitous or ambiguous propensity, and not its inner or autonomous force, makes the ejaculation of the wet dream so extraordinarily productive, generating the whole of *Lost Time* from its elided occurrence.

TWELVE

GOSSAMER THREAD

THE SECOND SCENE OF EJACULATION in *In Search of Lost Time* is anticlimactic to the extreme; imagine a playing record that comes screeching to a halt. It takes place in the little room smelling of orrisroot, that essentially Proustian locus, situated under the roof of the summerhouse introduced at the beginning of *Combray*. The same room forms the setting for a short fragment on masturbation from *Against Sainte-Beuve*, entitled "Solitary Pleasure."

Though the room is described by Proust in more or less the same terms on both occasions (a more than decorative blackcurrant changes into a lilac), the view from its always half-opened window varies considerably. That is why I will treat the two scenes separately before I consider what they have in common. If the wet dream taken up in the previous chapter implicates the double beginning of the novel, suspended between ejaculation and gestation, creation and evolution, exaltation and deception, the ejaculation at stake in this chapter is literally split between two texts, *Combray* and "Solitary Pleasure."

The two scenes offer little by way of sexual fantasies propelling young Marcel's masturbatory pleasure. Instead, his desire and pleasure self-reflexively negotiate and play with his bodily occupancy of the room and its viewpoints. Hence, the room and its views do not form the background, setting, or décor of Marcel's solitary pleasures. Rather, they are its tenuous objects, its constitutive elements. In that way, the scenes pose the question of the place of ejaculation in relation to the masculine subject and his body, their emplacement and displacement with respect to each other. They partake of the dynamic and dense relationship between the space inhabited by the Proustian subject-body, Marcel in the little room, and the reality "out there" that he perceives. Indeed, the question these scenes incessantly pose is whether ejaculation emplaces or displaces the subject who comes.

"GOSH, GOSH, GOSH, GOSH!"

Though the passage from *Combray* ends up in the confines of the little room in a mood of utter frustration, it starts with buoyant, exhilarating wanderings along the Méséglise way. With his parents preoccupied with the formalities following Aunt Léonie's death, Marcel is for the first time allowed to go for walks on his own (1:184). Autumn mornings are spent with leisurely reading, but, in the afternoons, the same boy who before had to be chased into the garden now sets out enthusiastically for the countryside with a plaid thrown over his shoulder. "[M]y body, which in a long spell of enforced immobility had stored up an accumulation of vital energy," Proust writes, "now felt the need, like a spinning top wound up and let go, to expend it in every direction" (1:185).

The interpunctions or markings of this extension of vital energy—walls of houses, the hedge of Tansonville, the trees of Roussainville's wood, and the bushes at Montjouvain—all receive the blows of Marcel's walking stick or umbrella, as well as the inarticulate exclamations of his bliss. A sudden reflection cast by a tiled roof on a pond provokes the provisional high point of this pleasure: "I cried aloud in my enthusiasm, brandishing my furled umbrella: 'Gosh, gosh, gosh, gosh!' " Marcel voices an exhilaration only qualified by the beginning writer's resolution to find more illuminating words for his rapture (1:186). Up to this point, Marcel's pleasure is perambulatory, sequential, syntagmatic. Soon, however, the same forest of Roussainville that is so far merely one part in the series of entertaining sights along the way will become the paradigmatic object of his desire.

This shift starts with Marcel's ostensibly casual consideration of "an alternative feeling" that accompanies the joy of walking alone, "stimulated by the desire to see appear before my eyes a peasant-girl whom I might clasp in my arms" (1:187). For a short while, this imagined company, another Eve in this Edenic setting, suffices to lend "additional merit" to "everything that was in my mind at the moment, in the pink reflection of the tiled roof, the grass growing out of the wall, the village of Roussainville into which I had long desired to penetrate, the trees of its wood and the steeple of its church." In turn, nature adds extra charm to the peasant-girl. With sensuality and imagination thus feeding into each other, the boy's "desire no longer had any bounds."

The "fresh emotion" brought up by the fantasy of the girl initially increases Marcel's vitality, filling his "sails with a potent, mysterious, and propitious breeze." On the same page, however, the stake is already raised. The imagined presence of the girl, it turns out, not only adds to an already existing pleasure, but also yields an epistemological gain, which again singles out Roussainville. For, the narrator notes, her embraces and kisses would "reveal to me the spirit of those horizons, of the village of Roussainville, of the books which I was reading that year."

As one begins to wonder how much weight an absent girl can carry, and how long Marcel can keep his imagination going, the deception manifests itself: "But to wonder thus among the woods of Roussainville without a peasant-girl to embrace was to see those woods and yet know nothing of their secret treasure, their deep-hidden beauty" (1:188). Ultimately, then, the presence of the girl has become epistemologically mandatory, essential. Furthermore, the syntagmatic and sequential extending of Marcel's pleasure on his walk starts to coalesce in the "secret treasure" and "deep-hidden beauty" of Roussainville, the allure of which arrests the previously haphazard and ambulatory tracing of his desire.

After that admission and a short essayistic intermezzo, the scenery suddenly shifts. We find ourselves in the little room smelling of orrisroot where Marcel masturbates to the point of ejaculation, described as "the moment when a natural trail like that left by a snail smeared the leaves of the flowering currant that drooped around me" (1:189). The motivation for this change in location is withheld for a page, until the narrator recounts the moment "when, unable to resign myself to returning home without having held in my arms the woman I so greatly desired, I was yet obliged to retrace my steps towards Combray" (1:190). The suddenness of this transition and its belated realistic motivation together raise doubt whether Marcel was actually anywhere else than in this particular room.

Once the scenery shifts, so does the mood that animates Marcel. The pastoral evocations of the lush beauty of nature are replaced by a sense of infertility and fatigue: "that sterile soil, that stale, exhausted earth." All vitality, fresh emotion, and potency are lost, and the boy's sensual imaginations are unmasked as "no more than the purely subjective, impotent illusory creations of my temperament." Biblically, this amounts to a fall: the paradise temporarily and imaginarily occupied by Marcel and his peasant-girl is irrevocably lost.

The text suggests three possible reasons for this extreme mood swing. First, and speaking realistically, a pubescent boy with expectations of hot sex in the countryside on his mind has returned home frustrated and disappointed. The same peasant-girl "whom I should not have failed to meet had I been with my grandfather and thus unable to engage her in conversation" has not materialized now that the absence of parental guidance would have offered opportunity and license (1:189).

Yet the description concerns not a single walk, but the condensation of a series of walks. Their failure thus is not so much accidental or circumstantial, but rather pinpoints the bankruptcy of a libidinal enterprise or stage. Even if he had met a peasant-girl from Méséglise or Roussainville, or a fisher-girl from Balbec, on any of these numerous walks, would, could, anything have really happened? Marcel asks, rhetorically, "And if she had appeared, would I have dared to speak to her?" (1:190). Most important, the full extent of his rage and frustration is directed not at the absent girl, but at another object: Roussainville, with its tantalizing secret treasure and deep-hidden beauty.

The second possible reason is situated on another level. Here, the process and psychology of writing impinge on the narration of the subject's childhood. Pointing out that *In Search of Lost Time* is to a large extent about a writer writing himself into being is hardly a surprising insight. Here one finds an apprentice writer at a loss for words. Preceding the account of the autumn walks is a short scene in which Marcel gloats over Françoise's inability to voice the extent of her bereavement over the death of Léonie. "I don't know how to *express* myself," she says. Marcel shrugs and says to himself, "It's really very good of me to discuss the matter with an illiterate old woman," by his own admission adopting "the mean and narrow outlook of the pedant" (1:185).

Marcel himself, however, cannot find the words for his rapture at the sight of the pink reflection in the pond, crying out "Gosh, gosh, gosh, gosh!" and not much more, while feeling "duty bound not to content myself with these unilluminating words" (1:186). The hypothesis must be that Marcel is able to voice frustration more eloquently than consummation at this stage of his development. Perhaps, then, the writing *requires* frustration in order to come into being as writing. Desperate and anticlimactic as it may be, the ejaculatory scene stretches over two pages; at any rate, a good deal further than another quadruple "Gosh!" can.

The third reason for the mood swing in the narrative concerns the implicit recalibration of desire in its course. This motivation goes to the underlying figuration of the drive that animates both the writing and the narration. Between the cheery "goshes" and the moody ejaculation in the little room lies a world of difference. It is as though the gravitational pull of Roussainville has reconfigured the way Marcel's desire is conceptualized. What has happened, nearly implicitly, gradually, and partially obfuscated by the fantasy figure of the peasant-girl, is the transformation of Roussainville from just another stop on the trajectory along which his desire expends or unwinds to the exemplary secret treasure or deep-hidden beauty, which must be "penetrated" in order to be known.

Hence, the figuration of Marcel's desire has changed its shape from an *extension of self* to the *penetration of what is other*. The desire that previously expended itself "in every direction" is now targeted with precision. A pleasure formerly "boundless" is now firmly object-bound; the free expenditure of vital energy has become locked to a definite object. A rapture that could initially be expressed through little more than "Gosh, gosh, gosh, gosh!" has given way to verbose frustration.

And whereas Roussainville originally welcomed the brandishing of Marcel's umbrella, it is now largely inaccessible. While his walks were described as healthy exercise to dispense with accumulated energy, his ravings in the room are draining and exhausting. In the first and extensive model, Marcel moves through the space that brings him pleasure. In the second and penetrative one, he is separated and removed from it. Nevertheless, the tower of the castle-keep of Roussainville remains teasingly visible through the half-opened window of the little room.

NATURAL TRAIL

As disappointed and frustrated as he may be, Marcel does come, albeit not without the refiguration of his desire for a third time. In the following passage, note the return of the ejaculatory tourism that Bowie suggests (see chapter 11). Moreover, the Roussainville castle-keep receives the confessions of Marcel's "earliest desires." Masturbation is described as an "untrodden path." To all intents and purposes, then, this is the first onanistic orgasm that Marcel enjoys:

> Alas, it was in vain that I implored the castle-keep of Roussainville, that I begged it to send out to meet me some daughter of its village, appealing to it as to the sole confidant of my earliest desires when, at the top of our house in Combray, in the little room that smelt of orris-root, I could see nothing but its tower framed in the half-opened window as, with the heroic misgivings of a traveller setting out on a voyage of exploration or of a desperate wretch hesitating on the verge of self-destruction, faint with emotion, I explored, across the bounds of my own experience, an untrodden path which for all I knew was deadly—until the moment when a natural trail like that left by a snail smeared the leaves of the flowering currant that drooped around me. (1:189)[1]

The strangeness of this ejaculation can hardly be overstated. An object fails to emerge, even phantasmicly. On the threshold of death or new experience, Marcel ejaculates, producing traces of sperm that look like a snail's trail. This untrodden path can either be read as the penetration of new territory, or as the opening up of a new road along which desire can unwind or extend.

But the ejaculation does little more than smear the blackcurrant's leaves. Since the drooping and soiled leaves offer little space for the completion of either penetration or extension, both these possibilities now turn out to be bankrupt.

Marcel's desire is not exhausted by the advent of orgasm. The passage that opens with "in vain," moves on with an "in vain" that is twice repeated after the ejaculation has already occurred. This repetition undoes the temporal hiatus that the English translation marks with a dash, and partakes of the same iterability that is already suggested by the four inarticulate "goshes." Hence, the process is still running its course: desire is completed somewhere else, if at all, and not with or in this ejaculation. What follows is a complex play with the views that the little room at the top of the house affords.

Marcel can "see *nothing but* [Roussainville's] tower framed in the half-opened window." This amounts to a severe reevaluation of this particular view, since he noted earlier in *Combray* that, from the same window, "I could see *as far as* the keep of Roussainville-le-Pin" (1:12; emphasis added). Presumably, it is not that tower Marcel now wishes to see, but a girl, even if "sensual pleasure" is already specified as one of the room's uses at its introduction. Moreover, it is primarily the secret and beauty of Roussainville that Marcel desires to penetrate.

Then, far beyond the vision granted by the window frame, Marcel sees everything: "In vain did I compress the whole landscape into my field of vision, draining it with an exhaustive gaze which sought to extract from it a female creature" (1:189). After this idle compression of the landscape, Marcel repeatedly stresses how far his eyes can travel. They go "as far as the porch of Saint-André-des-Champs"; he stares "at the trunk of a distant tree"; and he "scan[s] the horizon." Surveying this compressed landscape, his eyes apparently can as easily trace its horizon as single out a specific tree. In other words, the landscape has no traditional perspective. Subsequently, the trees of Roussainville's wood receive his sullen, raging blows. Stubbornly, Eve declines to make an entrance.

Finally, the visual itinerary of desire ends. Marcel returns home. But not without conceding that the chance of a peasant-girl appearing from behind the trees afar is as remote as her sudden materialization from behind a painting: "if they had been trees painted on the stretched canvas background of a panorama" (1:190). These, then, are the apparent terms of the third reconfiguration of Proustian desire: the flattening or stretching out of the desired image on a canvas, which repudiates the penetrable three-dimensionality of the deep and hidden secret or beauty of Roussainville.

I repeat the three steps traced so far: first, the extension of desire along the Méséglise way, "like a spinning top wound up and let go"; second, the desired but impossible penetration of the "secret treasure" and "deep-hidden beauty" of Roussainville; and, third, the wholly superficial play with the two-dimensional image-view, which enables the visual alternation between compression and stretching, between zoom (the trunk of a specific tree) and wide-shot ("panorama," "horizon").

The complex temporality of the passage, one paragraph to be exact, enables ejaculation to be narrated without climactic imperative, without bringing closure. In the preceding paragraphs, Marcel goes out for a walk, for the first time on his own, looking to solve a libidinal problem. The ejaculatory passage opens with a disappointing "Alas," taken up by the triple exclamations of "in vain." In this extended and iterative temporality of frustration, the moment of ejaculation occurs. It is presented as the possible destination of a voyage, though the journey continues until it stops short at the flat canvas of the landscape-as-painting. Only then does Marcel return home to install himself in the room where the masturbation takes place. At the end of the paragraph, the image of a traveler reading in a railway carriage reopens movement. Hence, the orgasm settles or ends nothing. At most, desire endlessly folds or circles back onto itself.

This is not to suggest, I hasten to add, that nothing has happened. The traces of sperm on the currant's leaves materially endure. I quote the description again in the original French:

> [J]e me frayais en moi-même une route inconnue et que je croyais mortelle, jusqu'au moment où une trace naturelle comme celle d'un colimaçon s'ajoutait aux feuilles du cassis sauvage qui se penchaient jusqu'à moi. (*À la recherche du temps perdu*, 1:144)

The semantic economy of the French is awesome. With an object ("une route inconnue"), *frayer* means "to carve (a way)." Without an object, however, it means "to spawn (fish-eggs)." *Frayer avec* denotes "to have (social) intercourse with." Thus, *en moi-même* doubly stresses the autoerotic, the autogenetic. While the English translation uses "smearing," a word that leaves little to the imagination, the French has *s'ajouter à*, for "join" or "are added to." *Ajouté* means "addition" or "supplement." Thus, what is produced by the boy, it seems, is the supplement of writing. What is added is the sperm-trace. Alternately, taking *supplement* literally, what is added is a "leaflet," a set of leaves, so that *s'ajouter* condenses both ink and paper, both the materiality of the writing-trace and the flat surface on which it is graphed.

The indexical proximity of the ejaculation and the leaves, of ink and paper, is underscored in the sentence by the repetition of *jusqu'à*: the timing of the former and the placement of the latter almost, impossibly, collapse.

They approach each other to such an extent that there is virtually no space left for the subject of ejaculation. Sandwiched between the two, he is removed from his central place. And, since *s'ajouter* is reflexive, the subject becomes an object: "Je me frayais en moi-même . . . jusqu'à moi." That notwithstanding, the alternative to both the extension of the self and the penetration of what is other is found: the superficial inscription and layering of/on what is both self and other, sperm on leaves, leaves marked by semen. Smeared and drooping, these leaves form the gravitational counterpart to the pleasured imagination that extends itself into space without limit.

What moves the scene, then, is not so much the anecdotal: what does or does not happen to young Marcel on his first walk alone, his first masturbatory experience. Instead, the text revolves around a boy just on his way to leaving behind the constraints of childhood, a subject in the making, who attempts to figure out possible constellations of desire—of subjectivity, objecthood, and their placement vis-à-vis each other—journeying from one to the next. Superimposed on and entangled with that project are the considerations of the adult writer who reflects on the material production of his writing, alternately conceived, in its double meaning, as the extension, the penetration, and the inscription of desire.

SOLITARY PLEASURE

The ejaculation scene from *Combray* finds its close counterpart in *Against Sainte-Beuve*. The fragment is titled "Solitary Pleasure." At the age of twelve, Marcel once more retreats to the room smelling of orrisroot high up in the Combray summerhouse, where he assumes divine provenance of the universe with his look through the window, tells the sun to make way for him, takes a seat, and comes.

"Solitary Pleasure" is analyzed by Serge Doubrovsky in *Writing and Fantasy in Proust: The Place of the Madeleine* and by Mieke Bal in *The Mottled Screen: Reading Proust Visually*. I will trace and contrast these interpretations in some detail, while proposing alternative possibilities. Though Doubrovsky's and Bal's respective projects are quite different, the former psychoanalytical, the latter narratological and visual, they both suggest readings centering on the notion of banality; on the Proustian poetic that waxes as lengthily and poetically on the prosaic details of daily life, ejaculation included, as it does, for instance, on the celebrated beauty of the hawthorn.

"I believe," Doubrovsky opens his book, "that Proust has been overly aestheticized, asepticized."[2] After that warning, the critic uncovers a series of sadistic, cannibalistic, and necrophiliac fantasies directed at the mother in *In Search of Lost Time*. Hence, Doubrovsky counters the aestheticized Proust with the sheer brutality of the unconscious fantasies he reads in and between the lines. The more delicately and poetically phrased a sentiment seems, the more horrific its underlying drives turn out to be. In this way, *Writing and Fantasy in Proust* does a splendid job in debunking and soiling the shrine of high literature and high modernity. Yet, unable to resist ample opportunity for provocation, Doubrovsky remains caught in the imperative of literary history that Proust is, above all, pretty. The impulse to debunk directly answers to the insistence of prettiness and preciousness.

"[F]or its insistent and ambiguous quality," Bal's book takes the term *platitude* as its framework or grid.[3] On the one hand, *platitude* points to the importance of the banal and the vulgar in Proust's writing. On the other, the notion suggests a visual flatness and superficiality, the absence of depth and volume in the image. The relevance of this flatness is already borne out by the two-dimensional description of Combray that opens the second chapter, of the peculiar view from the little room, stretching out and flattening against a canvas, and of the smearing of seminal traces on the blackcurrant's leaves. "The principal thesis" that *The Mottled Screen* develops "is that the tension *between* and the inharmonious resolution *of* the meanings of the word 'flatness' constitute a central impulse to Proust's literary project," Bal writes (3).

In addition, *platitude* entails a challenge for the subject: "Reduced to a flat surface, the image confronts the subject at the limits of vision" (6). This challenge especially bears on male subjects with culturally granted access to the aesthetic and the erotic that apprehend their objects in a "deep" perspective, which privileges penetration as the main means to get at them, to get to know them. As indicated, Marcel and the adult writer-narrator do consider, but finally repudiate, the epistemological, aesthetic, and erotic desire to "penetrate" the beautiful secret of Roussainville.

Doubrovsky and Bal also consider the materiality of writing, perhaps Proust's book's ultimate subject or theme. Doubrovsky problematizes the place of the writing subject, who cannot be said to "own" his writing. *In Search of Lost Time*, he argues, continuously poses "the simple, foolish question that every piece of writing poses to every writer: how is *that* (by, from) *me?*" Or, "The writing-sperm . . . is a trace belonging to *whom?*" (Doubrovsky, *Writing and Fantasy*, 134, 137).

Arriving at the inevitable suspension of writing between the mother who controls the input of food and language, and a son who strives to control the output of excrement, sperm, and other traces, thus forming a compromised positionality between other and self, Doubrovsky concludes with the general "*out-of-place place* of the subject" (139). Bal's "platitude" bears on writing, too. It forms the image and metaphor for an art that is "graphic" in both senses of the word: materially inscribed on a flat surface and explicitly embodied, concretely incarnated in ejaculation and semen, with respect to its production and its perception.

"Solitary Pleasure" opens with the classification of two kinds of masturbation. The one, occurring later in life, serves as the substitute for the real thing. As the next-best thing, it makes good for the absence of a specific woman ("to pass off the absence of a woman, imagining to ourselves that She is with us").[4] This type of masturbation Proust deems derivative and inferior. The other, however, which is more at stake in the fragment, is neither a complement nor a surrogate, but instead "unknown" and "original." Hence, the primary mode of masturbation does not relate to a fantasized object, but only to the self and its place in the world.

Both Doubrovsky and Bal deconstruct the hierarchy of primary and secondary masturbation. Doubrovsky connects the privileged type of solitary pleasure to "primary narcissism" (Doubrovsky, *Writing and Fantasy*, 7). As ever, however, Doubrovsky is quick to insert the maternal figure into the equation. He places "Solitary Pleasure" at the core of the madeleine episode in *Combray*, where a motherly figure serves her son tea and cakes (6). Bal's interpretation also takes up primary narcissism, but she, too, ascribes maternal significance to the breast-like hills and round clouds Marcel views from the window of the room (Bal, *The Mottled Screen*, 101–2). The "firm curve" of semen that the boy produces she reads as "the figuration of the absent woman," while the first paragraph's claim requires her to stay absent if the onanistic experience is to remain truly original and primary (151).

Nevertheless, the narrator repeatedly stresses the original and non-derivative nature of the masturbatory experience he recounts. "But when I was twelve years old, and for the first time, going upstairs to the top floor of our house at Combray, locked myself into the water-closet with its dangling garlands of orris root, it was an unknown pleasure that I went in search of, sufficient in itself and not a substitute for anything else" (Proust, "Solitary Pleasure," 30). Later, the narrator describes the event in similarly significant terms. Masturbation is compared to a "search of a pleasure that I did not know" (30). What is gained, then, is not only first-time pleasure but also original knowledge. To what object can this knowledge apply, if not to the mother, woman, or peasant-girl met before?

The setting of the proceedings is the familiar room under the roof of the Combray summerhouse. Now, however, the narrator gives more information as to its particular appeal. "[U]nusually spacious" as far as such rooms go, the room is situated at the top of the house: "So far aloft," that it is situated "in the attics of the house" (30). What becomes clear is that the room enables a positionality that is suspended between opposites: between what is interior and exterior, closed and open, private and public, safe and dangerous. The room closes perfectly, but the window is always partially open. A young lilac, replacing *Combray*'s blackcurrant, pushes its fragrant head through it. "I was completely alone," the narrator explains, "but this element of being out of doors added a delicious uneasiness to the sense of security which those sturdy bolts assured to my solitude" (30). Entangling opposites, the spatial correlates of the room remain ambivalent and unclear.

The room's particular charm can be evaluated in different ways. One could infer that the impression of being out in the open simply adds the kinky pleasure of a qualified exhibitionism. One may suspect that the "delicious uneasiness" entails the partial coming out of a pleasure usually firmly closeted. At the least, this boy's body partially transgresses the boundaries of privacy, solitude, and intimacy that are associated with the practice of masturbation. More intriguingly, however, this body can be seen to renegotiate what is interior and exterior to itself both through and in this space that it only obliquely inhabits.

From here, two possible routes open up: one further outside, the other further inside. Externality is suggested by the characterization of masturbation as an "exploration" or "search" in accordance with the theme of walking, travel, and tourism encountered above. However, a complementary consideration of interiority arrives as well in the description of masturbation as a "surgical" procedure: "performing a surgical procedure on my brain and marrow" (30). Primary masturbation, it seems, carries a momentum that potentially, simultaneously, pushes inside and outside, both further into space and deeper into the body.

GAZE

With pleasure on his mind, the boy whips up a frenzy of joy, omnipotence, and transcendence. Standing in front of the window and jerking off, he views a universe "in whose immensity and duration my everyday thoughts were resigned to claiming no more than a gnat's share [*une parcelle éphémère*]" (30). But not now, as his mind, "wider and more powerful," manages to span the totality of the universe—and possibly a little further than that. Clouds puffing up over the forest afar form the farthest reach of his view; yet, "I felt that my spirit extended a little further, was not quite filled by it, had a little margin to spare" (30). Apparently, the totalizing and exhaustive gaze of the subject still leaves open the stubborn supplement of a narrow margin left to be filled.

That notwithstanding, the externalizing momentum of masturbation opens up an infinity far beyond the frame of the window and the vision it accommodates. The exaltation of pleasure even conquers the mortality of the body. Earlier, the surgical procedure brings up the fear of dying ("I believed at every moment that I should die"). Now, who cares? "But what of that? [*Mais que n'importait!*]" And, stronger still: "I . . . could not die" (30). This willful negation of mortality amounts to the repression of the same body that produces the pleasure, which allows the gaze its extraordinary power to begin with. On the one hand, the body's pleasure lifts and projects the boy's gaze into totality and eternity. On the other hand, the mortality of that same body must be overcome for the subject to reach true transcendence. As a result, the mortal, ephemeral Marcel has become a god. The universe, immense and eternal, has become his dominion.

Subsequently and surprisingly, the body and its carnal mortality, temporarily overcome by the power and pleasure of the gaze, must serve as the resting place or ground for the vast view that is taken in. The sheer effort of inhabiting his dominion, it appears, starts to weigh down on the twelve-year-old divinity. He has to "carry" it; it all must "rest" on him: "I felt the lovely swelling hillsides that rose like breasts on either side of the river, supported, like mere insubstantial reflections, on the dominating stare of my pupils. All this world reposed on me . . ." (30). Immaterial as the view may be, the eyes must nevertheless support its enormity.

Initially, the nearly limitless extension of the subject in space is achieved visually, through the gaze, while the subject's body remains immobile and in place. However, the body and the mind cannot support the extension of the gaze for long. Totalized, yet ever leaving open the supplement of a narrow margin, the gaze is suddenly pulled back into the little room and reconnected to the mortal and material body that inhabits it. The pleasure that angles for completion and culmination reels or tumbles, in Barthes's words, into a bliss that interrupts and suspends it.

Consequently, the divinity buckles: he needs to take a seat. The masturbating body-mind, previously stretched to its outer limit, must now be resituated and reseated in the orrisroot room. The transition in the text is shocking. One moment the subject is an omnipotent god, the next he is a mere mortal in search of repose. What separates the two is a single intake of breath: "I paused to draw breath." In order to sit down, Marcel tells the sun whose rays warm a chair to move out of his way, draws the curtain, and takes a seat.

In the round clouds and breastlike hills that are part of the view that Marcel cannot quite own up to, Doubrovsky recognizes the shape of the maternal madeleine that haunts the narrator of *Combray*. Masturbating, the subject seeks to break away from motherly influence, only to see it return in the rounded clouds and hills, he argues. For Bal, too, the swelling forms are "clearly maternal" and persist as the counterpoint to the flat visuality suggested by the reflections without reality and volume (Bal, *The Mottled Screen*, 101).

However, I want to bracket such an Oedipal analysis a little longer, and stick with the fragment's claim that the masturbation it recounts is primary in the sense that it does not center on an absent woman, maternal or not. The view that the subject produces and takes in may be two-dimensional, but it is not still. Libidinal turmoil is signaled by the clouds that puff up above the forest and the hills that rise up on both sides of the river. This rising and rounding motion, I propose, implicates precisely the materiality of the body, the substantiality of the marrow and the brain that were the objects of the masturbatory surgical procedure, which formed the complementary and internalizing aspect of pleasure.

This "inner" corporeality seems to be long left behind as the gaze stretches to its external limit. Nevertheless, it morphs back into view as the image, the view that is observed, swells like the body. Hence, the external journeying of the gaze ultimately cannot overcome the mortal body that supports and fuels it. The elasticity of desire, its propensity to stretch out nearly indefinitely, nevertheless knows a point of resistance, when the extending trajectory of desire suddenly snaps back to its origin.

That instance of resistance turns out to be the body itself, particularly the penis. Rising and rounding itself, the material body infringes on the otherwise external view from the window; the inflation of the body, specifically the erection of the penis, resists the limitless stretching out of desire. Ultimately, the penis cannot support the gaze. The narrow margin of the view that cannot be filled, that cannot be covered by the gaze, precisely articulates the extent to which the penis, the organ of the body at stake in masturbation, cannot stretch indefinitely and infinitely. The boy's gaze, his body, and his pleasure break their externalizing course: he shuts the curtain, sits down, comes. The gravity of the body returns. Hence, the object to which the original knowledge brought about by primary masturbation pertains is the male body itself, its desire, and its pleasure.

Before seating himself on the chair, Marcel must negotiate the fact that this particular seat is already taken. Here, the fragment finally does become clearly Oedipal. To continue masturbating without being disturbed by the glare of the sun, Marcel orders the sun to make way for him: "Take yourself off, my boy, to make room for me [*Otetoi de là, mon petit, que je m'y mette*]" (Proust, "Solitary Pleasure," 31). Though ordering the sun around and calling it "my boy" seems a carry-over from the divine "ex-carnation" experienced a moment before, the Oedipal import of the statement becomes apparent once one realizes that it is surely a quote: the boy repeats an order given to him by his parents on numerous occasions. Thus the subject is not only physically resituated in the room in the summerhouse, but is also reframed in the family romance as a twelve-year-old boy. After all, the pleasures enjoyed on his walks and in the little room can only be forged by parental absence.

To Doubrovsky's mind, the madeleine scene from *Combray* works as a cover for the ejaculation of "Solitary Pleasure." The *Combray* ejaculation is its displaced remainder. He detects what he calls an "astonishing textual corroboration" between the two scenes, largely signaled by the affects of omnipotence, transcendence, and joy they have in common (Doubrovsky, *Writing and Fantasy*, 6). Remembrance and masturbation collide, and so do their respective settings: "the 'bedroom' where the Narrator remembers is the 'toilet' where he masturbates" (26–27). Ejaculation and defecation join in the attempt to "expulse" the mother. "For this reason," Doubrovsky explains, "the 'toilet' is the chosen place for the symbolic liberation. It's a question of knowing precisely by whom it is 'occupied' " (26). However, the father, not the mother, occupies the toilet. "In wanting to take his place in the 'sun,' " Doubrovsky writes, "the child wants *to put himself in his Father's place*" (103). This leads to what he calls a "masculine affirmation" when Marcel eventually ejaculates there.

As Bal writes, in a slightly different vein: "This little sentence [*Otetoi de là, mon petit, que je m'y mette*] signifies quite clearly and directly the suppression of the father-sun, since this literalizing psychoanalytic figuration means that to take the place of the father is concretely to sit in his seat" (Bal, *The Mottled Screen*, 101). Marcel's placement on the paternal seat remains qualified, however. The curtain will not shut properly. The lilac, earlier merely pushing its fragrant head through the window, has materialized in a "branch" that prevents the full closure of the curtain. Can this lilac prevent or reconfigure the masculine and paternal self-affirmation of Marcel when he, sitting on the father's seat, ejaculates?

THE LILAC

The reinforced seating arrangement in the room allows the body to release itself. At the start of the passage, ejaculation is a fountain. At the end, only little seedpods remain:

> At last [*Enfin*] a shimmering jet arched forth, spurt after spurt [*élans successifs*], as when [*au moment où*] the fountain at Saint Cloud begins to play—which we can recognise (since there is a personality in the untiring flow [*l'ecoulement incessant*] of its waters that their unyielding curve gracefully, incessantly, portrays) in the portrait

> Hubert Robert made of it, only there the admiring crowd had . . . which speckle the old master's picture with little seedpods [*valves*], pink, reddened, or black. (Proust, "Solitary Pleasure," 31; ellipsis in the text)

Triumph is tainted with anticlimax, already hinted at by the ambivalent *enfin* that sets up the moment. As "finally" or "at last," *enfin* indicates the success of the project. But in its meaning of "alas" or "anyhow," the word articulates the admission of a partial failure, following the frustrated attempt to shut the curtain. Moreover, this troubled *enfin* opens up a temporality that cannot time the ejaculation at a given moment. It skips from the momentary ("*au moment où*") to the serial or successive ("*élans successifs*"), to the endless ("*l'ecoulement incessant*"). Hence, the precise temporality of the ejaculation remains elusive, just like its placing.

For Doubrovsky, the Oedipal battle is nevertheless won at this exact yet paradoxical moment. In the shape of the recognizable individuality of the fountain's curve, the ejaculation finally delivers an identity unencumbered by parental constraints. "The ecstasy of ejaculation clearly grants the ipseity that has been mystically sought," he concludes (Doubrovsky, *Writing and Fantasy*, 26). Bal is more guarded. "Hardly has the father/sun been removed," she argues, "than the 'old master' takes his place. It is the painted fountain, and not the one that the little boy produces that possesses a particular individuality. Moreover, it is the painted fountain that has an 'endless flow.'. . . What should be inner essence is rendered through visible, external layers of paint" (Bal, *The Mottled Screen*, 151–52). The untenable window view of the landscape is merely replaced by another image: Robert's painting.

Thus, the triumphant ejaculatory fountain, allegedly delivering the autonomous individuality and masculine self-affirmation Marcel is seeking, is countered by its insecure timing, by the recourse to the painting that replaces the male body, and by its material remainder that disperses and crystallizes in the multicolored and crusty seedpods. So, what is the admiring crowd cheering for? As a metaphor for ejaculation, the fountain seems readily available and obvious. Yet, as Bal notes, its "acceptability could, in fact, be excessive, and, consequently, the object of an internal hostility and a flattening that are both specific to Proust" (155). No wonder, then, that the fountain is joined by two other figurations of male sexuality that bring in other considerations. These frame and follow the shimmering jet. The first concerns the strangely behaving lilac, the second centers on the sperm-trace encountered earlier in *Combray*.

Immediately after coming, the narrator perceives a tenderness surrounding him. The smell of the lilacs, unnoticed during the orgasmic excitement, returns to his senses. Another smell joins it: "a bitter smell, like the smell of sap [*sève*], was mixed with it, as though I had snapped the branch [*cassé la branche*]" (Proust, "Solitary Pleasure," 31). This acrid smell of the *sève*, for "plant's juice," "(life-)force" or "-juice," or "spunk," is obviously the smell of sperm. "As if I had snapped the branch": the same branch of the lilac that prevented the full closing of the curtain is now on the receiving end of a little violence.

The little margin that the gaze cannot fill and the small portion of the window that the curtain cannot close off form mirror images of each other. What prevents completion and totalization in both cases is the penis/branch. If the penis forms the stubborn obstacle to the limitless stretching out of desire in space, the branch precludes the complete self-enclosure of the subject in the room. The penis can neither accommodate the full occupation of external space nor safely anchor the body in inner and private space. Like a wedge, the organ prevents both the full exteriorization and the full interiorization of pleasure. Coming from the outside of the room, it insists on access like an alien interloper. The mystical ipseity that, according to Doubrovsky, the ejaculation of the penis prepares for the boy, then, does not include the penis. This cannot but qualify the "masculine affirmation" that this ejaculation is presumed to deliver.

At first, the young lilac pushes its "scented head" through the window. Climbing up along the exterior wall, it has found access through a chink. Following the swellings in the view from the room, it then materializes, hardens, into a branch that precludes the closure of the curtain. Finally, the branch is snapped, releasing an acrid smell with its juice. As a figure of masculine pleasure, the lilac is both profoundly exterior to the body and entirely superficial as it traces the outer wall. It does not penetrate outer space, but intrudes from outer space into the room that secures the subject.

Pleasure's exploratory drive nearly reaches the outer edges of space. At the same time, its interiorizing, surgical aspect reaches the marrow of the body, its deepest core. In both these motions, the lilac-penis cannot (em)place the ejaculating subject and his body. It forms the resistance to the limitless externalization of desire as well as the external remainder that troubles Marcel's privacy and solitude. The mottled jet of sperm that the boy produces from within as he comes quickly sets as externalized and alienated layers of paint. In contrast, the lilac moves outside-in. As I will show, the traces of sperm make a complementary journey inside-out.

SILVERY TRACE

The second and last figure of ejaculation, also alternative to the fountain, arrives in the shape of the "silvery trace" that is deposited on the lilac's leaves and the branch. A qualifying *seulement* counters the hydraulic grandeur of the fountain's jet and the accomplishment of Robert's painting:

> I had left a trail on the leaf, silvery and natural as a thread of gossamer [*le fil de la Vierge*] or a snail-track, that was all [*seulement*]. But on that bough, it seemed to me like the forbidden fruit on the Tree of Knowledge; and like the races [*les peuples*] that give non-human forms [*des formes inorganisées*] to their deities, for some time afterward it was in the guise of this almost interminably extensible silvery thread which I had to spin out of myself going widdershins to the normal course of my life that I pictured the devil. (31)

While the fountain carries a hydraulic momentum that rises up and away, and while the lilac comes from the outside and insists on access to the room, the seminal thread must be drawn out of the self.

"[B]y a remarkable coincidence," Doubrovsky observes, "the description of the masturbation act is, word for word, appropriate to the writing act" (Doubrovsky, *Writing and Fantasy*, 39). This approximation of ejaculation and writing, he continues, holds for their similar ends: the creation of a substance of one's own, unburdened by parental influences. It also concerns their joint materiality: threads of sperm and ink. As Bal writes, the silver thread is the "trace/writing on the flat leaf" (Bal, *The Mottled Screen*, 152). Finally, Doubrovsky argues that writing and ejaculation both take part in the deconstruction of autobiographical narrative from the conventional course of a "natural life" to the endlessly expanding series of novels (Doubrovsky, *Writing and Fantasy*, 40). Yet this deconstruction must then also implicate the individuality and masculinity that he grants the traces of sperm.

The snail's trail that smears the drooping leaves of the blackcurrant of the *Combray* scene here meets its ironic counterpart in the figure of the Virgin. The vertical hierarchy that is established between Mary and the snail, the immaculate and the viscous, the higher than high and the lower than low, is rotated horizontally, flattened into the materialization of the gossamer thread [*le fil de la Vierge*], which suggests both a fine fabric and the sticky excretions left on foliage by spiders. Hence, the gossamer thread takes up the same leveling of the high and the low, exaltation and deception, creation and evolution, ejaculation and gestation of the wet dream where the book energetically originates. No doubt it would have delighted Bataille.

Moreover, the gossamer thread condenses the traces of sperm with the ground or surface on which they are inscribed: flat leaves or sheets of paper inscribed with sperm or ink. Hence, the supplement or *ajouté* offered by ejaculation/writing, following on the brink of the totalization of space by the phallic gaze, condenses organ/pen, sperm/ink, and leaf/paper to such an extent that they can no longer be differentiated, together forming the fine and sticky substantiality of the gossamer thread. The seminal thread drawn from the body loops, knots, and strings itself to generate the fabric of gossamer.

Finally, the forbidden fruit and the devil make an appearance. Once more, ejaculation is narrated as a fall, which inevitably follows the near-apotheosis of the subject as the god who surveys all space with his gaze; a particularly masculine divinity without body, substance, or shape. At the top of the Combray summerhouse, Marcel shortly manages, through his gaze, to become the creator of the landscape visible through the window of the little room.

Immediately, however, an elusive corporeality insists on rematerialization in the swelling shapes in view, which then falls apart in the fountain, the lilac, the snail's trace, and the gossamer thread. Thus, taking his cue from the people who impart "disorganized shapes" on their gods, Proust insists on giving masculine pro-ductivity and writerly creativity concrete and material shapes, which all share the trope of ejaculation, disorganized as these shapes may be. That this masculinity must be given shape at all; that this masculinity further disperses in a plurality of possible shapes; and that this masculinity ultimately cannot order these shapes in a single image or concept is precisely the original and originating piece of knowledge that Proust and Marcel search in and through ejaculation.

According to Doubrovsky, the ejaculation that takes place in "Solitary Pleasure" lends the subject a "masculine affirmation" and a mystical ipseity or individuality. However, the fragment's subject, his pleasure, and the seminal and written trace he produces are—much like the thigh or rib of the wet dream—as misplaced as they are displaced. Temporarily, the scenes from *Combray* and "Solitary Pleasure" incessantly skid between a punctual, durative, and iterative rendering of the event, bringing up the "immanent mediality" that Derrida ascribes to orgasm. The spasmodic contractions and expansions of orgasm are intensely temporal, yet they cannot be situated in linear time. In the iterative mode, the ejaculation that suggests the textual materiality of the book, that sustains or affirms the subject who writes it, and that therefore should be able to be placed and timed at a single place and moment skips from the wet dream to the nightmare to the later scene in *Combray*, to then jump outside the book to *Against Sainte-Beuve*.

Spatially, the body and the little room smelling of orrisroot in which it is emplaced rhythmically expand to the outside and contract to the inside. The penis serves as the marginal supplement that prevents the completion of both moves, traveling in outside space or practicing a surgical procedure on the body's inner marrow. Visually, the power of the gaze to inhabit the world is briefly considered before it is fractured in a series of synesthetic perceptions: the fountain and the painting, the tender smell of the lilac intermixed with the acrid odor of sperm, the gossamer fabric that is sticky and delicate.

Materially, the writing and ejaculating body does not deposit its traces on a clean slate waiting to be filled with presence, but wraps itself up in the surface on which it inscribes itself, forming a folded and layered texture. Like Derrida's mime, the Proustian scriptor writes on the page he is, folding and layering himself out and in. In this intricate and ambivalent motionality, the subject, his penis, and his ejaculation cannot find a secure place.

THIRTEEN

A FEW DROPS THAT EXPRESS ALL

> I tried to pull [Gilberte] towards me, and she resisted; her cheeks, inflamed by the effort, were as red and round as two cherries; she laughed as though I was tickling her; I held her gripped between my legs like a young tree which I was trying to climb; and, in the middle of my gymnastics when I was already out of breath with the muscular exercise and the heat of the game, I felt, like a few drops of sweat wrung from me by the effort, my pleasure express itself in a form which I could not even pause for a moment to analyze; immediately I snatched the letter from her.[1]

UNLIKE THE TWO ORGASM SCENES discussed in the previous chapters, the ejaculation cited above takes place in public space, a park. The pleasure that expresses itself in the form of the "few drops" of semen continues the fashioning of the self, the sustained trying out of possible desires and pleasures through figurations of ejaculation, but now with explicit reference to social space.

Indeed, the project in which this ejaculation participates engages the question of how the narrator and Marcel, so far solitary and enclosed in the private bedroom and the orrisroot room, will relate to the external space that, like the chair in the room, may already be partially occupied by other men. Previously, when the desire of the Proustian subject expanded into outer space, that space was mostly empty, unpopulated. Now, however, the motions of pleasure begin to confront a series of other male subjects—familial, homosocial, and amicable—with an ambivalent mixture of rivalry and desire.

The occasion for the third ejaculation is a wrestling game between Marcel and Gilberte, playing together in the Champs-Elysées park. Yet the scene is not exclusively centered on Gilberte, the obvious object of desire. The letter Marcel snatches from her is addressed to her father, Swann, whom Marcel desperately wants to convince of his fine nature. Convinced by Gilberte of the futility of that attempt, Marcel retrieves the letter to prevent further damage to their relationship. The failure to ingratiate himself with Swann suffuses Marcel with anxiety.

On his way home from the park, Marcel remembers two other episodes from his young life in which he takes on the authority of older men: his precocious manipulation of his Uncle Adolphe through which he forges an encounter with an "actress" of his acquaintance, and his attempt to impress the elegant visitor Norpois, who severely condemns his first writings. Both these episodes end inconclusively or unsuccessfully, the latter even convincing Marcel of his "nullity."

However, the mood of anxiety and despair that characterizes Marcel's relations to older men, to Swann, Adolphe, and Norpois, is mitigated by a brief but crucial impression that gives him solace. When he visits the public lavatory in the park in the company of Françoise, the cool and musty smell emitted by the lavatory's exterior wall at once relieves Marcel of "the anxieties that Swann's words, as reported by Gilberte, had just awakened in me" (2:74). The olfactory sensation fills Marcel with a pleasure "that was solid and consistent, on which I could lean for support, delicious, soothing, rich with a truth that was lasting, unexplained and sure" (2:74). Though left unclarified, this extraordinary pleasure or truth helps Marcel to overcome his disappointment at Swann's disapproval, and sustains him in the subsequent confrontation with Gilberte, during which he both ejaculates and manages to retrieve the letter in one swift motion.

Thus, though the sudden ejaculation does not leave Marcel the required time to reflect either on the precise form that his pleasure has taken, or on the possible contents that this form expresses, the analysis is displaced to and woven through the immediate context of the occurrence. Framing and fanning out from the rapid ejaculation of the "few drops" is a gossamer texture of threads, which densely coalesce around Marcel's frustrated dealings with older, male authority figures, and around the delicious and enduring truth of the cool smell. As the figures of Swann, Adolphe, and Norpois suggest, what is at stake in the third ejaculation in *In Search of Lost Time* is the initiation of the boy into bourgeois society, his becoming-subject and becoming-man in its terms. The presence of not one but three possible models of identity, as well as the mysterious and inexplicable sensation of the smell that rivals all three, add to the complexity of the initiation, the becoming-subject, that Marcel achieves through this ejaculation. These complications form exactly what lends the few drops of semen their remarkable expressivity.[2]

ADOLPHE

The cool smell of the public convenience visited with Françoise just before the sudden ejaculation refers to Uncle Adolphe's room in the summerhouse in Combray. For, it "would never fail to emit that oddly cool odour," Proust writes, "suggestive at once of woodlands and the ancient régime" (1:84–85). Marcel used to be a frequent visitor of that room, but has not entered it for some time now because of an ongoing quarrel between Adolphe and the family, which arose largely through Marcel's fault. The motivation for this estrangement concerns one of the boy's earlier visits to Adolphe's Paris apartment.

These visits take place in his uncle's "study," a room lavishly decorated with prints of pink and fleshy goddesses. The narrator invariably assigns ironic scare quotes to the study, for there Adolphe primarily entertains another "class of acquaintance" (1:89). It consists of actresses, of "ladies of another class, not clearly distinguished from actresses in [Marcel's] mind," of "pretty widows (who had perhaps never been married)," and of "countesses (whose high-sounding titles were probably no more than *noms de guerre*)" (1:88). The sustained irony betrays the mixture of knowingness and naïveté that Marcel displays throughout the episode.

Subsequently, Marcel recalls the visit to Adolphe's study that formed the occasion for the disagreement between his parents and his uncle. At this point, the boy's love for the theater is still "Platonic," he specifies, "since my parents had not yet allowed me to enter one" (1:86). Yet Marcel schemes to force a meeting with one of Adolphe's actress friends, anticipating the event in a language that signals its theme of initiation:

> [T]hinking of the weary and fruitless novitiate eminent men would go through, perhaps for years on end, on the doorstep of some such lady who refused to answer their letters and had sent them packing by the hall porter, it struck me that my uncle could have spared from such torments a youngster like me by introducing him to the actress, unapproachable by all the world, who was for him an intimate friend. (1:88)[3]

Marcel will sidestep the competition of eminent men, cross the doorstep through a shortcut, and gain access to an otherwise unapproachable woman of ill repute.

Marcel visits his uncle at another time than the usual day and hour. The pretext: a change in the schedule of his lessons prevents him from seeing Adolphe that week. The opportunity: Marcel's parents have gone out for lunch earlier than usual (1:88). What follows is a high comedy of manipulation and embarrassment. Moving past the manservant who tries to send him off, he overhears a female voice: "Oh yes! Do let him come in, just for a moment; I should so enjoy it. . . . I should so like to see the little chap, just for a second" (1:89). Grumbling, Adolphe concedes.

Blushing from the "uncertainty whether I ought to address her as Madame or Mademoiselle," Marcel is introduced to a lady clad in pink. The woman compliments Marcel's beautiful eyes, which to her resemble his mother's. Adolphe mutters, "He takes most after his father." The lady remembers she has met his father on some or other occasion, saying, "He was so nice, so exquisitely charming to me" (1:91). Marcel immediately concludes that she must have turned "what must actually have been [a] brusque meeting" into an encounter more congenial in nature, ostensibly without entertaining the possibility that his father might have acted more elegantly and willingly toward the woman.

Adolphe has had enough and sends his nephew off. "With a blind, insensate gesture," Marcel kisses the woman's hand. She responds, "Isn't he delicious! Quite a ladies' man already; he takes after his uncle. He'll be a perfect 'gentleman,' " and even suggests the possibility of further contact: "Couldn't he come to me some day for 'a cup of tea,' as our friends across the Channel say?" Adolphe ushers Marcel out, who, in leaving, covers his "old uncle's tobacco stained cheeks with passionate kisses" (1:93). He promises his uncle the necessary and requested discretion, assuring him "that some day I would most certainly find a way of expressing my gratitude" (1:93). That moment arrives that same day, when Marcel tells his parents the story in detail. Predictably, words of a violent order ensue between Marcel's father and uncle; Adolphe will forever remain estranged from his family (1:93).

The initiation that is initiated by Marcel succeeds on all accounts. He gains access to an actress, bypassing the usual constraints preventing such a thing from happening. She is smitten by him and suggests a continuing acquaintance. In direct competition with older men for this woman's favors, he deals a shattering blow to his uncle, while his young age as well as his expert manipulation of pretext and opportunity allow him to maintain full innocence. The possibility that his own father could be among the lady in pink's friends is disclaimed, but goes some way toward explaining why Marcel first promises discretion, but then tells all to his parents. Hence, the Oedipal battle concludes in his favor, with the "ancient régime" of the family momentarily shaking on its grounds.

Nevertheless, several features of the scene signal an enduring trouble and ambivalence. Just as the lady invites Marcel for tea, he is "beginning to feel extremely tired" (1:92). Moreover, it may be disconcerting to venture out on one's own and make a new and illicit acquaintance, only to have her recognize in one nothing but family resemblances. In Marcel, the lady in pink recognizes first his mother and then his uncle, whereas Adolphe insists on a close resemblance to his father.

As the Platonic lover of the theater, finally, Marcel is left "in a state of troubled excitement, impotently and painfully trying to form a picture of her private life" by the face of any actress, while the names of actors are able to trigger the hyperbolic blossoming of his desire. With a school friend, Marcel composes lists of the best actors of the Parisian stage:

> And if, in his judgment, Febvre came below Thiron, or Delaunay below Coquelin, the sudden volatility which the name of Coquelin, forsaking its stony rigidity, would acquire in my mind, in order to move up to second place, the miraculous agility, the fecund animation with which the name of Delaunay would suddenly be endowed, to enable it to slip down to fourth, would stimulate and fertilise my brain with a sense of budding and blossoming life. (1:87)[4]

Taking up the false names and titles of the actresses, widows, and noblewomen of Adolphe's acquaintance, and the lady in pink who remains unnamed, the face of the anonymous actress fills Marcel with the impotent, troubled, and painful attempt to picture her "private life." In contrast, the volatile, agile, and fecund names of the actors do not bring up their private and intimate lives, but only relate to each other in their more-or-less arbitrary and changing ordering on the list.

These suggestive and persistent features in the account of the ostensibly successful initiation pinpoint a remainder of affects and concerns that cannot be solved in this type of initiation, however felicitous it may be. Doubtlessly, that is because it remains firmly entrenched in Oedipal and generational family politics, in which a young man is pitted against an older man, whom he cannot but emulate. If one succeeds, one will inevitably become the father whom Adolphe already recognizes in Marcel, and who may be part of the woman's circle of lovers. However, the sheer volatility and agility of the actors' names on the list allude to a dynamic beyond the "name of the father." Ultimately, then, the suggestion of the lady in pink for Marcel to become the "ladies' man" or "gentleman" she projects is refused.

NORPOIS

On his way home after the episode in the Champs-Elysées park that, owing to the impression of the smell of the public lavatory, brings to mind the Adolphe story, Marcel also recalls ambassador Norpois's visit to the family in the Paris house. He affirms the negative judgment Norpois meted out to his earliest literary ambitions on that occasion, because, he says, "a positive rapture had been conveyed to me, not by some important idea, but by a musty smell" (2:77). The association implicates a second initiation: Marcel's attempt to insinuate himself in the circle of learned connoisseurs over which the ambassador presides.

Norpois calls on the family for dinner. The visit triggers high anxiety in Marcel's mind, because he is set on impressing the old man, and even hands over a piece of writing of his own to submit to his aesthetic scrutiny. Displaying a world-weariness and sophistication in all matters of art, politics, and society, Norpois is a figure of indisputable authority and taste for the boy. He is described as "an old connoisseur," as the "best-disposed and most elegant of experts" (2:51, 54). While the earlier initiation succeeds in most, if not all, respects, this one will uncompromisingly fail.

At pains to ingratiate himself with the man, Marcel awkwardly tries to impress him with sophisticated conversation. When the boy argues for his literary preference for the writings of Bergotte, the expert's judgment turns out to be less than favorable: "it is all very precious, very thin, and altogether lacking in virility" (2:52). Detecting the unfortunate influence of Bergotte in Marcel's writing sample, Norpois characterizes "the few lines" as no more than a "childish scribble," adding insult to injury when he assures the fledgling writer that there is ample forgiveness in the word, especially "for the sins of youth" (2:52). Thus, the initiate fails to pass the test and is relegated to the position of a pre-initiate child or youth. Precious, thin, and lacking in virility as to character, Marcel will not take his place in the ranks of the men of letters to which he so desperately aspires.

The condemnation shatters Marcel, reconvincing him of his "intellectual nullity and [of the fact] that I was not cut out for the literary life" (2:53). This enforced nullity and unsuitability is rendered in an idiom that condenses fluidity and spatiality:

> I felt dismayed, diminished; and in my mind, like a fluid which is without dimensions save those of the vessel that is provided for it, just as it had expanded in the past to fill the vast capacity of genius, contracted now, was entirely contained within the straitened mediocrity in which M. de Norpois had of a sudden enclosed and sealed it. (2:54)[5]

Fluid, without dimensions, and vast, Marcel's mind is shut back and enclosed in the closet or little room of mediocrity.

As a last resort, Marcel hesitantly moves to kiss Norpois's "soft, white, wrinkled hands, which looked as though they had been left too long in water," continuing the hostility and revulsion for old age implied above by

Adolphe's tobacco-stained cheeks (2:56). Marcel does not follow through the gesture, hoping the urge will remain undetected. Parting flattery merely evokes a look of revulsion on the ambassador's side, which specifies and explains the effect of nullity that was experienced before.

"Flitting across the face of the Ambassador," Marcel observes "an expression of hesitating and displeasure, and in his eyes that vertical, narrow, slanting look (like, in the drawing of a solid body in perspective, the receding line of one of its surfaces)" (2:58). This perspectivized and perspectivizing look turns solid and immobile Marcel's previously plastic and fluid body-mind, alternately expanding and contracting, exteriorizing and interiorizing, in a fixed positionality that he experiences as annihilation. Through gossip, Marcel eventually learns that the aborted hand kiss was in fact noticed by the ambassador and met with stark disapproval (2:57).

The event plunges Marcel into gloom and depression, a hapless mood increased by the comments of his father, who, just after he has been pushed back to infanthood, nevertheless insists on his development into maturity. "In saying of me, 'He is no longer a child,' 'His tastes won't change now,' and so forth, my father had suddenly made me conscious of myself in Time" (2:63). The time at stake is specifically Oedipal: the temporal imperative ordering the boy to become a man who no longer lacks in virility, while at the same time designating him as an eternal child. The impossible event or moment that would magically transform the boy into a man remains elusive.

Marcel is put in his place through a judgment and a look. While he is trying hard to make the next step in his development, the novice is refused entry to the company of men of letters, power, and taste. The terms of this refusal merge gender and age with visuality and spatiality. The precocious and effeminate boy-child is on the receiving end of a perspectivizing look, vertical, narrow, and slanting, that repositions him in a space that is contracted, contained, enclosed, and sealed. Thus, neither the ambivalent, Oedipal initiation of the Adolphe episode, nor the failed homosocial initiation of the Norpois visit, both framing and fanning out from the ejaculation scene in the Champs-Elysées park, can motivate or explain the delicious, soothing, rich, lasting, and secure truth that Marcel gleans from his visit to the public lavatory. The text must suggest another solution to the problem of initiation. The outcome to Marcel's becoming-subject and becoming-man must take shape in other terms.

MEN IN CUBICLES

Despairing because of his failure to convince Swann of his good intentions and general worthiness, Marcel finds much-needed solace when he stands at the entrance of the public lavatory, awaiting Françoise, who has gone inside. The cool and fusty smell emitted by the lavatory's exterior walls relieves him of his anxiety. The olfactory sensation fills him with a pleasure, he notes, "that was solid and consistent, on which I could lean for support, delicious, soothing, rich with a truth that was lasting, unexplained and sure" (2:74). Though Marcel briefly considers "descend[ing] into the underlying reality which it had not yet disclosed to me," the soothing reality or truth of the smell is initially left unexplained.

Then the toilet lady, "an elderly dame with painted cheeks and an auburn wig," engages him in conversation (2:75). According to Françoise, the woman is a "proper lady," even a "marquise," who has fallen on hard times. "This 'marquise' now," Marcel recounts, "warned me not to stand outside in the cold, and even opened one of her doors to me, saying: 'Won't you go inside for a minute? Look, here's a nice clean one, and I shan't charge *you* anything' " (2:75). He weighs the favor, pondering whether the invitation is a bid for his seduction or an innocent offer. Marcel settles on the latter option, but nevertheless declines to go inside:

> In any event, if the "marquise" had a weakness for little boys, when she threw open to them the hypogean doors of those cubicles of stone in which men crouch like sphinxes, she must have been moved to that generosity less by the hope of corrupting them than by the pleasure which of all of us feel in displaying a needless prodigality to those whom we love, for I never saw her with any visitor except an old park-keeper. (2:75)[6]

The scene combines the terms of the two initiations that were considered above. Lacking a proper name and sporting a false title, the marquise refers to the class of acquaintance that Adolphe entertains in his study; her auburn wig and painted cheeks replace the attire of the lady in pink; and Adolphe is substituted for by the old park-keeper. The homosocial company of connoisseurs of whom Norpois represents the epitome finds its ironic counterpart in the men who crouch in the cubicles. The scene caricatures both earlier attempts at initiation, Oedipal and homosocial, and renders them moot. As Françoise returns, Marcel says his good-bye to her and the toilet keeper. Sustained by the comforting truth he cannot fully explain, the boy engages Gilberte in the play wrestling that brings about his ejaculation.

In the marquise's painted cheeks, Doubrovsky recognizes the mother: "We recognize the mother by her cheek" (*Writing and Fantasy*, 24). Furthermore, whoever says "sphinx" says both "Oedipus" and "sphincter," he observes, concluding that "the riddle of identity passes through the stage of defecation mastery . . . Sphinx-sphincter: being *yourself* begins here. The toilet is the battlefield, the battle being a struggle for identity" (24–25). Similar to Norpois, then, Doubrovsky effectively encloses Marcel in the Oedipal dimension of spatiality and temporality that the narrator has considered and rejected in the Adolphe episode, as well as through its caricatured reiteration in the toilet scene with the marquise and her park-keeper. For what Oedipal identity can be embodied by these numerous and crouching men?

Bal reads the passage as a sexual initiation that revolves on shut or closed spaces. The marquise, who presides over the enclosed men as an "old Python" or "sphinx," playing the part of the feminine monster in need of slaying, triggers the development of the subject: "The old Python, who is represented in mythical terms that justify an initiatory reading, obviously serves to provoke a development in the hero in which she plays no part" (*The Mottled Screen*, 167). Hence, the toilet keeper stands at the threshold between childhood and masculinity.

At once a playing child and an adolescent in love with Gilberte and corresponding with her father, Marcel is faced with a challenge that must resolve his identity in either of two ways: either to be shut in a closed space and risk nonemergence, or to decline the invitation and to risk nonmasculinity. Exactly Marcel's weighing of these options turns him into a man, Bal argues: "The boy is seen to mature into a man in the wisdom of his evaluation" (170). His refusal to go inside enables Marcel to "escape from the prepared schema" (171). For lining up alongside the men crouching in the cubicles would have implied the strong commitment or conformity to "the order of men" (171). "[F]aced with the binary choice between his position as child under his mother's wings and that of the men fastened into the 'normal' oedipal structure," Bal concludes, Marcel "is ready to leave, knowing what he wants" (172).

But what rigid conformity to Oedipal masculinity can be embodied by the crouching men, who have, as Bal writes, lost "all stature and mobility"? In a note, Bal proposes another reading that I want to pursue. "In the Proustian context, and in this specific context of a gathering of men in a public convenience," she writes, "the more obvious association seems to me to be that of certain homosexual practice" (268). Together with the failed homosocial initiation in the name of Norpois, this homosexual practice suggests Sedgwick's "male homosocial desire" that puts homosociality and homosexuality in an oxymoronic continuum.

As the image of that desire, the men who crouch in the cubicles pledge the possibility of the enduring entanglement of several Proustian oppositions. Combined with the crouching men, the aesthetic conversations of the connoisseurs are given libidinal weight. The solitude of Marcel in his bedroom and in the room smelling of orrisroot is mitigated by the likewise-inclined men who line up alongside him. These men are emplaced in their cubicles, but, crouching, they acquire some of the fecund and agile mobility that characterizes the actors' names on Marcel's lists. The motility of their desire does not relate to their respective private lives, but to their intimate yet separate placement with respect to each other. If their sphinx-like stature suggests the sphincter, then that muscle does not so much take part of the drama of toilet training that Doubrovsky swiftly assigns to Marcel, turning him into a child once more, but features as the common and plastic instance that relates the men to each other, thus countering the exclusive phallus. In contrast to the hierarchy of the Oedipal situation, which allows only the one older man to be on top at a given time, these men are both numerous and equal with respect to one another; they are lined up.

Hence, the consistent, supporting, delicious, soothing, lasting, and secure truth that Marcel gleans from his visit to the toilet in the park consists of the suggested possibility of a way of being in the world, of being among men, of being a subject among subjects, which cannot be reduced to the choice between *either* the inevitable heterosexuality of the Oedipal initiation, *or* the homosocial but nonsexual initiation of the Norpois episode. The reality that the image of the crouching men unveils for the boy is that, after all, it is possible to have it both ways.

The toilet keeper lords over a congregation of men who are equal to one another insofar as they jointly inhabit her domain. Indeed, the passage I have quoted above effortlessly moves from considering one boy, Marcel, to the marquise's possible "weakness for little boys," plural, to the crouching "men," both plural and adult. Thus her gaze apparently erases the relevance of those distinctions, singular and plural, child and adult. Her favoring of Marcel can serve as the medium through which the boy enters into an adulthood that does not submit to the Oedipal or connoisseurial interpellations of identity that were considered, but that turned out to be unsatisfactory or closed-off.

In that respect, the marquise mirrors the actress Berma, the object of Marcel's daydreams. In his imagination, Berma "must indeed have felt for many young men those desires which she confessed under the cover of the character of Phèdre" (2:68). "At the thought that [her face]," Marcel continues, "was no doubt at that very moment being caressed by those men whom I could not prevent from giving to Berma and receiving from her joys superhuman but vague, I felt an emotion more cruel than voluptuous, a longing that was presently intensified" (2:70). The intensification of the boy's voluptuous longing, it would appear, follows as much from the imagined young men who share her company as from the jealousy they inspire. Like the toilet keeper, Berma allows "many young men" to join ranks, forming a grouping in which Marcel desires to enlist. Whereas Phèdre loves but one man, Hippolyte, the son of her husband Thesée, Berma courts and is courted by many, quite irrespective of their familial status.

BEHIND THE CURTAIN WITH SWANN

The visual and spatial arrangement in which a plurality of men is lined up in close relation to each other also moves into focus at another and ostensibly incongruous juncture in Proust's text. In *Swann in Love*, the lovesick title character slowly makes his way through the palace of the Marquise de Saint-Ouverte to the ballroom, where a party takes place. On his way, he gives uncustomary attention to the beauty of the servants standing in wait in the entry rooms and on the stairway. In Swann's focalization, these servants appear "like saints in their niches," thus prefiguring the image of the men crouching in their cubicles (1:391).

Since his lover Odette has inexplicably cooled toward him, Swann's heartache shortly puts him through the looking glass. He will only regain his bearings when, making his way through the palace, he finally steps over to "the other side of the tapestry curtain" that is suspended at the entry of the ballroom, where he will join the other guests (1:392). Though Swann would usually make the journey in a few seconds, now a mood of "melancholy indifference" prompts him to notice the beauty of the footmen, lackeys, and attendants who stand around. "[F]or the first time," Swann observes "the scattered pack of tall, magnificent, idle footmen who were drowsing here and there upon benches and chests and who, pointing their noble greyhound profiles, now rose to their feet and gathered in a circle round about him" (1:389). These magnificent footmen form the first station in a sequence celebrating the beauty of the men in direct contradiction to Swann's sexual preference. In a series of lavish descriptions, paintings by Mantegna, Dürer, and others, wild animals, frescoes, and statues are all called upon by Swann to account for masculine beauty.

Then Swann mounts a monumental flight of stairs. Placed on the steps are yet more men, their "marmorean immobility" nearly turning them into statues (1:390). With awe, he observes

> on either side of him, at different levels, before each anfractuosity made in its walls by the window of the porter's lodge or the entrance to a set of rooms . . . , a concierge, a major-domo, a steward (worthy men who spent the rest of the week in semi-independence in their own domains . . .), [who] stood each in the arcade of his doorway with a pompous splendour tempered by democratic good-

> fellowship, like saints in their niches, while a gigantic usher, dressed Swiss Guard fashion like the beadle in a church, struck the floor with his staff as each fresh arrival passed him. (1:391)[7]

This three-dimensional arcade of beautiful men, standing like saints in their niches, semi-independent yet related to each other, solitary yet together, is of the same order as Marcel's men, who crouch in their cubicles.[8]

Though the passage can also be read as an aesthetic legitimation of servanthood, the "democratic goodfellowship" of the men suggests a fleeting vision of masculine subjects who can occupy social space together beyond the constraints of class and family that mark the ancient régime. Hence, Swann's perceptions briefly unburden him from the society in which he, as a nonaristocratic but rich Jew, remains ever misplaced, similar to the way in which Marcel, unable or unwilling to submit to Oedipal or connoisseurial identity, finds solace and an alternate truth in the image of the men in the toilet stalls. For Swann, at least, this other dimension is not maintained for long. As Swann crosses the curtain and reenters conventional society, he swiftly recovers, the narrator astonishingly notes, "his sense of the general ugliness of the human male" (1:392).

RE-SEARCHING MASCULINITY

In and through the three ejaculation scenes that I have discussed, a libidinally intelligent subjectivity searches for and researches possible forms of masculinity and pleasure. In contrast to Lacan, this experiential quest is not haunted by the anamorphic stretch between the phallus and castration, in which the metamorphic plasticity of the body can merely serve as a disturbing specter, but enchanted by the morphogenetic potential of embodied pleasures. Other than for Aristotle, the substantiality of the body and its products is not necessarily dead and formless without the divine spirit or psyche that gives both life and form, but is itself informative, suggestive, compelling. Proust's imaginative scrutiny of ejaculation and semen partakes of a comprehensive and continuous *recherche* into the forms that masculine pleasure and subjectivity might take. He attempts to figure out the relationship of the subject to what he creates, writes; the relationship between the bodily self and space, exterior as well as interior; and the subject's relationship to other men.

According to Doubrovsky, as I mentioned in chapter 12, traces of sperm incessantly pose a particular question to the Proustian subject: "how is *that* (by, from) *me?*" The ejaculation narrated in "Solitary Pleasure," Doubrovsky claims, finally supplies the answer to that question, offering the subject what he calls a masculine self-affirmation and a mystical ipseity. The three scenes, however, appear to feature more of a transformative, metamorphic subjectivity than a singularly formative one, let alone one that is fully formed. Rather than emplacing the subject, ejaculation displaces and misplaces it. Masculinity is the *object* of this quest not so much in the sense of being its "goal" or "destiny," but in the sense of being the "subject-matter" of the research.

Curiously and critically, Proust's narrator tries out, tries on, various constellations of corporeality, erotization, temporality, visuality, and sociality. The wet dream that opens the book suggests a writerly productivity that is suspended between creation and evolution, ejaculation and gestation, exaltation and deception. Precisely because of this entanglement of opposites, and not because of its inner or autonomous force, this ejaculation can achieve its hyperbolic generativity.

The ejaculations in the little room smelling of orrisroot spatialize pleasure, a dimension in which desire can take the shape of extension, penetration, or inscription. That latter, favored possibility finds its compelling image in the sperm-smeared leaves, the gossamer-fine and viscous textuality that supplies the model for the book as a whole. Both the spatial exteriorization and interiorization of desire, its stretching outward and inward, find in their course the marginalized penis that prevents the completion of both those moves.

Finally, the sudden orgasm enjoyed during the wrestling game with Gilberte fans out to implicate several ways of relating to other men. After considering, negotiating, satirizing, and rendering moot both Oedipal and homosocial/connoisseurial initiations into adult manhood, Marcel gleans an alternative, delicious, rich, supporting, and truthful possibility in the image of the numerous men who crouch in cubicles, separate yet related. Indeed, for Proust, ejaculation is not discrete but dense, not distinct but entangled and entangling, not climactic but endlessly reiterable, not formative but transformative, not singular but plural, not restricted but excessive.

EPILOGUE

Forcing the Issue

THE MEANINGS OF THE VERB AND NOUN "(to) issue" may clarify the conditions and aspects that make ejaculation such a dense topic of consideration and such a relevant issue for cultural analysis. First, the word suggests a performativity that externalizes or pro-duces, in Thomas's sense, something of the material body into visibility and materiality. "To go or come out," "to flow out," and "to sally out" are among the verb's intransitive meanings; "to give exit to," "to emit," and "to discharge" are synonyms for its transitive use.[1] In medical discourse, the noun denotes "a discharge of blood or other matter from the body." Masculinity must confront the issue of the externalized, material trace that the male body, the gender's presumed vehicle or form, discharges into visibility.

Second, "issue" also suggests the public reception and usage of what is, authoritatively or officially, produced or emitted, put into circulation. The seminal trace escapes the privacy or autonomy that would contain it. In this vein, the meanings of the word include "to 'come out' or be sent forth officially or publicly; to be published or emitted," "to give or send out authoritatively or officially; to send forth or deal out in a formal or public manner; to publish; to emit, put into circulation (coins, bank notes, stamps, and the like)." Because the word connects the bodily and the cultural, the intimate and the public, the issue of sperm is accorded public and cultural currency. Thus the masculinity that wants, or needs, to (re)claim the seminal trace as the sign for its unadulterated existence must come to terms with its public availability, akin to issued coins and stamps.

The third field of meanings that the term commands puts the connection between authoritative production and the public reception of the issue under strain. The (narrative) meaning for the noun of "the outcome of an action or course of proceedings or the operation of something; event, result, consequence" quickly segues to "a point or matter in contention between two parties," "a choice between alternatives, a dilemma." The public issuing becomes "at issue": "in controversy," "in dispute," "under discussion," "in question." "Issue" thus condenses the production, reception, and contestation of the produced trace; its meaning and relevance become debatable.

To these three meanings, the current pop-psychological usage of "having issues"—pressing matters in need of resolution—can be added, as can the usage of the term that suggests a questionable relevance: "What's the issue?" These two glosses on the term suggest that masculinity has yet to come to terms with liquid semen, as Irigaray suggests, and, simultaneously, that the issue might well be moot. So, one might ask, what are the issues that are at issue in the issue of sperm?

Let me summarize some of the issues that the preceding case studies on the representation of and reflection on ejaculation and sperm have brought up. If, in and through ejaculation and semen, masculinity must come to *matter*, that is, become both material and relevant, then that gender must take into account and negotiate the various issues that the fleeting instant and the substantial fluid bring up. All of these issues suggest a dense and ambivalent temporality and visibility that the bleak alternative between phallus and castration, subjectivity and lack, cannot accommodate and works to erase. As an intensely temporal occurrence, ejaculation disturbs the immediate switch from the phallus to castration; semen forms the indefinite but compelling stain that the economy of the phallus and castration cannot reabsorb or generalize.

Substantially, visually, and temporally extending and expending the masculine, ejaculation forces the issue: the need to come to terms, in a mixture of anxiety and fascination, with exactly the material considerations that conventional masculinity should overcome, or subsume into its incarnated form, in order for it to matter. Hence, ejaculation and semen threaten the self-containment and self-possession that the gender seeks out in representation. Once conceived through ejaculation, masculinity must either matter less by mattering more, or else come to matter differently.

COLOR

What color is sperm? Aristotle ascribes to semen a pure and even-toned white, which distinguishes it from the bulky and impure menstrual blood that forms its counterpart in reproduction. However, Aristotle also observes a temporally inflected difference in the color of the seed. For a limited time only, it is thick, hot, shiny, and frothy. Afterward, the substance goes transparent, runny, cold, dull, and flat. The specificity of the color of semen, its immaculate whiteness, then, is ever haunted by this entropic changeability. Metaphysically, sperm must be purely white; physically, this same white cannot but be impure. If sperm, in time, can go off, then its hue must be off-white rather than immaculate.

Hence, the color of sperm is imprecise, as Leiris noted with respect to saliva. Returning in the shape of the silvery and finely textured trace of semen that Proust describes, the hue of the seed is a milky, opalescent off-white. For Bataille, this off-white forms the occasion for the soiling and contamination of the distinct white of the sperm that, indiscriminately mixed up with urine and menstrual blood, becomes indiscrete. For Derrida, the color of sperm condenses an irregularly blotting, erasing whiteness, and a light-reflecting and refracting multiplicity or "lustre." This latter, pluralized whiteness returns in the baroque tone of white that, according to Bal, is decomposed or fractured into innumerable tiny convex mirrors, bouncing back the look that beholds it. Thus, the singularity of the form-giving spirit that, to Aristotle, gives the substance of sperm its white hue becomes overdetermined and dense: variable, contaminated, erasing, and multiplying.

SCALE

Serrano's monumental images of bodily liquids suggest a proportional vacillation in the perception of sperm between the cellular and the cosmological, the minute and the vast. Indeed, Serrano shows a jet of sperm that appears as the Milky Way, an inert pocket of semen as a prehistoric glacier. Aristotle compares the seed to the stars, and is yet able to make out minute pockets of air encapsulated in the liquid. Bataille's narrator compares his ejaculation to "that strange breach of astral sperm and heavenly urine across the cranial vault." Lacan's mythopoetic "vital flow" finds its marginal supplement in the slight appearance of "that mark." Barthes's *semina aeternatis* are textualized as *semences*, whose minute motion is unpredictable. And, finally, Proust imagines an ejaculatory fountain that can totalize space and then quickly set as little crusty seedpods of paint.

This incessant and sudden scale flipping between the very large and the very small may allude to the ambivalent place, both central and marginal, that sperm occupies in the economy of masculinity and meaning. Indecisively, semen is both hyperbolically augmented and belittled, rendered as apotheosis and as a negligible matter. Apparently, sperm forges the question of the proportional relation of masculinity to the male body that produces the substance, as well as to the space that that body inhabits. The few, small traces or drops of sperm must sustain a masculinity that is "universal" in scale, saturating space with its presence.

However, this flipping between and entanglement of the minute and the vast, below and above, suggests that masculinity cannot control and connect these two perspectives in its bodily form. Scaled up, the seminal Milky Way dwarfs the subject; scaled down, the marks, pockets, or traces of semen threaten his relevance and stature. The seed does not offer the subject a secure, proportional relation between the body and the space that it inhabits. Alternating between the larger than large and the smaller than small, semen cannot deliver a properly proportional shape to masculinity's incarnation of the male body. In both perceptual dimensions, sperm exceeds the bodily form that the gender must maintain.

PLANE

In ejaculation, semen spurts upward. When it does, it nevertheless eventually drops down again, and then viscously, determinedly, clings to the surface on which it lands. The consideration of sperm simultaneously triggers both vertical and horizontal elaborations. The semen that Aristotle deems divine and compares to the stars may end up as a dried-up wad of saliva in the street. If, in Lacan, the *Aufhebung*/erection of the phallus as well as the "vital flow" that suggests a hydraulic constancy map the penis and ejaculation onto a vertical plane, the connecting and separating bar or line and "that mark" rotate and flatten the vertical axis to a horizontal one.

This horizontalization returns in Bataille's "formless" that lowers and flattens vertically erected hierarchies, as well as in the murderous accidents that befall the men whose bearings, whether religious, corporeal, or gestural, are emphatically vertical. In turn, Proust's "misplaced thigh" encapsulates the high and the low, spirituality and materiality, creation and evolution, in a lateral, writerly creativity. Similarly, the appearance of semen as *le fil de la Vierge* [gossamer thread] knits together the Virgin, higher than high, and the snail's trail, lower than low. Moreover, the vision of the numerous men crouching in the cubicles of the public lavatory repudiates the Oedipal, hierarchical arrangement of father and son.

Additionally, the rigid, erect postures of the ambassadors in Holbein's painting are dissected by the diagonal line made up of the skull and the crucifix, and by the insecurely horizontal/vertical arrangement of the tassel and the dagger, which suggests the strange shape-shifting of the penis. In Leonardo's images, the vertical lines that allude to a heightened signification are crossed by the diagonal lines where, seductively, the body materializes. The frantic motion of the vertical axis that semen and ejaculation provoke—moving upside-down, tilting diagonally, and rotating horizontally—disturbs the rule that masculinity can only find an intelligible form when it elevates itself in the shape of the rigid posture that the phallus, erecting and hiding itself to become all the more significant, and all the less material and visible, mandates.

TEMPORALITY

Through its careful narrativization, ejaculation can possibly deliver what Barthes calls "the solution to the riddle, the revelation of fate" that the suspense of the story promises. As the "significant discharge" (Brooks), the cum shot of porn presents a timely and discrete image that instantiates, binds, and quantifies meaning and identity. In both cases, ejaculation must serve as the climax that is able to put to rest the tension that prompts the narrative.

However, representations of orgasm and ejaculation are often thick with the doubts and alternatives that their intense temporality brings up. Repetitive or arresting, the ejaculations in porn may also sidetrack or short-circuit the sense of an ending that their visibility should deliver. For Barthes, the pleasure of narrative suspense can be interrupted by a blissful untimeliness that suspends the story's progression to its ending, congealing and contracting its measured course.

Such a proliferation of possible temporalities characterizes some of the other representations of ejaculation as well. In his photographic images, Serrano ascribes to sperm the temporality of a slow but inexorable process, of a quasi-eternal, celestial phenomenon, of a fleetingness that is nearly impossible to capture, and of an inertia that freezes time. The motion of Proust's ejaculatory fountain modulates time by occurring both momentarily, successively, and endlessly. Much like convulsive "hiccups" or "guffaws," Bataille's ejaculations forgo any sense of an ending. Lacan's phallic "vital flow," appearing as an undeviating source of life and meaning, is set off by the precarious moment of its transmission that cannot be narrated, by the "latency" that stalls the emergence of meaning, by the persistence of "that mark," which the veil cannot cover, and by the strange and steady oscillation of the penis between its "developed" and "undeveloped" state.

Perhaps these excessive and contradictory temporalities can be explained by the "immanent mediality" that Derrida ascribes to the "supreme spasm" of orgasm. The orgasmic spasms are indeed intensely temporal. Yet this immanent temporality cannot be identified or known, and hence, cannot be mapped on linear time. Contracting and expanding, the spasms take place in what Derrida calls a "medium" temporality, entangling and knotting together the temporal line or thread. Thus, the reification of ejaculation as narrative climax and the proliferation of alternative temporalities both betray and attempt to make good for a temporality that ultimately eludes them.

PART/WHOLE

Both ejaculation and semen exceed the maintenance of a stable and meaningful relationship between the part(s) and the whole of the male body. Contracting and expanding, the motion of orgasm and ejaculation crosses the boundary between part and body. As a formless and sticky liquid, sperm cannot be apprehended as either the presence or the absence of the privileged part, as either the phallus or castration. Teeming with motile particles smaller than small, neither alive nor dead, semen invokes an excessive multiplicity. Whereas the phallus turns on a singular presence or absence, as well as on the substitution of a single part for a singular whole, or vice versa, ejaculation and semen exceed the measured alternation between absence and presence, part and whole, that ultimately works to recuperate masculinity's singularity.

For instance, dissemination, according to Derrida, parts the seed as it projects it. Consequently, the phallus is cut *up*, divided into numerous pieces, rather than cut *off*. For Derrida, reading implies entering into a textual machinery, which entrains textual and anatomical germs and members into a "series of displacements, slips, and recurrences" that, indefinitely, add or subtract a germ or member. In other considerations, the part that is privileged as signifying the (absence of the) whole is supplemented by another (the breast of Leonardo's *Angel in the Flesh*), doubled-up (the instrumental hand that joins the penis in porn), or marginalized (the Proustian lilac that prevents both the full interiorization and exteriorization of desire).

OPPOSITION/ENTANGLEMENT

Though a purely notional, spiritual, and immaterial ejaculation underpins the hierarchies and oppositions that sustain conventional masculinity, notably in Hegel's accreditation of insemination as nature's "highest fulfillment," a material ejaculation forms the juncture where these oppositions become entangled with each other rather than crisply distinguished.

This entanglement is confronted in the shape of the unfortunate "business" of reproduction, which requires the opposing principles of male and female, divine and earthly, form and matter, to make contact and mingle (Aristotle); of nature's cloacal or "naïve duplicity" in putting together procreation and urination in the same organ, as well as in combining picture-thinking and conceptual thought in the mind (Hegel); of the "concatenation" of the phallus and the signifiable in the production of the bastard, or hybrid, effect of meaning, as well as of the seminal juxtaposition of "the image of the vital flow" and "that mark" (Lacan); of the strategic "subtle subversion" or the happenstance "din" [*charivari*] that distinguishes and enfolds pleasure and bliss (Barthes); of the orgasmic and immanent "spasm" that returns oppositions as interdependent and reversible (Derrida); of the headless "débauche" that indifferently mixes up high and low, male and female, sperm and urine (Bataille); and of the "misplaced thigh" that condenses impregnation and gestation, creation and evolution, gods and lower organisms (Proust). Ejaculation places, displaces, and misplaces the oppositions through which masculinity should matter. For this entanglement, Serrano offers the most compelling images: flatly and horizontally, the two bodily liquids that Aristotle hierarchizes into an opposition enter into contact with each other, neither mixing nor separating, yet inexorably interacting.

CONCEPTION/INCONCEIVABLE

As a root metaphor, "conception" makes reproduction and cognition analogous to each other. Thus, the endeavor to think (through) semen can only render the substance as generative: as conceptually and procreatively productive. Consequently, the metaphor makes the "reckoning with the sperm *fluid*" that Irigaray advocates "inconceivable" in both the figurative and the literal sense of the word.

Hence, "conceivable," readily thinkable and legible, conceptualizations of sperm turn the substance into something that delivers significance and relevance, a principle that brings about meaning and value: the substance that ascribes form, and hence, intelligibility, to matter (Aristotle); the medium that serves for nature's "highest fulfillment" (Hegel); the narrative image of the "significant discharge" that binds and calibrates meaning (feature pornography); the phallic "vital flow" that generates the offspring of meaning (Lacan). These conceptualizations conceive of sperm only to the extent that it remains conceptual and conceptive.

At the same time, these examples of sperm-thinking also acknowledge semen's "contraceptive" potential: Aristotle's entropic wad of dried-up sperm; Hegel's exasperation over nature's duplicity in combining generation and waste in one organ; pornography's ambivalence vis-à-vis the visible stain that arrests rather than binds meaning; Lacan's indefinite "that mark" that supplements the seminal flow. Such "inconceivable" and "contraceptive" visions of ejaculation and sperm are followed through by Barthes, whose bliss suspends meaning and identity rather than reifying them; by Derrida, who multiplies and overdetermines semen, layering aspect on aspect; and by Bataille, who makes semen utterly indifferent and indiscrete. The conceptualization of semen is sandwiched between the conceptual accolade that is ascribed to it, which ordains that it cannot be "seen," and the visible scrutiny that makes the substance dense rather than discrete, so that, ultimately, it cannot support a distinct concept.

IMMINENT/IMMANENT

If anything, orgasm seems always imminent, mobilizing a temporality of postponement and ultimate arrival. Yet, once it happens, orgasm tips over this temporal plane into an immanence, where both temporal and spatial oppositions matter differently. In Proust, the nearly limitless exteriorization of desire, stretching into and occupying space, as well as its interiorization deep within the body are both stopped short and releveled, flattened, against the leaves mottled with sperm. According to Kristeva, the abject as such can only be "injoyed" in an immanent *jouissance*, which cannot be known, owned, or claimed. For Derrida, the orgasmic spasms happen in an "immanent medium," where spatial and temporal distinctions become reversed and entangled.

Bal's "white historiography" suggests an immanent temporality, in which "forms and things are morphogenetic, producing figures that are found in time," as well as the correlated temporality of viewing these timely and motile figures: the eye bouncing back, flipping between perspectives, being drawn in by the work. As Serrano's "squigglies and claret" indicate, orgasm and ejaculation urge a reading mode through which oppositions become motile and interactive differences: subject and object, form and color, form and formlessness, perspective and anamorphosis, singularity and plurality, discreteness and denseness, anticipation and retrospection, matter and spirit, white and off-white, the large and the small, wholeness and fragmentation.

GRAPHIC

Representing, writing (on), ejaculation and semen inscribes masculinity materially; it lends the gender a concrete, compelling, and anxiety-ridden sign or trace. For Thomas, writing is thus "(porno)graphic." Graphically, it exposes the body that does the writing; a body that, to some extent, stands askew in relation to the masculinity that is seeking out its form, its signature. Hence, lines of writing put masculinity "on the line."

Lacan conceives of signification through a graphic scene of copulation. Simultaneously, this scene circumscribes the typographic marker of the line, stripe, or bar, connecting and disconnecting. In turn, the discreteness of that signifier is rivaled by the dense "that mark." The white, seminal writing of Derrida's mime, writing on the blank page that he is, marks, blots out, and multiplies and fractures meaning into a scintillating "lustre." Mallarmé's numerous phallic penna stitch and scratch the hymen that enfolds them. Canceling out the masculine option between the spatial extension of the self or the penetration of what is other, Proust's flattened, gossamer-fine, and sticky traces on the leaves of the lilac or blackcurrant entangle subject and writing, self and other, ink and ground. Thus, ejaculation puts masculinity on the line. By making gender the issue, corporeally and conceptually, ejaculation puts masculinity at issue.

NOTES

INTRODUCTION

1. Fausto-Sterling, "How to Build a Man," 130.
2. In "The Egg and the Sperm: How Science Has Constructed a Romance Based on Stereotypical Male-Female Roles" (1991), anthropologist Emily Martin criticizes the scientific tendency to personify reproductive cells and to narrativize the processes in which they take part. "More crucial, then, than what kinds of personalities we bestow on cells is the very fact that we are doing it at all. This process could ultimately have the most disturbing social consequences," Martin concludes (501). I will return to Martin's article at the beginning of chapter 1.
3. Pinchbeck, "Downward Motility," 5; further citations are given in the text.
4. "Sperm Warfare," *FutureFeedForward*, February 11, 2001.
5. Irigaray, *This Sex Which Is Not One*, 113; further citations are given in the text. In the chapter "The 'Mechanics' of Fluids," Irigaray identifies a historical "lag" in the attention science and philosophy have given to fluids (106, 107). For rationality prefers solids. Hence, the primacy of the phallus in psychoanalysis betrays a "teleology of reabsorption of fluid in a solidified form" (110). In that same vein, Irigaray questions why excrement should figure as the most archaic object of desire: "The object of desire itself, and for psychoanalysts, would be the transformation of fluid to solid?" (113). Resisting adequate symbolization, fluids, she concludes, "have never stopped arguing" against the complicity between rationality and solid forms (113).
6. The narrator is the textual agent who presents the events; the focalizer is the agent who perceives the events; the character is the agent who experiences the events. For an introduction, see Bal, *Narratology*. Fracturing the monolingual prominence of the "speaking voice," this tiered and layered differentiation of the subjectivities operating in narrative, even when these bear one and the same name, makes possible the analysis of what Bal calls the "variability of interpretation and the difference of experience" in narrative (156).
7. Kimball, "Conceptions and Contraceptions of the Future," 73; further citations are given in the text.
8. Thomas, *Male Matters*, 40; further citations are given in the text.

9. Kristeva, *Powers of Horror*, 2; further citations are given in the text.
10. Bois and Krauss, *Formless*, 53; further citations are given in the text.
11. Winnett, "Coming Unstrung," 505. Winnett makes the claim that Peter Brooks's narrative model turns on the familiarity of male pleasure in its privileging of climax. Subsequently, she makes way for alternative, feminine rhythms as relevant for narrativity. See chapter 5.
12. Barthes, *The Pleasure of the Text*, 25.

1. SEMEN, BLOOD, STARS, AND ICE

1. Martin, "The Egg and the Sperm," 492. See also Tomlinson, "Phallic Fables and Spermatic Romance," who details the ways in which feminist writings cope with the "phallic fable" or "spermatic romance" that rule accounts of reproduction.
2. A recent popular documentary, *Life's Greatest Miracle*, featuring micro-photographic imagery of conception, seems highly attuned to the issue. From its transcript: "Sperm are often portrayed as brave little warriors forging their way through hostile terrain to conquer the egg. Nothing could be further from the truth. For every challenge the sperm face, success is, to a great extent, controlled by the woman's body and even the egg itself." Consequently, the text denies the sperm all agency: they are squeezed out, swept up, carried, guided through, propelled, released, and so on.
3. The press release for the exhibition of Serrano's works at the Barbican in London, titled "The Curve," describes the artist's Fluids works as "portraits of the era because blood and semen were vectors for the transmission of HIV, thereby becoming symbols of the public's fears of AIDS." See also bell hooks, "The Radiance of Red: Blood Work."
4. In interviews, Serrano often states the wish to blur the boundary between the abstract and the figurative, as well as the one between photography and painting. See Rosenberg's interview with Serrano and Ferguson, "Andres Serrano." The latter points out that Serrano deliberately uses the scale and lush colors of oil painting in his photography.
5. Goldberg, "Metallica's Rebel Yell"; the bracketed insertion is in the original.
6. In this sense, Serrano's works evoke the Bataillean (anti)category of the "formless," as taken up by Bois and Krauss. Two of the "operations" that they discuss are especially relevant here: "entropy" (as opposed to atemporal form) and "horizontality" (as opposed to a vertical sublimation); see Bois and Krauss, *Formless*, 73–78, 93–103. See also my introduction.
7. Aristotle allows for the possibility: "semen emitted under strain due to excessively frequent intercourse, has been known in some cases to have a bloodlike appearance when discharged"; *Generation of Animals* 1.19.
8. Ferguson, in "Andres Serrano," observes that Serrano presents the bodily fluids in a "quasi-scientific or abstract fashion."
9. For instance, according to Kristeva, *Powers of Horror*, both substances may prompt abject reactions to an equal extent, but Kristeva also observes that semen is gen-

erally taken as "pure" within religious hygiene rules, whereas specifically menstrual blood is seen as "unclean." In this puritanistic view, the *Semen and Blood* series may comprise the most abject image imaginable. Finally, blood has also been used to purify, to clear, or to remedy the abject, as in ritual sacrifice. The blood in Serrano's works has been connected by bell hooks to the devaluation of menstruation and to victims of political torture; she argues that the artist "shattered the cultural taboo that prohibits any public celebration of blood that is not an affirmation of patriarchy"; bell hooks, "The Radiance of Red: Blood Work." In the same book, Arenas notes that "in art, the sight of blood is often intolerable outside of a moralizing context," and connects the works to the bodily, creatural, and physical aspect of Christ; see Arenas, "The Revelations of Andres Serrano."

10. "Soul," in the Christian sense, does not quite translate Aristotle's *psyche*. Psyche denotes the principle of life or vitality. It gives matter its realization through a form or shape. The nutritive, sentient, appetitive, locomotive, and rational are its five aspects. Psyche is not, yet subsists in, substance, at best in pneuma. However, the specific connection of the rational psyche to matter is rather ephemeral —it "comes in over and above, from without"—and survives the death of the body (Peck, "Introduction," in Aristotle *Generation of Animals*, lviii). The oxymoron of woman as a "natural deformity" mingles two philosophical conceptions of nature: on the one hand, Peck's introduction to the treatise explains, "the male represents the full development of which Nature is capable" in Aristotle's thought. On the other hand, the "female is so universal and regular an occurrence that it cannot be dismissed out of hand as 'unnatural' " (xlvi). Hence, femininity's impossible place in nature.

11. For this process of "concoction," the Greek uses forms of the verb *pettein*, for "making soft." It denotes the "ripening (of fruit)," "cooking" and "baking," as well as "digesting" and "processing." In that last sense, as used by Aristotle, it designates the processing of food by heat, issuing from the heart, within the body. This processing produces all body substances, such as semen, milk, blood, marrow, fat, nails, hair, phlegm, excrement, and bile, depending on their respective state of processing. See *Generation of Animals* 8, note a, and Peck's "Introduction," lxiii.

12. See the "Introduction" to *Generation of Animals* for a note on "acquired" rather than "inherent" differences in Aristotle (lxvii), as well as one on graduality and analogy (lxviii).

13. See Aristotle *Generation of Animals* 1.18 for his remarks on sperm production in the fat, the young, the old, and the ill; see 4.1 for a note on eunuchs.

14. As the "Preface" to *Generation of Animals* explains, to Aristotle, "Form is not found apart from Matter . . . , nor is Matter found which is not to some extent 'informed' " (xii). Furthermore, for Aristotle, "action can only be exerted, change can only be brought about, by something that can come into contact with another thing." Hence, "something corporeal must be supplied by the male" (xiv). This something inhabits the pneuma that forms the vehicle for the soul or psyche, ultimately setting it apart from the menstrual blood that does not have it.

15. Aristotle distinguishes between four kinds of causes. The motive or efficient cause, delivered by the male in generation, is what sets in motion the process of formation; the material cause, embodied by menstrual blood, supplies its substance; the formal cause rules the shape of what is formed into being; and the final cause, or logos, determines the resulting organism's state of perfected being, its purpose. See *Generation of Animals*, "Introduction," xxxviii.
16. According to Aristotle, the soul is best transported in hot substances, and best of all in pneuma, its primary vehicle. Pneuma forms the terrestrial counterpart to the aither that is the element of the upper cosmos. Aither is the fifth and divine element, superior to air, water, earth, and fire. See the "Introduction" to *Generation of Animals*, lviii.
17. Aphrodite, the goddess of carnal love, is named after the sea spume from which she originates. In Greek, *aphros* means "foam," hence Aristotle's pun.
18. In this sense, the image mirrors Lacan's ejaculatory phrase, which pits the endurance of the "vital flow" against the fleeting moment of its transport ("as it is transmitted"). See chapter 2.
19. The Van Gogh's Ear exhibition was presented on the Web as if it actually had occurred. Web designer and artist Andrew Fish hosted the pages that were dedicated to it, but the pages presenting the exhibition (www.andrewfish.com/vangogh) are no longer available.
20. For an account of the scandals associated with Serrano, see Steiner, *The Scandal of Pleasure*, or Ferguson, "Andres Serrano." Ferguson argues that Serrano entered into the conservative climate of the culture wars as a "quicksilver catalyst." His works were appropriated as "counteradvertisements for politicians and religious groups lacking strong representations of their own."
21. As Serrano explains at the occasion of a question-and-answer session at a conference in 2005: "I had a technical problem here because at first I kept shooting and missing it. After ten times of getting films back that were completely black, I realized I needed a motor drive for the camera. So with a motor drive I was able to synchronize both actions; before I felt myself coming I started shooting, and I was able to photograph thirty-six exposures within twelve seconds—one of them would have the image. Only one. Sometimes the interesting part of being an artist is not only doing something but figuring out how to do it." See http://www.undo.net/cgi-bin/openframe.pl?x=/Pinto/Eng/eserrano.htm.
22. "[A] kind of liquid bone" is a simile from Methodius, *The Banquet of the Ten Virgins*, cited in Power, "Of Godly Men and Medicine," note 26.
23. Bataille, *Story of the Eye*, 42; further citations are given in the text.
24. For more on Bataille in relation to ejaculation and expenditure, see chapter 10.
25. Derrida, *Dissemination*, 322; further citations are given in the text. See chapter 9 for a more extensive reading of Derrida's book in relation to ejaculation, orgasm, and semen.
26. Thus, Derrida can be taken to counter the seminal "white mythology" of Aristotelian (meta)physics through Mallarmé, rendering rereadable the blotted-out "palimpsest" of its "production," in Thomas's sense: "White mythology—metaphysics has erased within itself the fabulous scene that has produced it, the scene

that nevertheless remains active and stirring, inscribed in white ink, an invisible design covered over in the palimpsest" (Derrida, *Margins of Philosophy*, 213). For a critical response, see Young, "Deconstruction and the Postcolonial."

27. Bal, *Quoting Caravaggio*, 45–75; further citations are given in the text. The works by Serrano she discusses are *Bloodscape V* (1998), *Piss Christ* (1987), *Memory* (1983), The Morgue series (1992), and The Church series (1991).
28. At two instances, Aristotle explicitly compares semen to paint. The final residue resembles the nourishment whence it originates, "just as (to take a common instance) the paint left over on an artist's palette resembles that which he has actually used" (1.18). If that simile implies a white that is composed of all other colors, another suggests its blotting propensity. Seminal "colliquescence" may occur when "a fresh secretion is decomposed into that which preceded it, just as when a fresh layer of plaster spread on a wall immediately drops away, the reason being that the stuff which comes away is identical with that which was applied in the first instance" (1.19).
29. In this way, *Frozen Sperm I* anticipates current anxieties about the uses of frozen semen when divorced from its living begetter. In the United Kingdom, these came to a head in the widely reported legal cases pursued by Diane Blood, who went to court to be granted permission to impregnate herself with the conserved sperm of her late husband four years after it had been collected from his dying and comatose body. Subsequently Blood sued to have her son Liam be officially recognized as her husband's child, and conceived again from the same sample in 2002.
30. For an account of white signifying both transcendence and a bleak and terrifying mortality, see the last chapter of Richard Dyer's *White*, titled "White Death." Dyer's cases include vampire, zombie, and science-fiction movies as well as Melville's *Moby-Dick*.

2. IMAGE OF THE VITAL FLOW

1. Lacan, "The Signification of the Phallus," in *Écrits*, 82 (emphasis added); further citations are given in the text.
2. On durative and punctual events, see Bal, *Narratology*, 93–94.
3. In *Bodies That Matter*, Butler remarks on the dubious productivity of defining the phallus by what it is not, by negation: "What is the character of this bind whereby the phallus symbolizes the penis to the extent that it differentiates itself from the penis, where the penis becomes the privileged referent to be negated? If the phallus must negate the penis in order to symbolize and signify in its privileged way, then the phallus is bound to the penis, not through simple identity, but through determinate negation. . . . And in that sense in which the phallus requires the penis for its own constitution, the identity of the phallus includes the penis, that is, a relation of identity holds between them" (85). For more on the phallus/penis distinction, see chapter 4.
4. Bakhtin, "The Heteroglot Novel," in *The Bakhtin Reader*, 112–20.
5. Macey, "Phallus," 319; further citations are given in the text.

6. Laplanche and Pontalis, *The Language of Psychoanalysis*, 313–14; further citations are given in the text.
7. Lacan, "The Signification of the Phallus," 79, 82, 85. However, the archaeological record has established an astonishing and casual omnipresence of penile imagery and sculpture in classical times—in cutlery, road signs, garden ornaments, and door handles, to name but a few examples—which does not tally with the highly charged veiling of the phallus in Lacan's account. See Atkins, *Sex in Literature, Volume 2*, 306–320.
8. Butler, *Bodies That Matter*, 80; further citations are given in the text. For a contrast to the Western economy of the single name for the penis, see the thirty-five names given to the organ in Shaykh Nefzawi's *The Perfumed Garden* (in Pitt-Kethley, *The Literary Companion to Sex*, 79–85), including *el teunnana*, the tinkler, *el fortass*, the bald, *el bekkai*, the weeping one, and *el mourekhi*, the flabby one.
9. As Bowie remarks in his engaging *Lacan*, "[T]he phallus and the entire 'masculinist' discourse that it unleashes . . . , are at odds with [the models of desire and meaning suggesting] perpetual mobility and incompletion, [which have] no particular bias on matters of gender" (141). Bowie explains the "nimbus" or "accolade" given to the penis/phallus in Lacanian theory on the basis of the organ's variability, detachability, apparential instability, and exteriority, which make it suitable as an intimation or articulation of structure (124–25).
10. For more on the notion of a "theoretical fiction" and a sustained attempt to read fictions theoretical and literary through and with each other, see Lord, *The Intimacy of Influence*.
11. As Silverman argues, "the male organ remains so emphatically in propria persona here that Lacan must have felt the need to put quotes around the whole passage"; "The Lacanian Phallus," 94.
12. On the notion of *Aufhebung*, Silverman offers the following gloss: "The rising motion invoked by this passage also works on two semantic registers: it refers on the one hand to the lifting of an object up and out of the real and into signification, and on the other to the penile erection whose contours can still be made out beneath the veil . . ."; "The Lacanian Phallus," 89. Bowie offers the imagination that underpins both aspects with a quote from Freud's *The Interpretation of Dreams*: "The remarkable phenomenon of erection around which human imagination has constantly played cannot fail to be impressive, involving as it does an apparent suspension of the laws of gravity"; quoted in *Lacan*, 129.
13. As Butler asks, "If Lacan claimed that the phallus only operates as 'veiled,' we might ask in return what kind of 'veiling' the phallus invariably performs"; *Bodies That Matter*, 85.
14. For a clear explanation of "demand" in relation to "need" and "desire," see Bowie, *Lacan*, 135–40.
15. For Lacan's interest in feminine, orgasmic pleasure as "beyond the phallus," see Bowie, *Lacan*, 140–52. I would argue that even male orgasmic pleasure is marginal to the phallus.
16. For a discussion of narrative rhythm, see Bal, *Narratology*, 104–5.

3. ANAMORPHOSIS / METAMORPHOSIS

1. *The Ambassadors* appears on the original French edition of *The Four Fundamental Concepts of Psycho-Analysis* of 1973, the English translation reissued by Penguin in 1994, and the 1995 edition by the State University of New York Press.
2. Lacan, *The Four Fundamental Concepts of Psycho-Analysis*, 85; further citations are given in the text.
3. For a recuperative critique of perspectivism for use in theater studies, see Bleeker, *The Locus of Looking*.
4. The Lacanian category of the real is not easily grasped. The real points to a dimension that eludes the imaginary and symbolic reality in which subjectivity and signification take shape. It can only be experienced when it encroaches upon that reality; Lacan compares its force with that of a sudden, loud knock on the bedroom door, which puts a sleeper in a state between dreaming and wakefulness; *Four Fundamental Concepts of Psycho-Analysis*, 57.
5. Laplanche and Pontalis explain that copulation is understood by the child as a brutal, anal rape; *The Language of Psychoanalysis*, 335.
6. Lacan, *Four Fundamental Concepts of Psycho-Analysis*, 70, emphasis added. In the case study on the Wolf Man, Freud analyzes the phobias and anxieties of a young man who at a tender age witnessed his parents' triple session of afternoon *a tergo* lovemaking from his cot; *Three Case Histories*, 222–23. One of the many lines Freud follows in the course of the analysis traces back elements of his patient's ordeal to the instances in the love scene when the paternal penis disappeared from sight, the *a tergo* position offering the child visual access to that fact. The Wolf Man asserts, Freud writes, "that he had observed the penis disappear, that he had felt sympathy with his father on that account, and had rejoiced at the reappearance of what he thought had been lost" (279).
7. Pieters, in "Facing History, or the Anxiety of Reading," contrasts the meanings given to Holbein's skull in readings by Greenblatt, *Renaissance Self-Fashioning*, and Lyotard, *Discours, figure*. Pieters characterizes the former in terms of the Barthesian studium, the desire to speak responsibly with the historic dead to garner knowledge. The latter he views in relation to the punctum: the fact that the deathhead *speaks* triggers an event of "figuration" that dislocates, dissolves, the discursive context in which Greenblatt's knowledgeable conversation with the dead takes place.
8. Foister, Roy, and Wyld consider the objects as emblems of wealth or learning; *Holbein's Ambassadors*, 30, 33. Yet, noting that the objects include portable instruments for measuring time and space, they settle on the symbolism of travel, which also indicates a world that is set in motion and out of joint (40).
9. Sauerländer, "The Art of the Cool."
10. Silverman, *The Threshold of the Visible World*, 177; further citations are given in the text.
11. Foister, Roy, and Wyld hazard several guesses as to how the historical viewer might have observed the skull in the painting: through an attached telescopic de-

vice, through a hole in a side wall, while descending a circling staircase, or with the help of a glass or other cylindrical object; *Holbein's Ambassadors*, 50–55.

12. Berger, *Ways of Seeing*, 109; further citations are given in the text.
13. Foister, Roy, and Wyld, *Holbein's Ambassadors*, 9; further citations are given in the text.
14. For a detailed account of the restoration, see the second part of Foister, Roy, and Wyld, *Holbein's Ambassadors*.
15. Of course, Holbein's portrait of Henry VIII is famous for its conspicuous codpiece.
16. "It has become clear," Foister, Roy, and Wyld comment, "that the skirt divided." Though "it has been suggested that originally a codpiece protruded through the divide in the skirt," the authors arrest further discussion: "The reconstruction of the codpiece . . . was not seriously considered"; *Holbein's Ambassadors*, 95.
17. Foister, Roy, and Wyld note that the diagonal line made by the skull and the crucifix negates and overshadows the vertical/horizontal organization of the scene; *Holbein's Ambassadors*, 43–44. They determine its significance as conveying death and salvation (9, 50).
18. Lacan, "The Mirror Stage as Formative of the Function of the I," in *Écrits*, 1–7, esp. p. 3.
19. Foister, Roy, and Wyld argue that *The Ambassadors* is a friendship painting in the style of a marriage or betrothal painting without art historical precedent. Friendship paintings would come in vogue much later (18).
20. Foister, Roy, and Wyld note that Dinteville (on the left) actually suffered from nervous illnesses and melancholia (57). That de Selve's "face is a little lacking in animation" is explained by the fact that he did not sit long for Holbein (62).
21. Harvey, *Men in Black*, 142.

4. THE PARTING VEIL

1. For an account of the drawing in its original context, see Zwijnenberg, *The Writings and Drawings of Leonardo da Vinci*, 102–6.
2. Above all, *Vitruvian Man* embodies the value of symmetry. In their entry on "Gestalt," Bois and Krauss bring in the asymmetries of the density of the human body—"subject to gravitation, ventrally sighted, dextrally favored"—in order to criticize the aesthetic of symmetrical form; *Formless*, 89.
3. Pedretti gives three reasons why *The Angel in the Flesh* is probably by Leonardo: the position of the figure, the liveliness of the figure's hair, and the fact that the face is drawn by a left-handed hand; "The Angel in the Flesh," 34–35.
4. In *Leonardo, Psychoanalysis, and Art History*, Collins deploys *The Angel in the Flesh* to bring out the sexuality of John the Baptist: "The sketch depicts an Angel of the Annunciation and is closely related to the St. John. The same type of grinning, longhaired boy turns his left hand to his chest and lifts his right arm in a pointing gesture. Leonardo, however, has made the angel more androgynous and feminine. And the angel holds to his chest a flimsy veil that seems ready to drop. But what definitely settles the matter of the erotic nature of this type of figure is a new

detail. As if to desublimate his own creation, Leonardo has endowed the figure with a large, erect penis" (88).

5. Butler, *Bodies That Matter*, 60; further citations are given in the text.
6. On personal and impersonal language situations, see Bal, *Narratology*, 47–48.
7. Silverman, *Male Subjectivity at the Margins*, 2; further citations are given in the text.
8. Silverman, "The Lacanian Phallus," 89; further citations are given in the text.
9. Boyarin, "Feminism Meets Queer Theory," 55; further citations are given in the text.
10. Bernheimer explains what the reassociation of the phallus with the penis can contribute to theory: "The most evident effect of penile reference on the transcendental phallus is the onslaught of temporality and the consequent variability of the penis between its rigid and limp states"; "Penile Reference in Phallic Theory," 119. As a thought experiment, Bernheimer conjures up images of the penis, and notes that those must come with a series of "salient differences." These are dependent on gender, race, class, experience; on size, state, and color; on particularity and genericness; on invested affects like pain, pleasure, delight, disgust; and on framing: "What parts of the body (testicles, skin, navel, buttocks, belly) form its background, if any?" (118).
11. Jane Gallop argues that the attempt to control the meanings of the phallus is, in the end, precisely phallic: "The Lacanian desire clearly to separate phallus from penis, is precisely symptomatic of desire [of commentators] to have the phallus, that is, their desire to be at the center of language, at its origin. And their inability to control the meaning of the word phallus is evidence of what Lacan calls symbolic castration"; quoted in Butler, *Bodies That Matter*, 57.
12. Bramly, *Leonardo*, 263; further citations are given in the text.
13. Zerner, "The Vision of Leonardo."
14. "We begin to suspect the possibility," Freud writes in his biographical monograph on Leonardo da Vinci, "that it was his mother who possessed the mysterious smile—the smile that he had lost and that fascinated him so much when he found it again in the Florentine Lady"; quoted in Silverman, *Male Subjectivity at the Margins*, 370. For an account updating recent developments in psychoanalysis, biography, and art history in relation to Leonardo, see Collins, *Leonardo, Psychoanalysis, and Art History*.
15. Both Collins and Pedretti call attention to the sketches of two-legged, walking penises in the Codex Atlanticus; see Collins, *Leonardo, Psychoanalysis, and Art History*, 81, and Pedretti, "The Angel in the Flesh," 35.

5. SIGNIFICANT DISCHARGE

1. The third moniker of the shot follows from the fact that the actors get paid extra for executing it; see Williams, *Hard Core*, 95.
2. The dominance of the figure is perhaps best attested by the fact that its exceptions, inadvertently or advertently internal ejaculations, are subject to a specialized or cult following under the heading of "cream-pie."
3. Dyer, "Male Gay Porn," 28; further citations are given in the text.

4. A reference to Kermode, *Sense of an Ending*.
5. The notion of homosociality is derived from Sedgwick, *Between Men*. Sedgwick coins the oxymoron "male homosocial desire" to analyze the thin boundary between and the continuum of homosociality or male bonding and homosexuality. When the boundary between the two is felt to be threatened, a "homosexual panic" ensues. See Sedgwick's Introduction, 1–20.
6. The imperative visibility of ejaculation overrules consistency, if need be. Sascha Alexander's *9½ Days, Part Two* (1993), offers an example. The female protagonist reminisces about her lovemaking with her late husband, an encounter visualized as flashback. In voice-over, she comments, "When he wanted to come, he preferred to do so in my clean-shaven pussy. *Und dann war es so weit* . . ." Upon which words one sees that her husband grunts, hastily withdraws, repositions his body, and ejaculates in her face, with unintentional comic effect.
7. In the Frequently Asked Questions compiled by the newsgroup rec.arts.movies.erotica, or rame (http://rame.net), director Jim Gunn remarks on the facial or "mug shot" as follows: "What you are really seeing is a classical 'cutaway' shot used as a transition between the ending of the sex action and the facial splash. Typically the sex scene ends in a medium shot that was being captured ten minutes earlier, before the director yelled, 'Ok, we've got enough footage,' and the male talent took a swig of water and mechanically jerked himself off onto the girl's face in a very deliberate way for the all-important cum shot." Though any image could serve as the cutaway shot, Gunn continues, "the man's facial expression is just so much more logical."
8. In another article, Dyer remarks on the "worked-for-quality betrayed in much porn by the sudden cut to an ejaculation evidently uninspired by what the performer was doing in the immediately preceding shot"; "Idol Thoughts," 51.
9. The ejaculation shown in the cum shot does not necessarily belong to the male performer participating in it. Editing may link up an ejaculation and a face that actually belong to different performers.
10. In this respect, feature porn differs from other pornographic sub-genres. "Gonzo" porn dispenses with the story line and frames its numbers in the elaborated exploits of the cameraman/director, whose actions from behind the camera—soliciting women to undress for him, directing their performances, voicing his pleasure, and the like—form its rudimentary plot. Compilation tapes offer numbers taken from various feature films without their embedding plot lines.
11. For a discussion on "The Sounds of Pleasure," see Williams, *Hard Core*, 121–27.
12. Dyer mentions point-of-view shots, shot/reverse shot patterns, and location shots; "Idol Thoughts," 50. In contrast, the hard-core sequences or numbers are marked by "spatial liability": "Very often the editing of these sequences betrays gaps in spatial and temporal continuity, ignored, and caused, by the 'frenzied' (to use Williams' suggestive term) will to see" (53).
13. The entry on the verb "to come" in the *Oxford English Dictionary Online* (2002) suggests the relevance of the differentiation of coming between act, event, and effect. The first meaning is "to move towards," "to approach," "to become present

at any place or point." Here, coming is an act performed by the subject. Yet the second meaning contests that agency, turning coming into an event that happens to the subject. The synonyms are "to receive," "to occur," "to befall," and to "have it coming to one." In a third set of meanings, agency is lost entirely; coming becomes an effect. The synonyms are "to come undone/unput/unstuck," "to become disintegrated," "to fall to pieces," and "to come to grief."

14. Doubrovsky, *Writing and Fantasy in Proust*, 134. Doubrovsky's reading of Proust is discussed in chapter 12 of this study.
15. Justine is not a run-of-the-mill porn movie. It received no less than eight awards at the 1994 Adult Video News Awards (the industry's own "Oscars" ceremony), and qualified for a five-star "superior" rating. Reportedly, director Paul Thomas has invigorated the genre with high production values and inventive story lines. The film is marketed for more than solitary consumption; the box-jacket announces that Justine is "a film for couples." A review by Natalie Dawn judges the film "a landmark for our generation," adding that "Director Paul Thomas . . . is the master of the everyday, always able to capture some essence of reality that eludes his colleagues." Another review, by dumblonde, comments on Simon's failed cum shot as follows: "There is one scene where [actor] Mike Horner doesn't pull out at all [when he comes], and this astounded me. Did I feel 'cheated'? Please . . ."
16. Brooks, *Reading for the Plot*, 107; further citations are given in the text.
17. Winnett, "Coming Unstrung," 505–6; further citations are given in the text.
18. With respect to the term "binding," Laplanche and Pontalis stress notions such as cohesion, demarcation, fixation, and quantification; *The Language of Psychoanalysis*, 52.
19. The main argument of Winnett's article is that Brooks allows masculinity to be a specific thematic as well as a matter of general narrative form, whereas femininity can only be a particular thematic. She argues "that male narratology conceptualizes narrative dynamics in terms of an experience it so swiftly and seamlessly generalizes that we tend to forget that it has its source in experience—in fact, in experience of the body"; "Coming Unstrung," 508. Subsequently, Winnett forges the recognition of "analogously representable female" dynamics for narrativity, centering on the "radically prospective" rhythms of giving birth and breastfeeding, thus qualifying the structuring accolade usually given to the ending, to climax. However, I would object to Winnett's implicit claim that the "significant discharge" covers and exhausts the recognizability of narratable male pleasures ("We all know what male orgasm looks like," 505). If male orgasm is readily recognizable in the narrative climax that Brooks describes as the "significant discharge," then the privileging of that formation for narrativity must also render invisible and irrelevant *other* formations of male pleasure.
20. Brooks, *Reading for the Plot*, 103, cf. 85. Compare Brüner's insistence that "deviance" is what sparks or triggers narrativity, the attempt to make an irritant fit into a story; *Acts of Meaning*, 97.
21. Williams, *Hard Core*, 92, 110; further citations are given in the text.

22. As Thomas writes, "in fact both participants [male and female] are excluded from the 'uncontrollable' pleasure that the money shot purports to display: his ejaculation becomes the verifiable sign of the orgasm she is not really having (and could not visibly prove even if she were), while her performed convulsions signify the uncontrollable *jouissance* to which he, as a man, has no access (except through watching her)"; *Male Matters*, 20.
23. Dolce, "Editor's Letter," 44, emphasis added; further citations are given in the text.
24. Heath, "A Hard Man Is Good to Find," 270. Martin Amis's essay on the adult industry, "A Rough Trade," offers a second typical example: "[G]enerally speaking," Amis writes, "men are the also-rans of porno." Amis then quotes the following musing from a character from Updike, *Rabbit at Rest*: "The trouble with these soft-core movies . . . [is that] they show tits and ass and even some pubic hair but no real cunt and no pricks, no pricks hard or soft at all. It's all very frustrating. It turns out pricks are what we care about, you have to see them. Maybe we're all queer . . ."
25. Williams, *Hard Core*, 107. Williams's analysis of the cum shot appears to wed traditional iconophobia ("a poor substitute") to that other, and mutually exclusive, dominant discourse on the visual image: positivism ("visual evidence"). Apparently, the image shows the truth and substitutes it for a mere semblance.
26. Kermode, *The Sense of an Ending*, 67.
27. Smith, "Vas," 107, cf. 106; further citations are given in the text.
28. Slade, "Flesh Need Not Be Mute," 127, 129; further citations are given in the text.
29. Similarly, de Lauretis writes that the movement of narrative folds back onto what it seeks to overcome: "[I]ts 'sense of an ending' remains inseparable from the memory of loss and the recapturing of time"; *Alice Doesn't*, 25. Johnson, in her reading of Melville's *Billy Budd*, states that to end is to repeat, and to repeat is to "be ungovernably open to revision, displacement, and reversal"; *The Critical Difference*, 81. The ending in question is Budd's execution by hanging. To the shared amazement of the congregated onlookers, Budd's corpse does not show the signs of the mechanical ejaculation expected to accompany his manner of death.

6. LEVERING EJACULATION

1. Faludi, "The Money Shot."
2. For a note on working-class iconography in gay porn, see Dyer, "Idol Thoughts," 56.
3. As I explain in the Introduction, Thomas coins the concept of production to analyze the "production anxiety" that he sees as typical for modern masculinity. He appropriates the term from Baudrillard, who describes it as "to render visible, to cause to appear and be made to appear"; quoted in Thomas, *Male Matters*, 34. For Thomas, the concept stresses the materiality and visibility of masculine agency and writing. "[M]asculinity," he writes, "cannot represent its supposedly immaculate self-construction without giving itself over to discursive productions in

which the always potentially messy question of the body cannot fail to emerge" (13). Thus, the notion theorizes a male anxiety over the differential between symbolic self-presentation and material, visible trace.

4. In its sense of "container," Smith's choice of *vas* might also point to uterus-envy, a point that I will not pursue.
5. Van Alphen criticizes Smith's reading: "The visibility of the ejaculation turns it into a sign of action and production. These two qualities seem to be pursued in order to cancel out the idea of the death of the body that could be evoked by an ejaculation inside the body"; *Francis Bacon and the Loss of Self*, 184.
6. Thomas argues that the reception of the sperm by the female star serves "to bolster male hyperbole by taking on the role of the discarded, humiliated self"; *Male Matters*, 22.
7. Kristeva, *Powers of Horror*, 5. For a searing critique of the essentialization of the abject as maternal lining, see Krauss's conclusion to Bois and Krauss, *Formless*, "The Destiny of the *Informe*," 235–52. Krauss blames Kristeva for the continuation of the association between the "slimy" and the feminine interior, imagined as limp, moist, clinging, and dark, and hence, as threatening to the autonomy of the (male) subject (238–39). In contrast to Kristeva's abject, she argues, Bataille's "formless" [informe] is not a substance, an essence, or a theme, but an operative function, a process (249).
8. Both van Alphen and Mitchell associate a visual fixation in narrative with trauma. Van Alphen, in "Caught by Images," views the repetition of "visual imprints" in a story as enacting rather than recounting traumatic memory. These imprints impede the mastery and comprehension of an event that narrativization may afford. Mitchell observes a descriptive excess in slave narratives, which threatens the "progress toward an end," paralyzing that progress through "the endless proliferation of descriptive detail"; *Picture Theory*, 201, 194. I will entertain the excess or the fixation of the visual in hard core in relation to the story line as possibly both haunting and enchanting.
9. Dyer notes the same in general: "The moment of coming is sometimes shot simultaneously from three different camera positions, which are then edited together, sometimes one or more in slow motion"; "Idol Thoughts," 53.
10. Dyer, "Idol Thoughts," 49. "According to much twentieth-century critical theory," Dyer adds, "this ought not to be so. It has long been held that work that draws attention to itself—cultural constructs that make apparent their own constructedness—will have the effect of distancing an audience. A film that draws our attention to its processes of turning us on ought not to turn us on; you shouldn't be able to come to what are merely terms" (60). Whether it turns on the viewer or not, the self-reflexivity of these cum shots does forge a coming to terms with the fact that ejaculation is not inherently or self-evidently climactic, and hence privileged, for the narrative of sexuality. If "the show is the event," as Dyer argues, then ejaculation becomes considerably less eventful, less climactic (60).
11. Quoted in Burger, *One-Handed Histories*, 73.
12. Bersani, *Homos*, 103; further citations are given in the text.

13. LaBruce's own Web site offers choice cuts from reviews by way of recommendations; see http://www.brucelabruce.com. The London *Daily Mail* calls the film "the most disgusting motion picture . . . ever seen." The reviewer not only objects to *Hustler White*'s sexuality and violence, but also laments that "it is not even well-made pornography."
14. For an engaging overview of thoughts on female ejaculation and the controversies that surround it, see Sprinkle, "The G Spot?"
15. Johnson's "Excess and Ecstasy" compares constructions of female pleasure in mainstream straight pornography and woman-made and lesbian hard core. According to Johnson, the former displaces female pleasure through a surplus of imagery (facial close-ups) and sounds (screams and moans) situated at some remove from the body, whereas the latter seeks out representations of pleasure that are anchored to the body (31). The female ejaculations in these films partake of that endeavor, also working to marginalize the penis, because the stimulation by a finger or a dildo of the G-spot accommodates fully visible squirting (37). Additionally, Johnson notes an eroticization of the male body in these films, the potential pleasures of which can only appear "in the form of ejaculatory punctuation" in mainstream hard core (31). In one of her cases, she observes a male orgasm that is not shown in extreme close-up, as is the case of the standard cum shot, but is instead reframed "in the broader context of the body's responses," so that the viewer is allowed to witness the "convulsive reactions of the male body in orgasm" (40).

7. "NOW TAKE ONE OF ME AS I COME"

1. On the relations between femininity, representation, and mortality, see Bronfen, *Over Her Dead Body*.
2. Eco defines the sign as "anything that can be used in order to lie"; *A Theory of Semiotics*, 10.
3. Eco, "How to Recognize a Porn Movie," 207; further citations are given in the text.
4. Barthes, "The Reality Effect," 138; further citations are given in the text.
5. *Adult Video News* frequently publishes feature articles on trends in the genre. For a discussion of gonzo porn, see Austin, "Gonzo in the Year 2000"; for amateur porn, see Thompson, "Porn by the People, for the People"; for nasties, see Wyke, "Exploiting the Many Markets of Adult."
6. This statement was made in an *Adult Video News* interview; see Wyke, "Exploiting the Many Markets of Adult."
7. Williams, "Porn Studies," 3; further citations are given in the text.
8. Schaefer, "Gauging a Revolution," 371; further citations are given in the text.
9. Patterson, "Going On-line," 117; further citations are given in the text.
10. Genette, "*Vraisemblance* and Motivation," 240; further citations are given in the text.
11. This ejaculation scene is the topic of discussion in a thread of postings to the newsgroup rec.arts.movies.erotica, headed "Pedro Almodóvar's 'Kika': Money

Shot??" (October 30–31, 2002). "However, it wouldn't be what I think of when referring to a money shot," poster randyripoff concludes the exchange.

12. For an introduction to the Peircean sign typology of icon, index, and symbol, see Bal, with coauthor Norman Bryson, *On Meaning-Making*, chapter 8, especially 165–71. Bal and Bryson argue against the conflation of iconicity and visuality, making all three semiotic modes for visual analysis available to an equal extent. Briefly, the icon suggests a partial and hypothetical similarity to its object, the index brings up a contiguous relationship to what it points to, and the symbol relies on a cultural convention to signify it.

8. THE SUSPENSE AND SUSPENSION OF BLISS

1. Generally, the term *jouissance* is used in two different ways. One stems from Lacanian psychoanalysis and suggests a feminine pleasure as "beyond" the phallus. The other refers to the experience of the pre-Oedipal child. For a helpful introduction, see the entry on the term in Wright, *Feminism and Psychoanalysis*. Here, I am concerned with Barthes's distinct and idiosyncratic use of the term.
2. Eagleton, *Literary Theory*, 82, 141; further citations are given in the text.
3. Lentricchia, *After the New Criticism*, 145; further citations are given in the text. For an illuminating view on the enduring difficulty of what he terms "left puritanism" with pleasure, see Helmling, "Marxist Pleasure." Helmling rereads both Eagleton's and Jameson's commentaries on Barthes, to contrast their opposing judgments with Eagleton's own pleasured reading of Jameson. "Insofar as Eagleton's own pugilistic wit," Helmling writes, "invites us to pleasures that feel distinctly masculine, his aversion to Barthesian *jouissance* might seem almost a residual, unwitting homophobia: the revolutionary band of brothers, apparently, is to enjoy collective pleasures, but not collective ecstasies" (no pagination). Jameson recuperates Barthes by linking pleasure, through its association with fear, to the serious "sublime," Helmling argues, "a passion of 'fear' prompted by 'History,' by 'what hurts.' " Things get complicated as Eagleton promotes carnavalesque enjoyments of his own, and must admit to pleasure in his reading of Jameson.
4. Barthes, *The Pleasure of the Text*, 22–23; further citations are given in the text.
5. The little room smelling of orrisroot, the solitary pleasures that it accommodates, and the ejaculation that takes place there will be discussed in the second chapter on Proust, chapter 12.
6. Bataille's quasi-heroic view on ejaculation as a form of expenditure will be at stake in chapter 10 of this study.
7. For a careful consideration of the nexus between homosexuality and (post)colonialism in relation to utopian desire in Barthes's work, see Knight, *Barthes and Utopia*. Knight contrasts Barthes's relentless debunking of colonial myth in *Mythologies* with his own unwitting sexual-colonial exploits as related in the posthumously published *Incidents*, and traces Barthes's views on such oriental countries as Japan, Turkey, China, and Morocco. For an attempt to "out" a Barthes

ever hesitating on the closet's threshold in his lifetime writings, see Miller, *Bringing Out Roland Barthes*.

8. Stephen Heath objects to the use of "bliss" for *jouissance* because it lacks a verbal form, connotes religious and social dimensions in opposition to Barthes's usage, and forgoes the precise sexual meaning of "coming"; Heath, "Translator's Note," in Barthes, *Image Music Text*, 9. Jonathan Culler prefers "ecstasy"; *Barthes*, 83. In accordance with the translation I have studied I will continue to use "bliss." For a remark on Barthes's creative and loose use of terminological pairings, see Culler, *Barthes*, 6.
9. Moriarty, *Reading Roland Barthes*, 154.
10. According to Culler, Barthes's recourse to the body in the later work serves several functions, such as the estrangement of the self from consciousness, the avoidance of the question of the subject, and the emphasis on the materiality of the signifier. The attendant risk, Culler continues, is the renewed mystification of the source of signification as "natural substratum beyond . . . transient cultural features" (*Barthes*, 78). On the contrary, I would argue that Barthes's invocation of the body in *The Pleasure of the Text* alienates and textualizes what may seem most "natural" to both masculine sexuality and narrative: the urge for climax.
11. Perhaps the least "masculine" appearance of pleasure is the following one: "it can be an act that is slight, complex, tenuous, almost scatterbrained: a sudden movement of the head like a bird who understands nothing of what we hear, who hears what we do not understand"; Barthes, *The Pleasure of the Text*, 24–25.
12. Another reading infers father-son incest; see Eilberg-Schwartz, *God's Phallus*, 86. Eilberg-Schwartz connects the Noah story to God's own act of exposure to Moses in Exodus, and reads both in terms of a homosexual/erotic "panic" brought about by the worshipping of a male god by a fraternity of men. The repudiation of the visual and the abstraction of the deity's bodily form are twin effects of that "panic," he argues.

9. DISSIMULATING THE SUPREME SPASM

1. Derrida, *Dissemination*, 172, 286; further citations are given in the text.
2. Compare Derrida's remark on *brisure* as both "crack" and "joint"; *Dissemination*, 302–3.
3. Such a "disseminal throw" also comes up in Derrida's piece on gender and Heidegger, "Geslecht: Sexual Difference, Ontological Difference." "There is no dissemination," Derrida claims, "that does not suppose such a 'throw' [*jetée*], Da of Dasein as thrown [*jetée*]. Thrown 'before' all the modes of throwing that will later determine it: project, subject, object, abject, trajectory, dejection"; 395–96. Da as ejected, as ejaculated?
4. Quoted in Culler, *On Deconstruction*, 309; further citations are given in the text.
5. Derrida, *The Ear of the Other*, 103; further citations are given in the text. I am indebted to Hent de Vries for alerting me to this reference.
6. "Since 1972, Derrida's work has continued to proliferate and diversify," writes

Barbara Johnson in her "Translator's Introduction" to *Dissemination* (viii). Note how easily "proliferate and diversify" can be replaced by "disseminated."

7. In her interview with Derrida, McDonald points to the same footnote, saying: "It seems to me that while the extensive play on etymologies . . . effects a displacement of these terms [hymen], it also poses a problem for those who would seek to define what is specifically feminine. That comes about not so much because these terms are either under- or over-valued as parts belonging to woman's body. It is rather that, in the economy of a movement of writing that is always elusive, one can never decide properly whether the particular term implies complicity with or a break from existent ideology"; "Choreographies," 71. Derrida does not quite answer this critique.
8. With respect to this statement, Thomas, criticizing Derrida for always making writing out to be something less or more than "just" material, than "graphic" in the sense of "explicit," infers a specific kind of womb-envy, "not for its reproductive capacities, but rather—and quite conspicuously in regard to the material question of dissemination—for the capacity of that sex . . . for a jouissance without visibilized or perceptible remains"; *Male Matters*, 150) I will attend to Thomas's critique at the end of this chapter.
9. The strategy of *entamer le phallus*, of "redistributing" the phallus rather than negating it, is proposed in Derrida's critique of Lacan in "Le facteur de la vérité": "Here dissemination threatens the law of the signifier and of castration as the contract of truth. It broaches, breaches [*entame*] the unity of the signifier, that is, of the phallus"; *A Derrida Reader*, 469. *Entamer* does not suggest the "cutting off" of the phallus, but a "cutting into" and "cutting up," much as one does with a cake.
10. For an extensive reading of this seminal white in relation to Aristotle and Serrano, see chapter 1.
11. This image constitutes yet another way of reconceiving of Plato's glittering Father-Sun.
12. The number four has added significance for Derrida, because it is the first number available for counting beyond philosophy's attachment to the one of monocentrism, the two of binarism, and the three of a dialectic that moves back to one. See, for instance, Derrida, *Dissemination*, 24–25.

10. ANXIETY AND INTIMACY OF EXPENDITURE

1. For this reason I hesitate before a blanket endorsement of Bataille, which Thomas, for instance, expresses under the vague heading of "Bataille's Postmodern Prodding"; see Thomas, *Male Matters*, 61.
2. Bataille, "The Notion of Expenditure," 167; further citations are given in the text.
3. David Bennett reads Bataille with and against texts by Freud and D. H. Lawrence that betray the tenacity and tenuousness of a dominant economic model that, since the "masturbation phobia" beginning in the early 1700s, anxiously concerned itself with the undue "spending" of energy, desire, money, time, and

semen: "The 'economizing' of sex and the eroticizing of money, it seems, are two sides of the metaphoric coin" (288). Bennett also notes that Bataille's apparent belief that "reckless spending" would repudiate capitalism now sounds only "quaint" in a consumption-driven culture (289).

4. For a transparent and befuddled attempt to restrict meaning within the narrowest of economies, see Umberto Eco's *Interpretation and Overinterpretation.*
5. Richman in *Reading Georges Bataille* offers a careful reading of Bataille's concepts in relation to Marcel Mauss's anthropological work on the "gift" and Derrida's textual "general economy."
6. Bataille, "The Use-Value of D. A. F. de Sade (An Open Letter to My Current Comrades)," 147; further citations are given in the text.
7. Susan Rubin Suleiman frames Bataille's concept in the history of the 1930s, which necessitated the transition from a virility based on outward action in the political sphere toward an internalized violence, a kind of "inner sundering," when the effectiveness of such a course of action had become moot; "Bataille in the Street," 79. Bataille's politics, then, would imply a restorative move in the face of impotence and powerlessness. Ultimately, Suleiman faults Bataille for his obsession with masculinity, since it cannot but lock "him into values and into a sexual politics that can only be called conformist, in his time and ours. Rhetorically, 'virility' carries with it too much old baggage" (43). In contrast, I will argue that it is exactly the obsessiveness of Bataille's engagement with masculinity that supplies the occasion for its "unpacking."
8. Michaels, "Talking Blue . . ."; see also "Zero Gravity Sex Film Up for Award."
9. See the product review at http://www.blissbox.co.uk/store/detail.asp?productid =3871. *Adult Video News* reports that Private Media has continued its efforts to produce spectacular cum shots. Michael Ninn's *Perfect* shows a cum shot in bullet-time, the special effect pioneered by *The Matrix.* The film presents an ejaculation as if frozen in time, while the camera seemingly makes a full circle around it, thus showing the ejaculation from all possible angles. See Kernes, "With Perfect, Ninn Takes Porn to a New Level."
10. Barbara Gallagher in "No Space Sex?" reports that NASA, usually squeamish about sexual experiments, may soon be forced to include sex in its research, as the possibility of the lengthy habitation of spacecrafts and space stations becomes imaginable.
11. Bataille, "Base Materialism and Gnosticism," 160; further citations are given in the text.
12. Wilson, "Fêting the Wound," 177.
13. Sontag, "The Pornographic Imagination," 87; further citations are given in the text.
14. Barthes, "The Metaphor of the Eye," 126; further citations are given in the text.

11. MISPLACED THIGH

1. I use the revised and updated edition of the Scott Moncrieff and Kilmartin translation published in 1996 by Vintage. Longer quotations are accompanied by

notes giving the French text from the Éditions Robert Laffont version of 1987. Citations are given in the text.

2. Bowie, *Proust Among the Stars*, 211; further citations are given in the text.
3. "Quelquefois, comme Ève naquit d'une côte d'Adam, une femme naissait pendant mon sommeil d'une fausse position de ma cuisse. Formée du plaisir que j'étais sur le point de goûter, je m'imaginais que c'etait elle qui me l'offrait. Mon corps qui sentait dans le sien ma propre chaleur voulait s'y rejoindre, je m'éveillais"; *À la recherche du temps perdu*, 1:26.
4. In I Timothy 2:12–13, Paul asserts: "But I suffer not a woman to teach, nor to usurp authority over the man, but to be in silence. For Adam was first formed, then Eve" (King James Version).
5. Bal, *Lethal Love*, 113; further citations are given in the text.
6. Bal's larger concern in the fifth chapter of *Lethal Love* is to arrive at a narratological understanding of the category of "character" without overlooking what she terms "semiotic chronology" (107). This chronology has nothing to do with character development, but with the gradual construction of a character out of textual building-blocks. Adam and Eve only exist from the beginning of Genesis on the basis of a "retrospective fallacy," which entails the "projection of an accomplished and singular named character onto previous textual elements that lead to the construction of that character" (108). This approach triumphs fully fledged characters over a text, Genesis, where the making of character is exactly the point. As a result, character-construction work, the divine, semiotic job of figuring out what it takes for a character to emerge, is lost from view.
7. "Car, d'images incomplètes et changeantes, Swann endormi tirait des déductions fausses, ayant d'ailleurs momentanément un tel pouvoir créateur qu'il se reproduisait par simple division comme certains organismes inférieurs; avec la chaleur sentie de sa propre paume il modelait le creux d'une main étrangère qu'il croyait serrer et de sentiments et d'impressions dont il n'avait pas conscience encore, faisait naître comme des péripéties qui, par leur enchaînement logique, amèneraient à point nommé dans le sommeil de Swann le personnage nécessaire pour recevoir son amour ou provoquer son réveil"; *À la recherche du temps perdu*, 1:314.

12. GOSSAMER THREAD

1. "Hélas, c'était en vain que j'implorais le donjon de Roussainville, que je lui demandais de faire venir auprès de moi quelque enfant de son village, comme au seul confident que j'avais eu de mes premiers désirs, quand au haut de notre maison de Combray, dans le petit cabinet sentant l'iris, je ne voyais que sa tour au milieu du carreau de la fenêtre entr'ouverte, pendant qu'avec les hésitations héroïques du voyageur qui entreprend une exploration ou du désespéré qui se suicide, défaillant, je me frayais en moi-même une route inconnue et que je croyais mortelle, jusqu'au moment où une trace naturelle comme celle d'un colimaçon s'ajoutait aux feuilles du cassis sauvage qui se penchaient jusqu'à moi"; *À la recherche du temps perdu*, 1:144.

2. Doubrovsky, *Writing and Fantasy in Proust*, 1; further citations are given in the text.
3. Bal, *The Mottled Screen*, 3; further citations are given in the text.
4. Proust, "Solitary Pleasure," in *Against Sainte-Beuve*, in *Marcel Proust on Art and Literature, 1896–1919*, 29–30; further citations are given in the text.

13. A FEW DROPS THAT EXPRESS ALL

1. Proust, *In Search of Lost Time*, 2:76. The translation: "Je tâchais de l'attirer, elle résistait; ses pommettes enflammées par l'effort étaient rouges et rondes comme des cerises; elle riait comme si je l'eusse chatouillée; je la tenais serrée entre mes jambes comme un arbuste après lequel j'aurais voulu grimper; et, au milieu de la gymnastique que je faisais, sans qu'en fût à peine augmenté l'essoufflement que me donnaient l'exercice musculaire et l'ardeur du jeu, je répandis, comme quelques gouttes de sueur arrachées par l'effort, mon plaisir auquel je ne pus pas même m'attarder le temps d'en connaître le goût; aussitôt je pris la lettre"; *À la recherche du temps perdu*, 1:419.
2. Bowie reads the scene as another Ovidian metamorphosis. Like Daphne, Gilberte becomes a tree as Apollo-Marcel takes her. She escapes, leaving him only "an objectless inward rapture"; *Proust Among the Stars*, 242. Bal stresses Marcel's superficial and epidermic consummation of Gilberte in accordance with the "singular absence of penetration" in Proust. The drops of semen-sweat feature as the "mark of writing, the signature" left by the subject on the tree, similar to the scene from "Solitary Pleasure"; *The Mottled Screen*, 172–73.
3. "[J]e pensais que le stage que peut-être pendant des années des hommes importants faisaient inutilement à la porte de telle femme qui ne répondait pas à leurs lettres et les faisait chasser par le concierge de son hôtel, mon oncle aurait pu en dispenser un gamin comme moi en le présentent chez lui à l'actrice, inapprochable à tant d'autres, qui était pour lui une intime amie"; *À la recherche du temps perdu*, 1:80.
4. "Et si, à son avis, Febvre ne venait qu'après Thiron, ou Delaunay qu'après Coquelin, la soudaine motilité que Coquelin, perdant la rigidité de la pierre, contractait dans mon esprit pour y passer au deuxième rang, et l'agilité miraculeuse, la féconde animation dont se voyait doué Delaunay pour reculer au quatrième, rendaient la sensation du fleurissement et de la vie à mon cerveau assoupli et fertilisé"; *À la recherche du temps perdu*, 1:80.
5. "Je me sentais consterné, réduit; et mon esprit comme un fluide qui n'a de dimensions que celles du vase qu'on lui fournit, de même qu'il s'était dilaté jadis à remplir les capacités immenses du génie, contracté maintenant tenait tout entier dans la médiocrité étroite où M. de Norpois l'avait soudain enfermée et restreinte"; *À la recherche du temps perdu*, 1:405.
6. "En tous cas, si la 'marquise' avait du goût pour les jeunes garçons, en leur ouvrant la porte hypogéenne de ces cubes de pierre où les hommes sont accroupis comme des sphinx, elle devait cherches dans ses générosités moins l'espérance de les corrompre que le plaisir qu'on éprouve à se montrer vainement prodigue

envers ce qu'on aime, car je n'ai jamais vu auprès d'elle autre visiteur qu'un vieux garde forestier du jardin"; *À la recherche du temps perdu*, 1:418–19.

7. "[D]'un côte et de l'autre, à des hauteurs différentes, devant chaque anfractuosité que faisait dans le mur la fenêtre de la loge ou la porte d'un appartement . . . un concierge, un majordome, un argentier (braves gens qui vivaient le reste de la semaine un peu indépendants dans leur domaine . . .) se tenaient sous l'arcature de leur portail avec un éclat pompeux tempéré de bonhomie populaire, comme des saints dans leur niche"; *À la recherche du temps perdu*, 1:272.
8. The gorgeous oddity of the scene is perhaps best attested by the film adaptation of *Swann in Love* by Volker Schlöndorff. Though the film opens with this exact scene, it manages to censor virtually all of its appeal through two changes. First, Swann narrates his own story in voice-over, so that the irony is entirely lost on him: the affair with Odette becomes deadly serious. Second, Charlus accompanies Swann on his journey to the ballroom, so that his lustful glances motivate the attention the camera pays to the lackeys, footmen, and servants (in the book, he leaves Swann to make a visit to Odette in order to evaluate her demeanor for Swann). Meanwhile, Swann completely ignores them.

EPILOGUE

1. The definitions cited here and below are from the *Oxford English Dictionary Online*, 2003.

BIBLIOGRAPHY

BOOKS AND ARTICLES

Amis, Martin. "A Rough Trade." *Guardian Unlimited*, March 17, 2001. Available at: http://books.guardian.co.uk/departments/politicsphilosophyandsociety/story/0,,458058,00.html.

Arenas, Amelia. "The Revelations of Andres Serrano." In Serrano, *Andres Serrano: Body and Soul*, n.p.

Aristotle. *Generation of Animals*. Translated by A. L. Peck. Loeb Classical Library. London and Cambridge, Mass.: William Heinemann and Harvard University Press, 1963.

Atkins, John. *Sex in Literature, Volume 2: The Classical Expression of the Sexual Impulse*. London: Calder and Boyars, 1973.

Austin, Steve. "Gonzo in the Year 2000." *Adult Video News*, December 1999.

Baker, James. *Sperm Wars: The Science of Sex*. New York: Basic Books, 1996.

Bakhtin, Mikhail. *The Bakhtin Reader: Selected Writings of Bakhtin, Medvedev, Voloshinov*. Edited by Pam Morris. London: Edward Arnold, 1994.

Bal, Mieke. *Lethal Love: Feminist Literary Readings of Biblical Love Stories*. Bloomington: Indiana University Press, 1987.

———. *On Meaning-Making: Essays in Semiotics*. Sonoma, Calif.: Polebridge Press, 1994.

———. *The Mottled Screen: Reading Proust Visually*. Translated by Anna-Louise Milne. Stanford, Calif.: Stanford University Press, 1997.

———. *Narratology: Introduction to the Theory of Narrative*. 2nd ed. Toronto: University of Toronto Press, 1997.

———. *Quoting Caravaggio: Contemporary Art, Preposterous History*. Chicago: University of Chicago Press, 1999.

Barthes, Roland. *A Barthes Reader*. Edited by Susan Sontag. New York: Hill and Wang, 1982.

———. *Image Music Text*. Essays selected and translated by Stephen Heath. London: Fontana Press, 1987.

———. "The Metaphor of the Eye." 1963. In Bataille, *Story of the Eye*, 119–27.

———. *Le plaisir du texte*. Paris: Éditions du Seuil, 1973.

———. *The Pleasure of the Text*. Translated by Richard Miller. With a Note on the Text by Richard Hower. New York: Hill and Wang, 1983.

———. "The Reality Effect." In *Realism*, edited by Lilian R. Furst, 135–41. London and New York: Longman, 1992. Originally published as "L'effet de Reél," in *Essais critiques IV: Le Bruissement de la langue* (Paris: Éditions du Seuil, 1984), 167–74.

Bataille, Georges. "Base Materialism and Gnosticism." In *The Bataille Reader*, 160–66.

———. *The Bataille Reader*. Edited by Fred Botting and Scott Wilson. Oxford: Blackwell, 1997.

———. "The Notion of Expenditure." In *The Bataille Reader*, 167–82.

———. *Story of the Eye*. Translated by Joachim Neugroschal. 1928; Harmondsworth, Eng.: Penguin, 1982.

———. "The Use-Value of D. A. F. de Sade (An Open Letter to My Current Comrades)." In *The Bataille Reader*, 147–59.

Bennett, David. "Burghers, Burglars, and Masturbators: The Sovereign Spender in the Age of Consumerism." *New Literary History* 30, no. 3 (Spring 1999): 269–94.

Berger, John. *Ways of Seeing*. 1972; Harmondsworth, Eng.: Penguin, 1990.

Bernheimer, Charles. "Penile Reference in Phallic Theory." *differences: A Journal of Feminist Cultural Studies* 4, no. 1 (Spring 1992): 116–32.

Bersani, Leo. *Homos*. Cambridge, Mass.: Harvard University Press, 1995.

Bhabha, Homi K. *The Location of Culture*. London: Routledge, 1994.

Bleeker, Maaike. "The Locus of Looking: Dissecting Visuality in the Theatre." PhD diss., University of Amsterdam, 2002.

Bois, Yve-Alain, and Rosalind E. Krauss. *Formless: A User's Guide*. New York: Zone Books, 1997.

Bonito Oliva, Achille, and Danilo Eccher. *Appearance*. Milan: Edizioni Charta, 2000.

Bowie, Malcolm. *Lacan*. London: Fontana Press, 1991.

———. *Proust Among the Stars*. New York: Columbia University Press, 1998.

Boyarin, Daniel. "Feminism Meets Queer Theory at the Sign of the Phallus; or Philo *mit/avec* Lacan." In *ASCA Brief: Intellectual Traditions in Movement*, 41–83. Amsterdam: ASCA Press, 1997.

Bramly, Serge. *Leonardo: Discovering the Life of Leonardo da Vinci*. Translated by Siân Reynolds. New York: HarperCollins, 1991.

Bronfen, Elizabeth. *Over Her Dead Body: Death, Femininity, and the Aesthetic*. Manchester, Eng.: Manchester University Press, 1992.

Brooks, Peter. *Reading for the Plot: Design and Intention in Narrative*. 2nd ed. 1984; Cambridge, Mass.: Harvard University Press, 1992.

Brüner, Jerome. *Acts of Meaning*. Cambridge, Mass.: Harvard University Press, 1990.

Bryson, Norman. "Géricault and 'Masculinity.' " In *Visual Culture: Images and Interpretations*, edited by Norman Bryson, Michael Ann Holly, and Keith Moxey, 228–59. Hanover, N.H.: University Press of New England, 1994.

Burger, John R. *One-Handed Histories: The Eroto-Politics of Gay Male Video Pornography*. New York: Harrington Park Press, 1995.

Butler, Judith. *Bodies That Matter: On the Discursive Limits of "Sex."* New York: Routledge, 1993.

Collins, Bradley I. *Leonardo, Psychoanalysis, and Art History: A Critical Study of Psychobiographical Approaches to Leonardo da Vinci*. Evanston, Ill.: Northwestern University Press, 1997.

Culler, Jonathan. *Barthes: A Very Short Introduction*. Oxford: Oxford University Press, 2002.

———. *On Deconstruction: Theory and Criticism after Structuralism*. London: Routledge and Kegan Paul, 1983.

"The Curve" (press release). 2001. Previously available at http://www.barbican.org.uk/information/press/pressitem.asp?releaseID=44.

Dawn, Natalie. Review of *Justine 2: Nothing to Hide*, directed by Paul Thomas. Undated. http://www.dvdpornreviews.com/reviews/read_review.asp?sku=282.

de Lauretis, Teresa. *Alice Doesn't: Feminism. Semiotics. Cinema*. Bloomington: Indiana University Press, 1984.

Derrida, Jacques. *A Derrida Reader: Between the Blinds*. Edited by Peggy Kamuf. New York: Harvester Wheatsheaf, 1991.

———. *Dissemination*. Translated by Barbara Johnson. Chicago: University of Chicago Press, 1981. Originally published as *La Dissémination* (Paris: Éditions du Seuil, 1972).

———. *The Ear of the Other: Otobiography, Transference, Translation*. Edited by Christie McDonald. Translated by Peggy Kamuf and Avital Ronell. Lincoln: University of Nebraska Press, 1988.

———. "Geslecht: Sexual Difference, Ontological Difference." 1987. In *A Derrida Reader: Between the Blinds*, 378–403.

———. *Margins of Philosophy*. Translated by Alan Bass. 1972; Chicago: University of Chicago Press, 1982.

Dolce, Joe. "Editor's Letter." *Details*, September 1996.

Doubrovsky, Serge. *Writing and Fantasy in Proust: The Place of the Madeleine*. Translated by Carol Mastrangelo Bové, with Paul A. Bové. Lincoln: University of Nebraska Press, 1986.

dumblonde. Review of *Justine 2: Nothing to Hide*, directed by Paul Thomas. Undated. http://www.adultdvdtalk.com/reviews/read_review.asp?sku=2266.

Dyer, Richard. "Idol Thoughts: Orgasm and Self-Reflexivity in Gay Pornography." *Critical Quarterly* 36, no. 1 (Spring 1994): 49–62.

———. "Male Gay Porn: Coming to Terms." *Jump Cut* no. 30 (March 1985): 27–29.

———. *White*. London: Routledge, 1997.

Eagleton, Terry. *Literary Theory*. Minneapolis: Minnesota University Press, 1982.

Eco, Umberto. "How to Recognize a Porn Movie." In *How to Travel with a Salmon and Other Essays*, translated by William Weaver, 206–210. London: Minerva, 1995.

———. *Interpretation and Overinterpretation*. Edited by Stefan Collini. Cambridge, Eng.: Cambridge University Press, 1992.

———. *A Theory of Semiotics*. Bloomington: Indiana University Press, 1976.

Eilberg-Schwartz, Howard. *God's Phallus: And Other Problems for Men and Monotheism*. Boston: Beacon Press, 1994.

Faludi, Susan. "The Money Shot." *The New Yorker*, October 30, 1995.

Fausto-Sterling, Anne. "How to Build a Man." In *Constructing Masculinity*, edited by Maurice Berger, Brian Wallis, and Simon Watson, 127–34. New York: Routledge, 1995.

Ferguson, Bruce. "Andres Serrano: Invisible Power." In Serrano, *Andres Serrano: Body and Soul*, n.p.

Foister, Susan, Ashok Roy, and Martin Wyld. *Holbein's Ambassadors: Making and Meaning*. London: National Gallery Publications, 1997.

Foucault, Michel. *The Use of Pleasure: The History of Sexuality, Volume 2*. Translated by Robert Hurley. 1984; New York: Vintage Books, 1990.

Freud, Sigmund. *Three Case Histories*. Edited by Philip Rieff. The Collected Papers of Sigmund Freud, 7. New York: Collier Books, 1963.

Gallagher, Barbara. "No Space Sex?" *Scientific American*, January 2000.

Genette, Gérard. "*Vraisemblance* and Motivation." *Narrative* 9, no. 3 (October 2001): 239–53.

Goldberg, Michael. "Metallica's Rebel Yell." July 1996. Available at: http://www.addict.com/issues/2.08/html/hifi/Features/Metallica.

Halperin, David M. *One Hundred Years of Homosexuality and Other Essays on Greek Love*. New York: Routledge, 1990.

Harvey, John. *Men in Black*. London: Reaktion Books, 1995.

Heath, Chris. "A Hard Man Is Good to Find." *Details*, September 1996.

Helmling, Steven. "Marxist Pleasure: Jameson and Eagleton." *Postmodern Culture* 3, no. 3 (1993). Available at: http://muse.jhu.edu/journals/postmodern_culture/v003/3.3helmling.html.

hooks, bell. "The Radiance of Red: Blood Work." In Serrano, *Andres Serrano: Body and Soul*, n.p.

Irigaray, Luce. *This Sex Which Is Not One*. Translated by Catherine Porter with Carolyn Burke. Ithaca, N.Y.: Cornell University Press, 1985.

Johnson, Barbara. *The Critical Difference: Essays in the Contemporary Rhetoric of Reading*. Baltimore, Md.: The Johns Hopkins University Press, 1980.

Johnson, Eithne. "Excess and Ecstasy: Constructing Female Pleasure in Porn Movies." *The Velvet Light Trap* 32 (1993): 30–50.

Kermode, Frank. *The Sense of an Ending: Studies in the Theory of Fiction with a New Epilogue*. 1966; Oxford: Oxford University Press, 2000.

Kernes, Mark. "With Perfect, Ninn Takes Porn to a New Level." *Adult Video News*, January 2002. Available at: http://www.adultvideonews.com/bone/by0102_09.html.

Kimball, A. Samuel. "Conceptions and Contraceptions of the Future: *Terminator 2*, *The Matrix*, and *Alien Resurrection*." *Camera Obscura* 17, no. 2 (2002): 69–107.

Knight, Diane. *Barthes and Utopia: Space, Travel, Writing*. Oxford: Clarendon Press, 1997.

Kristeva, Julia. *Powers of Horror: An Essay on Abjection*. Translated by Leon S. Roudiez. New York: Columbia University Press, 1982.

Lacan, Jacques. *Écrits: A Selection*. Translated by Alan Sheridan. New York: W. W. Norton, 1977.

———. *The Four Fundamental Concepts of Psycho-Analysis*. Edited by Jacques-Alain Miller. Translated by Alan Sheridan. 1973; Harmondsworth, Eng.: Penguin, 1994.

Laplanche, J., and J.-B. Pontalis. *The Language of Psychoanalysis*. London: Karnac Books and the Institute for Psycho-Analysis, 1988.

Lentricchia, Frank. *After the New Criticism*. London: Athlone Press, 1980.

Lord, Catherine. *The Intimacy of Influence: Narrative and Theoretical Fictions in the Works of George Eliot, Virginia Woolf, and Jeanette Winterson*. Amsterdam: ASCA Press, 1997.

Macey, David. "Phallus." In *Feminism and Psychoanalysis: A Critical Dictionary*, edited by Elizabeth Wright. Oxford: Blackwell, 1992.

Martin, Emily. "The Egg and the Sperm: How Science Has Constructed a Romance Based on Stereotypical Male-Female Roles." *Signs: Journal of Women in Culture and Society* 16, no. 2 (1991): 485–502.

McDonald, Christie V. "Choreographies: Jacques Derrida and Christie V. McDonald." *Diacritics* 12, no. 2 (Summer 1982): 66–76.

Michaels, Dave. "Talking Blue . . . ," March 16, 2000. Available at http://www.excaliburfilms.com/pornlist/eroticanews/talkingbluemar14.htm.

Miller, D. A. *Bringing Out Roland Barthes*. Berkeley and Los Angeles: University of California Press, 1992.

Miller, J. Hillis. *Reading Narrative*. Norman: University of Oklahoma Press, 1998.

Mitchell, W. J. T. *Iconology: Image, Text, Ideology*. Chicago: University of Chicago Press, 1986.

———. *Picture Theory*. Chicago: University of Chicago Press, 1994.

Moriarty, Michael. *Reading Roland Barthes*. Cambridge, Eng.: Polity Press, 1991.

Ovid. *Metamorphoses*. Translated by Mary M. Innes. Harmondsworth, Eng.: Penguin Classics, 1955.

Oxford English Dictionary Online. Available at http://dictionary.oed.com.

Patterson, Zabet. "Going On-line: Consuming Pornography in the Digital Era." In *Porn Studies*, edited by Linda Williams, 104–23. Durham, N.C.: Duke University Press, 2004.

Pedretti, Carlo. "The Angel in the Flesh." *Accademia Leonardo da Vinci* 4 (1991): 34–51.

Pinchbeck, Daniel. "Downward Motility." *Esquire*, January 1996.

Pitt-Kethley, Fiona. *The Literary Companion to Sex*. New York: Random House, 1992.

Power, Kim E. "Of Godly Men and Medicine: Ancient Biology and the Christian Fathers on the Nature of Women." *Woman-Church* 15 (Spring 1994): 26–33.

Proust, Marcel. *Against Sainte-Beuve and Other Essays*. Translated by John Sturrock. Harmondsworth, Eng.: Penguin, 1988.

———. *À la recherche du temps perdu*. Paris: Éditions Robert Laffont, 1987.

———. *In Search of Lost Time*. Translated by C. K. Scott Moncrieff and Terence Kilmartin. Revised by D. J. Enright. London: Vintage, 1996.

———. *Marcel Proust on Art and Literature, 1869–1919*. Translated and edited by Sylvia Townsend Warner. Greenwich, Conn.: Meridian Books, 1958.

rame.net. "The Adult Movie FAQ." 1994–2000. http://www.rame.net/faq.

Rich, Frank. "Naked Capitalists." *New York Times*, May 20, 2001.

Richardson, Michael. *Georges Bataille*. London: Routledge, 1994.

Richman, Michelle H. *Reading Georges Bataille: Beyond the Gift*. Baltimore, Md.: The Johns Hopkins University Press, 1982.

Rosenberg, Adriana. Interview with Andres Serrano. Undated. http://www.proa.org/exhibicion/serrano/exhibi-fr.html.

Sauerländer, Willibald. "The Art of the Cool." *New York Review of Books*, April 13, 2000. Available at: http://www.nybooks.com/articles/article-preview?article_id=160.

Schaefer, Eric. "Gauging a Revolution: 16 mm Film and the Rise of the Pornographic Feature." In *Porn Studies*, edited by Linda Williams, 370–400. Durham, N.C.: Duke University Press, 2004.

Sedgwick, Eve Kosofsky. *Between Men: English Literature and Male Homosocial Desire*. New York: Columbia University Press, 1985.

Serrano, Andres. *Andres Serrano: Body and Soul*. With essays by bell hooks, Bruce Ferguson, and Amelia Arenas. Edited by Brian Wallis. New York: Takarajima Books, 1995.

Silverman, Kaja. "The Lacanian Phallus." *differences: A Journal of Feminist Cultural Studies* 4, no. 1 (1992): 84–114.

———. *Male Subjectivity at the Margins*. New York: Routledge, 1992.

———. *The Threshold of the Visible World*. New York: Routledge, 1996.

Slade, Joseph W. "Flesh Need Not Be Mute: The Pornographic Videos of John Leslie." *Wide Angle* 19, no. 3 (1997): 115–48.

Smith, Paul. "Vas." *Camera Obscura* 17 (May 1988): 89–112.

Sontag, Susan. "The Pornographic Imagination." In Bataille, *Story of the Eye*, 83–118.

"Sperm Warfare 'Realistic Threat,' Study Concludes." *FutureFeedForward*, February 11, 2001. Available at: http://futurefeedforward.com/archive.php.

Sprinkle, Annie. "The G Spot?" Available at http://www.anniesprinkle.org/html/writings/g_spots.html.

Steiner, Wendy. *The Scandal of Pleasure: Art in an Age of Fundamentalism*. Chicago: University of Chicago Press, 1995.

Suleiman, Susan Rubin. "Bataille in the Street: The Search for Virility in the 1930s." *Critical Inquiry* 21 (Autumn 1994): 61–79.

Thomas, Calvin. *Male Matters: Masculinity, Anxiety, and the Male Body on the Line*. Urbana: University of Illinois Press, 1996.

Thompson, Ellen. "Porn by the People, for the People." *Adult Video News*, June 2000.

Tomlinson, Barbara. "Phallic Fables and Spermatic Romance: Disciplinary Crossing and Textual Ridicule." *Configuration* 3, no. 2 (1995): 105–34.

van Alphen, Ernst. "Caught by Images: On the Role of Visual Imprints in Holocaust Testimonies." *Journal of Visual Culture* 1 (August 2002): 205–21.

———. *Francis Bacon and the Loss of Self*. London: Reaktion Books, 1992.

"Van Gogh's Ear." Exhibition/Installation hosted on the Web. Introduced by Jeff Bourgeau. Undated. http://www.andrewfish.com/vangogh.

Williams, Linda. *Hard Core: Power, Pleasure, and the "Frenzy of the Visible."* Expanded paperback ed. Berkeley and Los Angeles: University of California Press, 1999.

———. "Porn Studies: Proliferating Pornographies On/Scene: An Introduction."

In *Porn Studies*, edited by Linda Williams, 1–26. Durham, N.C.: Duke University Press, 2004.

Wilson, Sarah. "Fêting the Wound: Georges Bataille and Jean Fautrier in the 1940s." In *Bataille: Writing the Sacred*, edited by Carolyn Bailly Gill, 172–92. London: Routledge, 1995.

Winnett, Susan. "Coming Unstrung: Women, Men, Narrative, and Principles of Pleasure." PMLA 105, no. 3 (May 1990): 505–18.

Wright, Elizabeth, ed. *Feminism and Psychoanalysis: A Critical Dictionary*. Oxford: Blackwell, 1992.

Wyke, Andrew. "Exploiting the Many Markets of Adult." *Adult Video News*, September 2000.

Young, Robert J. C. "Deconstruction and the Postcolonial." In *Deconstructions: A User's Guide*, edited by Nicholas Royle, 187–210. Basingstoke, Eng.: Palgrave, 2000.

Zerner, Henri. "The Vision of Leonardo." *New York Review of Books*, September 25, 1997. Available at: http://www.nybooks.com/articles/article-preview?article_id=1093.

"Zero Gravity Sex Film Up for Award." May 16, 2000. Available at: http://www.space.com/sciencefiction/movies/uranus_experiment_000516.html.

Zwijnenberg, Robert. *The Writings and Drawings of Leonardo da Vinci*. Cambridge, Eng.: Cambridge University Press, 1999.

FILMS

Assault on the Male: The Estrogen Effect. Written and produced by Deborah Cadbury. 1993; London: British Broadcasting Corporation, 2004.

Caracas Adventure, The. Directed by Kristen Bjorn. Miami: Kristen Bjorn Productions, 1994.

Chase, The. Directed by Jane Waters. Private Productions, 1996.

Flyin' Solo. Directed and written by Paul Barresi. Chatsworth, Calif.: US Male/In-X-Cess, 1998.

Hustler White. Directed by Bruce LaBruce and Rick Castro. Screenplay by Bruce LaBruce and Rick Castro. Dangerous to Know Swell Co. and Hustler White Productions, 1996.

Justine 2: Nothing to Hide. Directed by Paul Thomas. Metro Home Video, 1992.

Kika. Directed by Pedro Almodóvar. Screenplay by Pedro Almodóvar. Madrid: El Deseo S.A., 1993.

Life's Greatest Miracle (documentary). Medical photography by Lennart Nilsson. Written by Julia Cort. PBS airdate: November 20, 2001. A NOVA Production (#2816) in association with WGBH/Boston and ZDF Germany, ARTE France and Germany, RAI 3 Italy, NHK Japan, BBC Open University England, SVT1 Sweden, NRK Norway, DR TV Denmark, YLE1 Finland, RUV Iceland. Boston: WGBH Educational Foundation, 2001. Companion Web site: http://www.pbs.org/wgbh/nova/miracle.

Lunch Hour. Directed by Josh Elliot. Catalina Video, 1990.

Manwatcher. Directed and written by Kristen Bjorn. Miami: Kristen Bjorn Productions, 1998.

9½ Days, Part Two. Directed by Sascha Alexander. Sascha Alexander Productions, 1993.

Restoring The Ambassadors. London: British Broadcasting Corporation, April 29, 1996.

Swann in Love [Un Amour de Swann]. Directed by Volker Schlöndorff. Bioskop Film, France 3 Cinema, Les Films du Lasange, Société Française de Production, Société des Etablissements L. Gaumont, 1984.

Uranus Experiment, The. Directed by John Millerman. Barcelona: Private Media, 1999.

INDEX

MURAT AYDEMIR
is assistant professor of
comparative literature and
cultural analysis at the
University of Amsterdam.